Health Research in Developing Countries

Heiko Becher · Bocar Kouyaté (Eds)

Health Research in Developing Countries

A collaboration between Burkina Faso and Germany

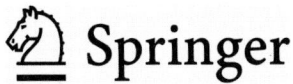

Professor Dr. Heiko Becher
Universitätsklinikum Heidelberg, Hygiene Institut
Abt. Tropenhygiene und Öffentliches Gesundheitswesen
Im Neuenheimer Feld 324
69120 Heidelberg
Germany

email: heiko.becher@urz.uni-heidelberg.de

Dr. Bocar Kouyaté
Centre de Recherche en Santé de Nouna
BP 02 Nouna
Burkina Faso

email: bocar.crsn@fasonet.bf

ISBN 3-540-23796-8

Library of Congress Control Number: 2004116207

This work is subject to copyright. All rights are reserved, whether the whole or part of the material is concerned, specifically the rights of translation, reprinting, reuse of illustrations, recitations, broadcasting, reproduction on microfilm or in any other way, and storage in data banks. Duplication of this publication or parts thereof if permitted only under the provisions of the German Copyright Law of September 9, 1965, in its current version, and permission for use must always be obtained from Springer. Violations are liable to prosecution under the German Copyright Law.

Springer is a part of Springer Science+Business Media
springeronline.com
© Springer-Verlag Berlin Heidelberg 2005
Printed in Germany

The use of general descriptive names, registered names, trademarks, etc. in this publication does not imply, even in the absence of a specific statement, that such names are exempt from the relevant protective laws and regulations and therefore free for general use.

Cover design: Erich Kirchner, Heidelberg
Coverphoto: Pitt Reitmaier
Typesetting and layout: By the authors. Final layout by EDV-Beratung Frank Herweg

Printed on acid free paper 40/2242/xo – 5 4 3 2 1 0

Foreword

The Institute of Tropical Hygiene at the University of Heidelberg has a long and fruitful tradition concerning health research in developing countries. Since the foundation of the Evaluation and Project Consulting Working Group (EVA PLAN) in 1987 many health research projects in numerous developing countries world wide have been carried out including baseline studies, controlling and evaluation of projects, teaching and education in health measures . These activities were supported by the German Association of Technical Cooperation and the Credit Bank for Reconstruction of the German Federal Ministry of Development.

Already in 1986 a first health project was started in cooperation with Burkina Faso and others followed in the further years which led to a very fruitful continuous collaboration. A highlight was the establishment of the "Sonderforschungsbereich 544: Control of Tropical Infectious Diseases" by the German Research Foundation (DFG) at the University of Heidelberg in 1999. With this a basic financial sponsorship of the Nouna Health Research Center could be realized.

Based on the great experience of the scientists of the Institute for Tropical Hygiene of the University of Heidelberg in health projects in developing countries since 1986 and the intensification of the cooperation with highly acknowledged scientists in Burkina Faso in the last years not only single research projects but already a whole programme of health research could be developed . A highly remarkable scientific outcome of these efforts has been arranged in the submitted commemorative publication, edited by Heiko Becher and Bocar Kouyaté. I want to congratulate all authors of this publication. This is for me a wonderful demonstration of collaboration between scientists in the international field which is concerned with health problems that urgently have to be solved . I hope this will not only motivate those scientists who are already committed to go ahead working in this field but will also activate young scientists to go into this important field of research.

October 2004

Hans-Günther Sonntag , Dr. med. Dr. h.c.
University Professor for Hygiene and Medical Microbiology
Dean of the Medical Faculty, University of Heidelberg

Foreword

Ce document que vous avez entre vos mains est le témoin d'une coopération scientifique et technique exemplaire dans le domaine de la recherche en santé entre le Ministère de la santé de mon pays et l'Université de Heidelberg en Allemagne. Cette coopération autour du Centre de Recherche en Santé de Nouna (CRSN) a permis non seulement de créer de la capacité dans le domaine de la recherche en santé mais aussi et surtout de fourniture régulièrement des informations aux décideurs pour mieux orienter notre politique de santé. Les publications contenues dans ce document illustrent la richesse et la qualité de la production scientifique du CRSN de 1999 à 2004.

C'est pourquoi, je voudrais exprimer ma gratitude à toutes les institutions de coopération scientifiques aussi bien nationales que bilatérales ou multilatérales qui ont apporté leur contribution à l'édification de ce centre de recherche qui constitue aujourd'hui une référence au Burkina Faso et dans la région . Je ferais une mention spéciale pour le réseau des sites de surveillance démographique dans les pays en développement appelé INDEPTH. Par son dynamisme, INDEPTH a permis un échange scientifique fructueux entre le CRSN et d'autres institutions similaires en Afrique, en Asie et bientôt en Amérique Latine.

Enfin, j'exprime le vœux qu'à l'instar du Centre de Recherche en Santé de Nouna, notre volonté de faire de la recherche en santé un outil au service du développement devienne une réalité de tous les jours.

Prof. Jean Gabriel OUANGO

Secrétaire Général du Ministère
de la Santé du Burkina Faso   Octobre 2004

Foreword

The CRSN is a remarkable success story. Hundreds of kilometers away from the capital or any other major city, the Center was built up from scratch through the firm commitment of the Burkinian Ministry of Health and the University of Heidelberg. With the generous and far-sighted support of the Land of Baden Württemberg, it has established itself as a regional center of excellence for health research. It has assumed a leading role in the network of some 30 similar research institutions from the south (INDEPTH). The research output described in this book speaks for itself.

More than any other comparable research center we know Nouna has consequently pursued a holistic view of research, combining disciplines that rarely "talk" to each other: anthropology and molecular biology, geography and economics, mathematics and sociology, demography. The term from the improving health: from gene to society is not a euphemism but has become a strong leitmotif for the Center. The demographic surveillance system, meticulously and rigorously refined over the years not only provides a precise population denominator for studies, but also serves as a platform bringing different strands of research together.

Setting up research capacity in many relevant disciplines might be considered in our modern days as "lack of focus". However, it was done not only by choice, but also dictated by necessity, since the health problems poor countries face cannot and will not be solved through single "silver bullet" interventions, but only through the carefully orchestrated innovations in health systems and interventions. Since the research focus "Tropical Medicine" (TMH) and the special research grant (SFB) "Control of Tropical Infectious diseases (SFB 544)" at Heidelberg University try to achieve a similar interdisciplinary approach to health research, there clearly is a meeting of the minds. There is also a strongly personal aspect to this collaboration: many researchers on both sides became friends over the long years of collaboration. This adds the dimension of the heart to that of the mind and makes this collaboration so durable and creative.

We would like to thank the staff of the Center, particularly Dr. Bocar Kouyaté; its visionary leader, congratulate them on their success against many odds and look forward to an ever closer cooperation.

Heidelberg, October 2004

Prof. Rainer Sauerborn
Speaker of TMH Research Focus

Prof. Hans-Georg Kräusslich
Speaker of the SFB Collaborative grant

Preface

The constitution of the WHO states in the first article: "The objective of the World Health Organization shall be the attainment by all peoples of the highest possible level of health". In few places of the world this aim has been achieved. For Sub-Saharan Africa in particular, there is a long way to go. And within Sub-Saharan Africa some countries are better off than others. Burkina Faso is one of the poorest countries with high population density and limited natural resources resulting in poor economic prospects for the majority of its citizens.

Fortunately, there are efforts of various kinds to improve the situation. In the course of globalisation, most of these efforts are international. This book describes the results of a collaboration between health scientists in Nouna / Burkina Faso and Heidelberg / Germany. It gives an example of systematic efforts to develop research partnerships and structures for capacity building between an institution in the north (University of Heidelberg, Germany) and a developing country in the south (Burkina Faso). It shows how such a collaboration can contribute to achieve the objective of the WHO as stated above. Some practical difficulties that arise for research institutes in developing countries are described in a letter to THE LANCET in the year 2000:

CORRESPONDENCE

Sir—In response to Richard Horton's report on building research capacity in less-developed countries,[1] we draw on our collaborative experience with a health research centre of rural west Africa.

Burkina Faso is one of the poorest countries in Africa, and research is not very high on the national agenda. There is generally little motivation for physicians to engage in research, and channels for south-south exchange of scientists remain poorly developed. Thus, we are encouraged by the decision of the Ministry of Health of Burkina Faso to create and support the Centre de Recherche en Santé de Nouna (CRSN), a national centre of excellence for biomedical and health-systems research.

The CRSN was established in October, 1999, in the small town of Nouna in north-western Burkina Faso. The centre is financially, logistically, and educationally supported through a twinning arrangement with an alliance of scientific groups working on tropical-disease control at the University of Heidelberg, Germany. Electricity reached Nouna only 3 years ago and access to telephone lines is limited. Although the capacity of the CRSN has grown substantially to roughly 60 staff members, including nine national senior scientists and several regularly visiting scientists from collaborating institutions in Europe, the communication conditions remain largely inadequate. People working at the centre and all their activities rely on only one telephone line, which is generally busy from the early morning to the late evening. Moreover, electricity supply and internet access are frequently interrupted, and new machinery can only become established in the existing limited technical infrastructure of the region. Thus, in reality, our scientists usually have access to the internet only during night hours, if at all. Finally, most scientists from French-speaking countries face major language barriers that could be overcome only by English-language courses, as well as funding for participation in international conferences on research.

We agree that the internet and, especially, access to e-mail has greatly improved the working conditions of scientists in sub-Saharan Africa. However, there remains substantial room for improvement of technical infrastructures and refinement of the contents of joint ventures in research before scientists in less-developed countries have roughly equal opportunities for research and publication to those in more-developed countries, and before a truly mutual exchange of information is possible.

*Bocar Kouyaté, Corneille Traoré, Karine Kielmann, Olaf Müller

*Centre de Recherche en Santé de Nouna, POB 02, Nouna, Burkina Faso; and Department of Tropical Hygiene and Public Health, Ruprecht-Karls-University, Germany
(e-mail: bocar.crsn@fasonet.bf)

1 Horton R. North and South: bridging the information gap. *Lancet* 2000; 355: 2231–36.

Reprinted with permission from Elsevier (**The Lancet**, 2000, Vol. 356, p. 1035)

Five years after the official founding of the Nouna Health Research Center (CRSN) it is time to look back, and to look forward for new projects to come.

What has been achieved so far was only possible with the technical support of INDEPTH Network and the financial support of institutions and foundations. The Ministry of Research, Sciences and Art of the federal state Baden-Württemberg, Germany, generously contributes to maintain the infrastructure of the CRSN. A special research grant by the German Research Foundation (DFG) with the title "SFB 544 - Control of Tropical Infectious Diseases" has been in place for almost sixth years. It greatly helped to conduct projects in different fields of health sciences such as clinical research, epidemiology and health systems research.

This book is structured into five chapters beginning with an introductory chapter. In the first section of this chapter, the leading persons who build up and maintained the collaboration between Nouna and Heidelberg describe the history from 1970 until today. This is followed by a brief description of the data and information exchange between both institutions. The next section describes the INDEPTH network in which Nouna is embedded. The last two sections of this chapter give a more general overview on specific ethical issues which arise in health research in developing countries, and on routine health information systems. Chapter two is devoted to clinical research and begins with an overview on studies on malaria and AIDS which were performed or are ongoing. The other subsections are reprinted papers form this area, presented in chronological order of publication. Similarly, chapter three deals with epidemiological studies, with an introduction and subsequent reprints of scientific publications, and chapter four which gives scientific results on health system research. Finally, chapter five presents results of and ongoing studies on biochemistry-based health care research which will gain further importance in the next future of this collaboration.

We thank our colleagues from both institutions who supported us in all stages of this project and they are too many to be mentioned here by name. The secretarial support of Ms Elke Braun van der Hoeven is gratefully acknowledged, as well as the editorial support by the Springer Verlag, and the excellent collaboration with the editor, Mr. Clemens Heine. We also thank the publishers of the articles reprinted in this volume who generously allowed the reproduction. We hope this book will motivate others to build up, to maintain and to further develop collaborations of similar nature.

BOCAR KOUYATÉ, NOUNA, BURKINA FASO

HEIKO BECHER, HEIDELBERG, GERMANY

OCTOBER 2004

Contents

Forewords V

Preface
Becher H., Kouyaté B. XI

1. Introduction 1
1.1 History of the CRSN: from a project to an institution 1
1.1.1 Twenty years of collaboration Heidelberg-Nouna
Diesfeld H.-J. 1
1.1.2 Transformation into a national research center:
The CRSN 1999 to today and the Heidelberg – Nouna collaboration
Kouyaté B., Sauerborn R. 7
1.2 Nouna DSS Data structure, data exchange
and routine epidemiologic procedures
Becher H., Stieglbauer G., Yé Y. 17
1.3 INDEPTH Network:
Generating Empirical Population and Health Data
in Resource-constrained Countries in the Developing World
Sankoh O., Binka F. 21
1.4 Ethics of biomedical research in developing countries
Müller O., Kouyaté B. 33
1.5 Health information systems
Krickeberg K. 43

2. Clinical Research 51
2.1 Clinical Research 51
2.1.1 Malaria studies in Nouna, Burkina Faso
Müller O. 51
2.1.2 Introduction of a program for prevention of transmission of human
immunodeficiency virus from mother to infant in rural Burkina Faso:
first operative results
*Böhler T., Sarker, M., Ganamé, J., Coulibaly, B., Hofmann, J., Nagabila, Y.,
Boncoungou, J., Tebit, D.M., Snow, R.C., Kräusslich H.-G.* 55
2.2 Effect of zinc supplementation on malaria and other causes of morbidity
in west African children: randomised double blind placebo controlled trial.
BMJ. 2001 Jun 30;322(7302):1567.
*Müller O., Becher H., van Zweeden A.B., Ye Y., Diallo D.A., Konate A.T.,
Gbangou A., Kouyaté B., Garenne M.* 65
2.3 Evaluation of a prototype long-lasting insecticide-treated mosquito net
under field conditions in rural Burkina Faso.
Trans R Soc Trop Med Hyg. 2002 Sep-Oct;96(5):483-4.
Müller O., Ido K., Traoré C. 73

2.4   Severe anaemia in west African children: malaria or malnutrition?
      Lancet. 2003;361(9351):86-7.
      Müller O., Traoré C., Jahn A., Becher H. 77

2.5   Clinical efficacy of chloroquine in young children with uncomplicated
      falciparum malaria – a community-based study in rural Burkina Faso.
      Trop Med Int Health. 2003 Mar;8(3):202-3.
      Müller O., Traoré C., Kouyaté B. 79

2.6   The association between protein-energy malnutrition, malaria morbidity
      and all-cause mortality in West African children.
      Trop Med Int Health. 2003 Jun;8(6):507-11.
      Müller O., Garenne M., Kouyaté B., Becher H. 83

2.7   Effect of zinc supplementation on growth in West African children:
      a randomized double-blind placebo-controlled trial in rural Burkina Faso.
      Int J Epidemiol. 2003 Dec;32(6):1098-102.
      *Müller O., Garenne M., Reitmeier P., Baltussen van Zweeden A., Kouyaté B.,
      Becher H.* 89

2.8   Efficacy of pyrimethamine-sulfadoxine in young children
      with uncomplicated falciparum malaria in rural Burkina Faso.
      Malar J. 2004 May 11;3(1):10.
      Müller O., Traoré C., Kouyaté B. 95

3   Epidemiological Studies 99

3.1   Epidemiological Studies, Introduction
      Becher H., Hammer G., Kynast-Wolf G., Kouyaté B., Somé F. 99

3.2   Clustering of childhood mortality in rural Burkina Faso.
      Int J Epidemiol. 2001 Jun;30(3):485-92.
      Sankoh O.A., Ye Y., Sauerborn R., Müller O., Becher H. 105

3.3   Community factors associated with malaria prevention by mosquito nets:
      an exploratory study in rural Burkina Faso.
      Trop Med Int Health. 2002 Mar;7(3):240-8.
      Okrah J., Traoré C., Pale A., Sommerfeld J., Müller O. 115

3.4   Mortality patterns, 1993-98, in a rural area of Burkina Faso, West Africa,
      based on the Nouna demographic surveillance system.
      Trop Med Int Health. 2002 Apr;7(4):349-56.
      Kynast-Wolf G., Sankoh O.A., Gbangou A., Kouyaté B., Becher H. 125

3.5   Patterns of adult and old-age mortality in rural Burkina Faso.
      Journal of Public Health Medicine 2003 Dec;25(4):372-6.
      Sankoh, O.A., Kynast-Wolf G., Kouyaté B., Becher H. 135

3.6   Malaria morbidity, treatment-seeking behaviour, and mortality in a cohort
      of young children in rural Burkina Faso.
      Trop Med Int Health. 2003 Apr;8(4):290-6.
      Müller O., Traoré C., Becher H., Kouyaté B. 141

3.7   Risk factors of infant and child mortality in rural Burkina Faso.
      Bull WHO 82(4): 265-274.
      Becher H., Müller O., Jahn A., Gbangou A., Kynast-Wolf G., Kouyaté B. 149

4	**Health System Research**	159
4.1	Introduction	159
4.2	Measuring the local burden of disease. A study of years of life lost in sub-Saharan Africa. Int J Epidemiol. 2001 30(3):501-8. *Würthwein R., Gbangou A., Sauerborn R., Schmidt C.M.*	161
4.3	Examining out-of-pocket expenditure on health care in Nouna, Burkina Faso: implications for health policy. Trop Med Int Health. 2002 7(2):187-96. *Mugisha F., Kouyaté B., Gbangou A., Sauerborn R.*	171
4.4	Perceived quality of care of primary health care services in Burkina Faso. Health Policy Plan. 2002;17(1):42-8. *Baltussen R.M., Ye Y., Haddad S., Sauerborn R.*	183
4.5	Informal risk-sharing arrangements (IRSAs) in rural Burkina Faso: lessons for the development of community-based insurance (CBI). Int J Health Plann Manage. 2002 17(2):147-63. *Sommerfeld J., Sanon M., Kouyaté B.A., Sauerborn R.*	191
4.6	Obtaining disability weights in rural Burkina Faso using a culturally adapted visual analogue scale *Baltussen R., Sanon M., Sommerfeld J., Würthwein R.*	209
4.7	Gender's effect on willingness-to-pay for community-based insurance in Burkina Faso. Health Policy. 2003 May;64(2):153-62. *Dong H., Kouyaté B., Snow R., Mugisha F., Sauerborn R.*	219
4.8	A comparison of the reliability of the take-it-or-leave-it and the bidding game approaches to estimating willingness-to-pay in a rural population in West Africa. Soc Sci Med. 2003 May;56(10):2181-9. *Dong H., Kouyaté B., Cairns J., Sauerborn R.*	231
4.9	Willingness-to-pay for community-based health insurance in Burkina Faso. Health Economics 2003 Oct;12(10):849-62. *Dong H.J., Kouyaté B., Cairns J., Mugisha F., Sauerborn R.*	241
4.10	Differential willingness of household heads to pay community-based health insurance premia for themselves and other household members. Health Policy Plan. 2004 19(2): 120-6. *Dong H., Kouyaté B., Cairns J., Sauerborn R.*	257
4.11	The two faces of enhancing utilization of health-care services: determinants of patient initiation and retention in rural Burkina Faso. Bull WHO 82 (8), August 2004, 572-579 *Mugisha F, Kouyaté B, Dong H, Chepng'eno G, Sauerborn R.*	265
4.12	The feasibility of community-based health insurance in Burkina Faso Health Policy 69 (2004) 45-53 *Dong H., Mugisha F., Gbangou A., Kouyaté B., Sauerborn R.*	275

5	**Biochemistry-based health care research**	285
5.1	Introduction *Coulibaly B., Eubel J., Gromer S., Schirmer H.*	285
5.2	Methylene blue as an antimalarial agent. Redox Rep. 2003;8(5):272-5. *Schirmer R.H., Coulibaly B., Stich A., Scheiwein M., Merkle H., Eubel J.,* *Becker K., Becher H., Muller O., Zich T., Schiek W., Kouyaté B.*	293
5.3	Pharmacogenomic strategies against resistance development in microbial infections *Ziebuhr W., Xiao K., Coulibaly B., Schwarz R., Dandekar T.*	299

Author index 303

Adresses of authors of chapters 305

1   Introduction

1.1 HISTORY OF CRSN: from a project to an institution

In early 1970's, the institutions in charge of the cooperation between Germany and Upper Volta (Burkina Faso) were working closely to improve the health conditions of the population in Burkina. It was an intensive collaboration to assess the intervention through health system research. Before 1990, it was an evaluation of the intervention. In 1992, a collaborative research project between the Ministry of Health in Burkina Faso and the Department of Tropical Hygiene and Public Health of Heidelberg University in Germany was established. It was named Projet de Recherche Action pour l'Amélioration des Services de santé (PRAPASS); the Centre de Recherche en Santé de Nouna (CRSN) is a research institution, which started in early October 1999 by a transformation of PRAPASS into a national research institution. In the following sections of this chapter, the history of this collaboration is outlined.

1.1.1 Twenty years of collaboration Heidelberg-Nouna

HANS-JOCHEN DIESFELD

Leopoldstr. 6, 82319 Starnberg, Germany

Tel: 00 49 8151 12143
Fax: 00 49 8151 773780

Email: h-j.diesfeld@urz.uni-heidelberg.de

Since 1975, in the framework of Burkina Faso – Germany cooperation in the health sector, the German Volunteer Service (DED) has actively participated, in collaboration with the German Technical Cooperation (GTZ), in the improvement of basic health services. Over the years, a growing number of rural hospitals (Centre Médical) were equipped by German medical doctors and nurses, during a period where only very few Burkinan doctors were available and when there was still no Medial Faculty. Those German doctors and nurses got their specific preparatory training at the Department of Tropical Hygiene and Public Health, Heidelberg University, where they were given information about the latest internationally discussed and recommended health policies and - programmes. This was the time, when the health policy of Burkina Faso (then Upper Volta), following the implementation of the principles and strategies of the WHO/UNICEF -"Alma Ata Declaration" of 1978 on "Primary Health Care", experienced a radical change from a rather curative, hospital-centred to a more decentralised, population-based comprehensive health care concept of health policy.

By 1982 15 Health Districts with their Rural Hospitals and their peripheral health stations and village health posts in Western, North and Northwest Provinces of Burkina Faso were participating in this "Programme Amelioration des Services Sanitaires Ruraux", under the Ministry of Health of Burkina

Faso with assistance of DED and GTZ. The District Hospital Nouna, Kossi province was one of the very first to be included in this programme. The first German physician, *Dr. Habicht* with the German theatre nurse *Mrs. Rosemary Kempers* arrived in Nouna already some years earlier in 1974 before he was followed by a sequence of German physicians from the German Volunteer Service. In November 1982, at the request of the Ministry of Health of Burkina Faso and the German Volunteer Service an evaluation mission was carried out by the Department of Tropical Hygiene and Public Health, University of Heidelberg, headed by me in collaboration with the late *Dr. A. K. Pangu* and *Dr. A. Stroobant*.

The objective of this mission was not only to look into the performance, efficacy and effectiveness of this Burkinan-German collaboration but also to identify problems of utilisation of health services and their possible reasons. One of the recommendations of this mission was to intensify the interaction between the Medical Districts supported by DED as a kind of pilot region and the Ministry of Health through an iterative process of monitoring, feed back, planning and adjustment process. The German Voluntary Service agreed to assign one medical officer to concentrate on this process.

At this point of time, 1983/84, the European Parliament had decided to establish a Programme for Science and Technology for Development with special emphasis on cooperation between European research institutions with partners in developing countries with the particular aim to strengthen research capacities. One of the main topics was health research, at that time rather ill-defined. The European Commission, Directorate for Research and Technology (DG XII) was put in charge of this programme and the first calls for research proposal were published in 1984. Having been somehow involved in this conceptual discussion as a scientific representative of Germany, member state of the European Union, I had the chance to plead a case for including Health Systems Research into the scope of the research profile.

This gave us the chance, together with the Burkinian Ministry of Health and in partnership with the Department of Public Health, Faculty of Health Sciences, University of Ouagadougou to formulate a number of research questions on the efficiency, efficacy and utilization of mother and child health services and the primary health care programmes in Burkina Faso. The objectives of the research were the measurement of the quality, effectiveness and utilization of preventive and curative health services at the district and community level. The main hypotheses were that the actual provision of services is not in line with the need of high risk groups and that the coverage of programs and acceptance by the population is deficient. The aim of the study was to provide empirical data for a better adaptation of health programs to local needs. This implied the personal feed back of the results and their discussion at central and local levels in order to help to improve the performance of services as well as to design subsequent intervention studies jointly with the local authorities.

The research proposal was intensely discussed between members of the "Departement des Etudes et Planification" of the Ministry of Health and the Department of Tropical Medicine and Public Health of Heidelberg University and the Department of Public Health of the University of Ouagadougou. The Ministry of Health decided that the research area should be in the Kossi Province (Fig. 1) and in the catchment area of Solenzo Medical Centre, where Nouna was the next reference hospital, and where one of the researchers from Heidelberg University, *Dr. Rainer Sauerborn* had been Médecin Chef from 1979 to 1982. Finally the research proposal was accepted by the Ministry of Health and submitted to the European Commission, DG XII.

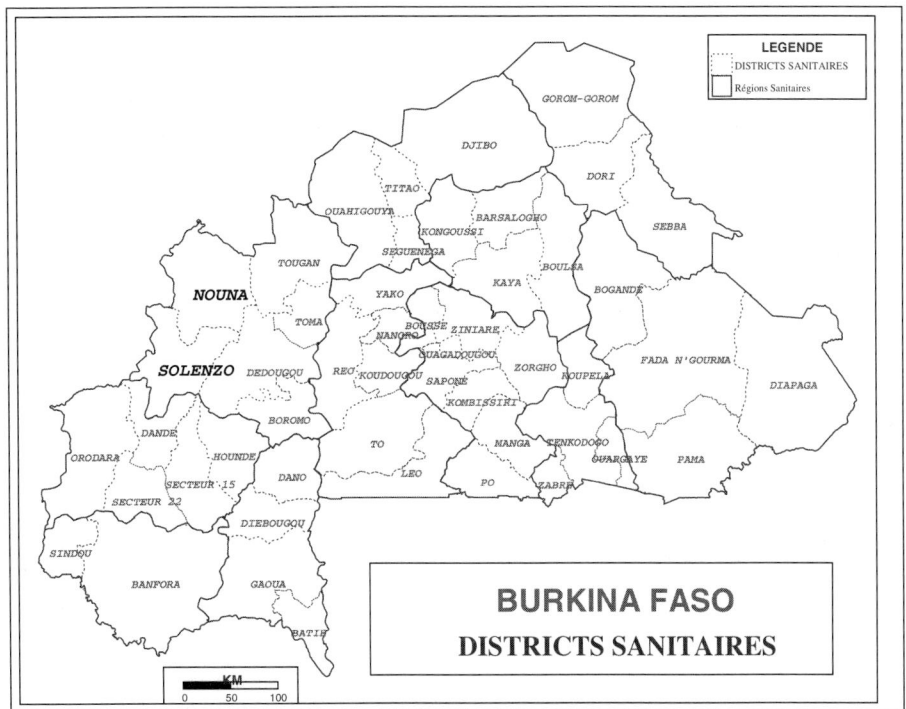

Figure 1: "Districts Sanitaires" with Solenzo and Nouna

This was a time when Health Systems Research was still in its infancies and the discussion on appropriate research methods was still ongoing. Qualitative versus quantitative methods and the triangulation of different methods was still not at all an accepted approach, in particular by epidemiologists.

At last, the research proposal was accepted by the European Commission and the Regional Panel [under STD 1 – TDS –M-053-D(B)] for the period 1984 – 1988 and the study took off immediately. A conceptual framework was developed to investigate determining factors influencing perception of health problems by the population and the respective healer choice and their interaction with the chosen health care system. In order to examine the provider and user of services and their interaction as well as the potential non-user the study design comprised the following elements: a representative stratified household survey in the catchment area Solenzo Centre Medicale of different strata of health services in order to describe the socio-economic status, health and health seeking behaviour, the strata being chosen according to accessibility to various levels of health services. User survey in various strata of health services, provider survey in the respective health units by non-participatory observation, description of services and interviews with health personnel was performed.

There was a tripartite collaboration from the beginning: Ministry of Health seconded *Dr. Adrien Nougtara* as the national researcher, the Faculty of Health Sciences had been very interested and its then Dean, *Professor R. M. Ouiminga* had been very helpful in encouraging three medical students, *Gaston Sorgho, Joseph Bidiga* and *Lougousse Tiebelesse*, to join as junior researchers under the supervision of the then Head of the Department of Public Health, *Professor Francois Cannone*. The University of Heidelberg seconded *Dr. Rainer Sauerborn* from the Pediatric Department of the University Hospital as the German field researcher and myself as the Principal Investigator, responsible towards the European Commission.

DED and GTZ were extremely helpful in providing technical assistance and transport, beyond the means at our disposition through the research grant. The personal commitment and untiring support by *Dr. Cornelius Oepen* and *Dr. Eberhard Koob* has to be gratefully acknowledged.

The field research was completed by 1985 and the analysis of the data as a kind of participatory evaluation of results with the health services at peripheral and central level took place in two seminars in 1986. This was a specific methodological approach of action research where all parties concerned were involved.

On December 13, 1986, even before the final report of the research was compiled, the three medical students from Burkina Faso defended their theses successfully before the Faculty of Health Sciences, myself serving as the "président du jury". This was the first time in Burkina Faso, that medical students attempted to do their thesis work "in the field" of day to day basic health care up country and not within the protected area of the University Hospital. In the course of this event a "Faculty Partnership" between the Faculty of Health Sciences in Ouagadougou and the Medical Faculty of Heidelberg was inaugurated officially and the Dean, *Professor Ouiminga* was invited and took part as an official representative of his University at the ceremonies commemorating the 600th anniversary of the University of Heidelberg on October 14, 1986. From then onwards, for a number of years there was a fruitful collaboration between the two faculties, in different clinical fields, beyond the health systems research area. Encouraged by this experience, the Department of Public Health of the University Ouagadougou established until to date, observational field research by medical students as part of their curriculum. As a consequence of the evaluation seminars the Ministry of Health summoned in December 1988 a seminar in order to plan a project for action research for the next three years, again submitted to the European Commission and approved [STD 2 TS2-0306 (DB)] in 1990 under the title "Action research on the utilization of health services in Burkina Faso". Projet Recherche Action pour l'Amélioration des Soins de Santé (PRAPASS). A "Comité de Coordination de la Recherche-Action" (Fig. 2) was formed at the Ministry of Health which this time was the principal investigator answerable to the research funding European Commission. This time the Ministry of Health chose the catchment area around the Centre Médical Nouna as the study site.

The study aimed to assess the output and outcome of newly organized rural health services. The major health policy changes to be tested were:

- the participation of the target population in the financing and management of health services
- the enhancement of service quality through standardization of medical tasks
- an increased attraction by better integration of services,
- the introduction of a delivery system of essential generic drugs,
- the strengthening of mother's skills in treating key childhood illnesses.

The study population comprised of all households in the catchment area of Nouna hospital and three health centres (excluding Nouna town), altogether 6000 households with approx. 30.000 individuals. Health impacts were monitored in terms of changes in age and cause specific mortality using annual censuses and monthly vital events registration and verbal autopsy of all deaths of children during the survey period. A subsample of 600 households was studied by periodic household surveys. They yielded information on any change in health service utilization, health care expenditure and in time lost due to illness.

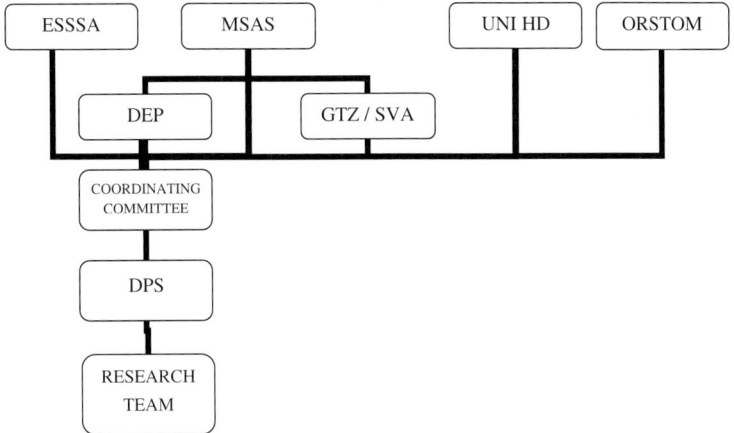

MSAS: Ministère de la Santé et d'Action Sociale (Principal investigator)
ESSSA: Ecole Supérieure des Sciences de la Santé (Université de Ouagadougou, Faculté de Médecine, Dépt. De Santé Publique)
UNI HD: Université de Heidelberg, Département d'Hygiène Tropicale et de la Santé Publique, Germany
ORSTOM: Office de Recherche Scientifique et technique outremer, Paris, Ouagadougou
DEP: Direction des Etudes et de la Planification du MSAS
GTZ/SVA: Deutsche Gesellschaft für Technische Zusammenarbeit / Deutscher Entwicklungsdienst
DPS: Direction Provinciale de Santé (Nouna, Province de Kossi)

Figure 2: Comité de Coordination de la Recherche-Action

This Demographic Surveillance System (DSS) exists till today and enables the Ministry of Health to become in November1998 part of the INDEPTH Network (International Network of Demographic Evaluation of Populations and Their Health) which has today 36 members from 19 countries in Africa, Asia, Oceania and Latin America covering a population of 1.2 million in Africa alone (see chapter 1.3).

In 1992 during a contract holder meeting of the Commission of the European Communities, Directorate XII, Science, Research and Development the two EC funded research projects, the completed and the ongoing one, were presented and methodology and relevance of health systems research was discussed in a large international scientific forum. The new research programme studied a number of different topics. Several new full time and part time research assistants were engaged in executing the different research topics and running the more and more expanding research station in Nouna. Two full time physicians, formerly medical doctors under DED working in Burkina Faso *Mathias Borchert* and *Justus Benzler* could be gained to run the field station and executing and supervising the various field activities and managing the data processing. They were supported by a Physician, seconded from DED, *Dr. Rolf Heinmüller*. Specific studies were carried out by and together with burkinian colleagues such as *Dr. Hien Mathias, Dr. Nougtara Adrien, Dr. Ibrango or Mrs Nikiema-Heinmüller*. Interim researchers from ORSTOM, *Prof. Michel Garenne*, from the Department of Tropical Hygiene and Public Health, Heidelberg University, like *Gérard Krause, Ulrike Hornung* or *Ulrich Wahser*. The Ministry of Health provided a suitable building complex within the compound of the District Hospital of Nouna, a former epidemiological field station. Field investigators, interviewers and data entry clerks had to be recruited and trained.

During the first years there was the problem of only sporadic public electricity supply, supported by a generator, which made the increasing demand by upcoming modern information technology rather difficult and cumbersome. Telephone and facsimile communication with the Heidelberg Tropical Institute were quite difficult. The maintenance of laptops for the registration and monitoring of all the incoming data from the DSS under the prevailing climatic and environmental conditions was quite stressful for the researchers and the growing number of specifically trained data collectors and computer operators. Transport was still a problem which thanks to the support of DED and GTZ could be overcome.

Research topics aiming at improving child health, equity and efficiency implications of prepayment schemes and health insurance in Burkina Faso were compared with similar experiences in Ghana, the capacity and willingness to pay for health services was studied in cooperation with GTZ/DED, the effect of quality assurance on utilisation in rural health services or drug utilisation patterns and quality of prescription with the introduction of the Governments Essential Drug Programme (MEG) were all based on the functioning DSS.

The list of publications in the annex is impressive. The iterative process between Ministry of Health and Research Station in Nouna and its team and the growing number of successfully completed research projects led to an increasing acceptance of this kind of scientific cooperation by the Ministry of Health. This and the continuous efforts from the researchers side to look for further funds and sponsors and favourable developments in the process of acceptance of Health Systems Research internationally, within the University of Heidelberg and within the German scientific and research sponsoring community (EU-INCO-DC and DFG) as well as the Ministry of Higher Education of the Federal State of Baden Württemberg paved the way towards a very important and visionary move by the Government of Burkina Faso to establish the "Centre de Recherche en Santé de Nouna (CRSN)" in October 1999 in close partnership with the University of Heidelberg.

This is an example of consistent and persistent systematic efforts to build on the basis of scientific achievements, academic partnership between health research and health policy. This effort being totally in line with the health research funding policy of the European Community and the European Commission to develop research partnerships and structures for research capacity building between Europe and countries in Africa, Asia and Latin America (EC-INCO-DC), has helped over the past twenty years to secure sufficient project-specific research grants to develop this cooperative structure.

The constant and critical question asked by all international research funding organisations, in particular the European Commission, is what impact does health systems research have on national health policy, health research policy and national capacity building. This project, supported by an increasing number of externally funded research projects and increasing basic funding by the ministry of health, Burkina Faso, has become one of the very few positive examples and a showpiece of the European Commission's health research funding policy.

1.1.2 Transformation into a national research center: the CRSN 1999 to today and the Heidelberg – Nouna collaboration

BOCAR KOUYATE

Centre de Recherche en Santé de Nouna, BP 02 Nouna, Burkina Faso

Tel.: 00226-20-537043

Email: bocar.crsn@fasonet.bf

RAINER SAUERBORN

University of Heidelberg, Department of Tropical Hygiene and Public Health, Im Neuenheimer Feld 324, 69120 Heidelberg, Germany

Tel.: 0049-6221-565344

Email: rainer.sauerborn@urz.uni-heidelberg.de

In this chapter, we trace the quantum leap, the Nouna research site took when it was transformed from a bundle of assorted projects (PRAPASS) to a national research institution.

The institutional architecture

The way in which a research center, even more so, a research cooperation, is set up, tells a lot about its ownership, its efficacy and long-term sustainability.

In 1999 the Ministry of Health of Burkina transformed the project into a permanent research institution directly affiliated to the general secretariat. The initiative for this move came from the former Secretary General of the Ministry, *Bocar Kouyaté*, and *Rainer Sauerborn* who established a formal research cooperation between the nascent Center and the Department of Tropical Hygiene and Public Health, he chairs at the University of Heidelberg.

This was more than an organizational change and reflected the increasing ownership the Ministry took in the research. This step also meant that the national scope and relevance of the research carried out in Nouna was recognized. While the local communities, the district and the province in which Nouna is situated remained important stakeholders with whom the center engages and to whom the researchers feed-back their results, the main target for exchange and feedback would henceforth be the national level. Figure 1 illustrates the change in institutional affiliation from the district level (bottom right square) to the national level.

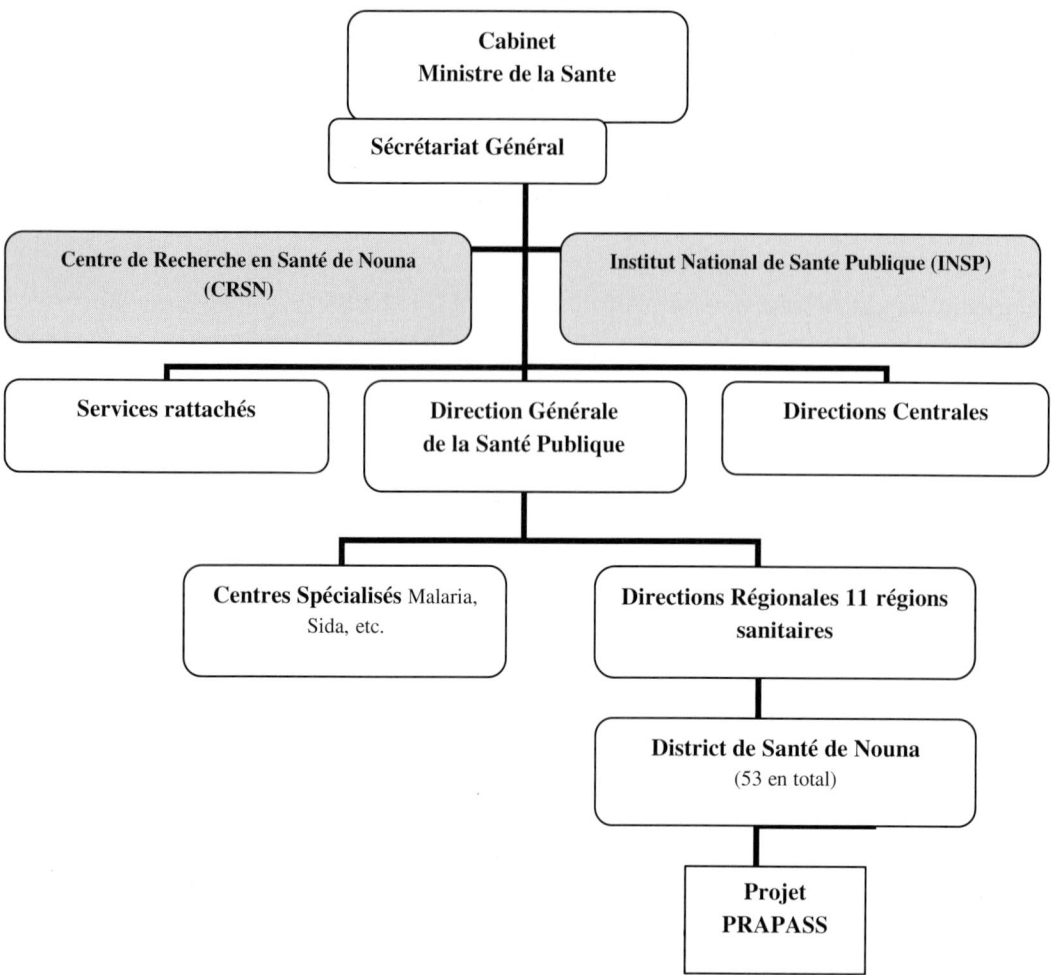

Figure 1: Institutional affiliation: From Project (see white box at the bottom) to a National Research Center directly reporting to the Secretary General of the Ministry of Health.

The interaction between researchers and decision-makers, a crucial element of health systems research, was greatly enhanced. In an iterative way, research results were communicated to and discussed with decision-makers, both local, regional and national, their feedback, in turn, influenced the direction of research, e.g. how new policies were formulated and then field tested.

Figure 2 illustrates this continuous and long-term exchange between decision-makers and scientists using as an example the topic of health care financing. Over a period of more than two decades, this dialogue led to several policy innovations which finally culminated in pilot testing a complex operation of community-based insurance.

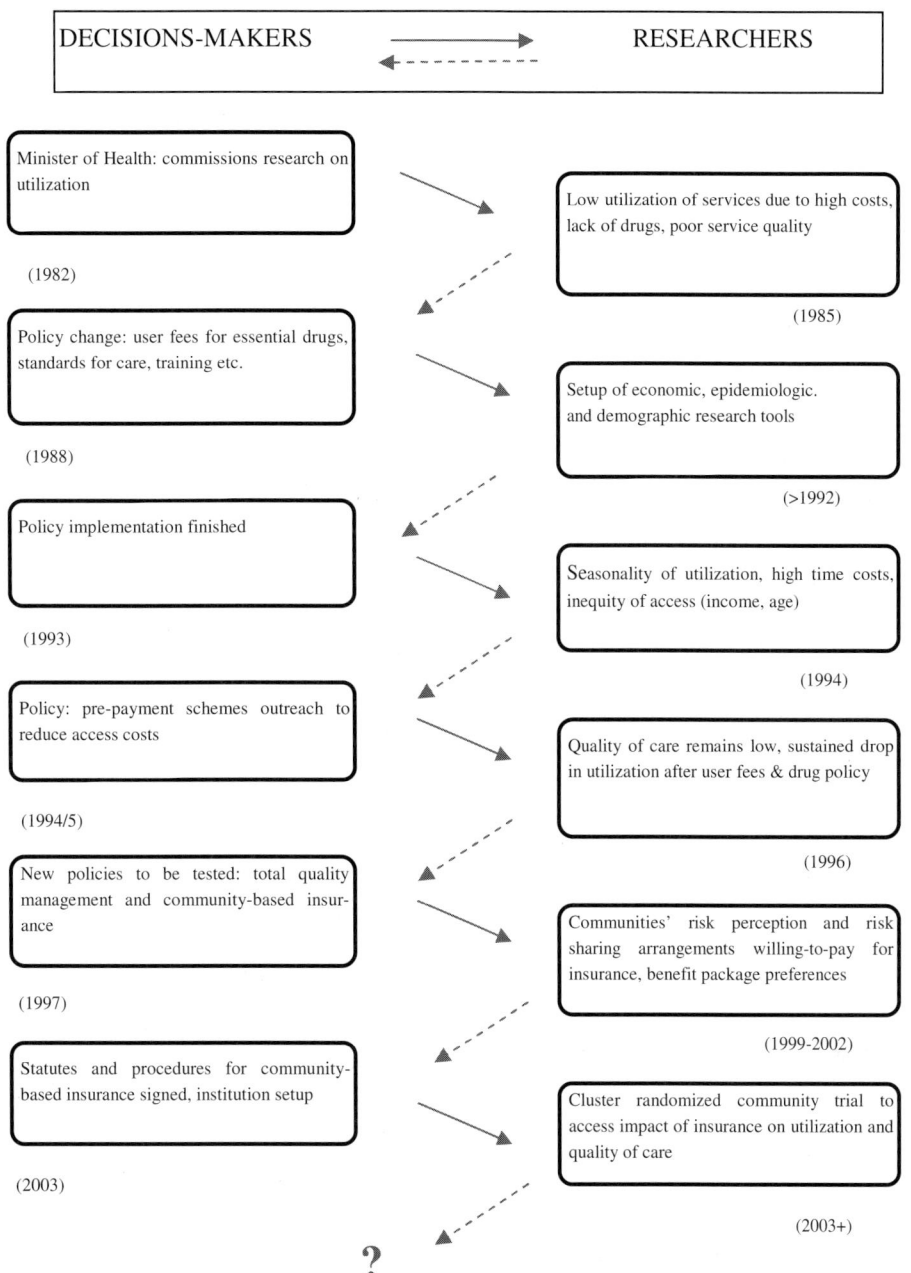

Figure 2: The iterative and long-term exchange between researchers and decision-makers, using the policy issues of health care financing and quality of care as examples.

Initial research, stimulated by the evaluation of a German development cooperation project (DED/GTZ) by *Jochen Diesfeld* and colleagues (see preceding chapter), had pointed to serious under-utilization of health services and its main cause: the high costs which the households of the sick had to bear to obtain care. In addition the timing of the costs, i.e. regardless of the season of the year, posed a great problem to households. In a joint workshop the Ministry of Health of Burkina Faso gave Nouna researchers the green light to explore prepayment systems, particularly health insurance. Based on evidence from a series of epidemiological, anthropological and economic studies, community-based insurance scheme was designed in a joint effort of Ministry, local community and research team. This insurance scheme is currently being implemented, accompanied by a randomized community trial to assess its effectiveness and to understand potential weaknesses in order to further improve the policy.

At the same time the link between the new CRSN and the University of Heidelberg was strengthened and formalized. An agreement of research cooperation was signed between the Ministry and the Department of Tropical Hygiene and Public Health. The Land Baden-Württemberg agreed to fund the core expenses of the Center as a support of the large collaborative grant (SFB544) which an interdisciplinary group of researchers from Heidelberg University had just been awarded.

Both the CRSN and the network of researchers in Heidelberg have been guided by international scientific advisory boards, each of whom invited an observer of the other board to their meetings to increase research coordination. Figure 3 shows the structure of the research cooperation, complete with the faculty partnership mentioned in the previous chapter.

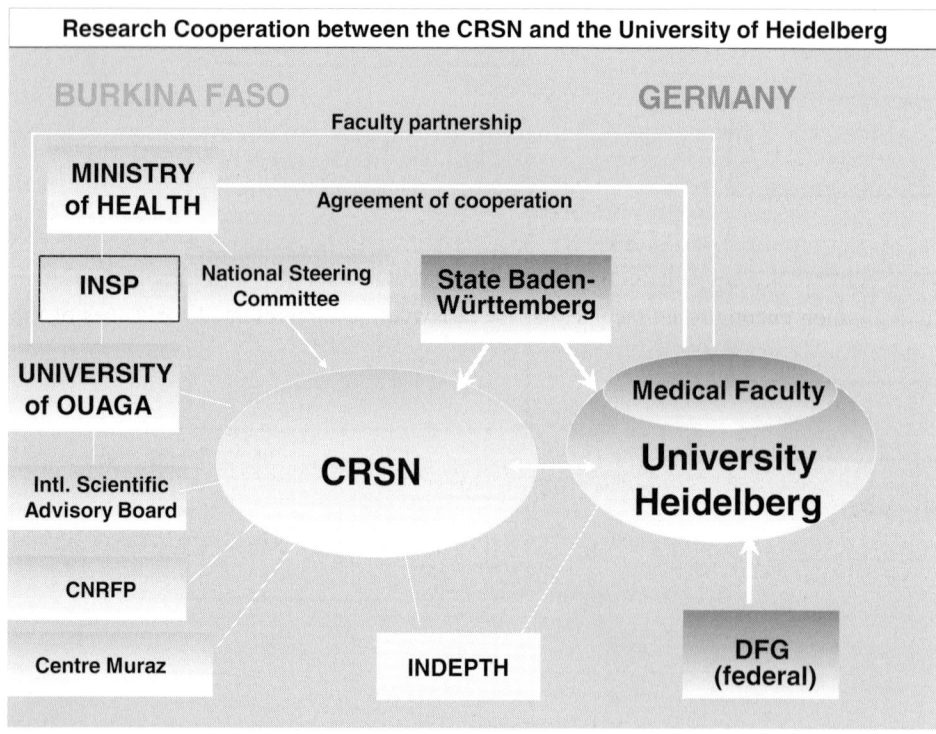

Figure 3: Institutional set-up of the research cooperation, both nationally and internationally

Strengthening the Center's scientific capacity

This is an essential ingredient of our cooperation. It aims at both the individual researcher and the research environment. There were three CRSN staff members trained in Heidelberg at the M.Sc. (Master of Community Health and Health Management in Developing Countries) level, and a number of colleagues have finalized their doctoral degree (Dr. med. or Dr. sc. hum.) or are currently working on it. Improving general research conditions is much more difficult to tackle, yet crucial for building capacity.

Courses held at Nouna have been another important part for capacity building. These courses covered important aspects in biostatistics, epidemiology, anthropology, programming, grant proposal writing, and others. They were held by scientists from Heidelberg and lasted between one and two weeks. The number of participants was an average ten to fifteen. Most of the participants were members of the CRSN, in some cases young researchers from Ouagadougou, or from the Kossi health district took part. The CRSN offered good facilities for such short courses, and usually the benefits of these courses exceeded the teaching subjects. The regular personal contact between researchers from both institutions was intensified leading to a better mutual understanding.

A lot has been achieved in terms of information access (internet access, establishment of a library with 5000 hardcopies of selected published papers). The challenge ahead lies in a closer integration in the national scientific community (university and extra-university research centers) through training of national students and through joint research. Opening up of national career paths for accomplished CRSN scientists is another issue that needs to be tackled.

The international scientific advisory board, composed of eminent scientists from Canada, Germany, Mali and Burkina Faso has been very helpful in guiding both the research agenda and the improvement of research skills of the team.

An integral part of research capacity of any Center carrying out population-based and clinical research is an active and vigilant ethics committee. In the absence of a national ethics committee, the Center created a local one which encompassed technical skills (a lawyer) and represented the values of the local communities through members from a wide range of religious, ethnic, gender and age groups.

National and international integration of the CRSN

Nationally, the CRSN is known as one of several cooperating health research centers, perhaps the one with the most comprehensive agenda. The link with the university is still weak and remains to be strengthened.

Internationally, the center cooperates with dozens of partners both in the north and the south which include Karolinska Insitut, Leeds University, London School of Hygiene and Tropical Medicine, Institut Pasteur, NIH, WHO, the International Labor Office and, of course, Heidelberg University. With other developing countries, the CRSN took the lead in initiating and in steering a network of 28 such research sites which is described in chapter 1.3.

Broadening the research agenda along four axes

The PRAPASS project had kept an exclusive focus on health system research (first axis). With the creation of the CRSN and the award of a large interdisciplinary research grant (SFB 544 "Control of Tropical Infectious Diseases") to its partners in Heidelberg, the research agenda broadened to comprise three additional axes:

The first addition in 1999 was lab-based biomedical research (second axis). A parasitological lab was equipped guided by Prof. M. Lanzer, biochemical and entomological lab facilities were soon added, including an insectarium which holds the complete life cycle of the malaria transmitting mosquito Anopheles gambiae.

The third research axis, clinical patient-oriented research, was only added recently (2004) guided by Drs Ali Sié and Thomas Junghanss. Both research partners agreed that the routine health facilities serving the study population needed to be improved. The Medical Faculty of Heidelberg University and the Ministry of Health each posted one senior physician to the health district of Nouna whose task has been to oversee and guide the quality improvement in the district hospital and its satellite health centers.

The forth axis is the most recent addition to the Center's portfolio: The environmental dimension of health. This involves mapping the changes of land cover (surface water, vegetation, i.e. mosquito breeding sites) and continuously recording meteorological data in order to track the environmental factors which influence malaria transmission.

Ground-based data are used to validate satellite data on land cover, temperature and rainfall which in the long run will serve as a cost-effective means to monitor and predict the transmission of selected infectious diseases on a national, perhaps regional scale.

Through new additions to the scientific team, the CRSN staff reflects this multidisciplinary approach. Today, the team comprises an impressive array of skills in public health, clinical medicine, demography, economics, sociology, anthropology, pharmacology, biology, geography, biostatistics, computer sciences and entomology.

The platform or backbone which holds the diverging research agendas together is the so-called demographic surveillance system (DSS). This means that the health and vital events of an entire population, as distinct form a sample thereof, is surveyed on a prospective and continuous basis. Each and every one of the 65 000 inhabitants in 44 villages of the research zone is registered and visited every three months. Every hut is displayed in a geographical information system linking the database up with an electronic map. Figure 4 shows the DSS as the centerpiece of the different research disciplines.

It provides an always up-to-date denominator for population-based research, allows individuals to be sampled for example for enrolment in clinical trials and to be unequivocally retrieved. The DSS forms a sampling frame for surveys and anthropological studies and links morbidity data to socioeconomic and environmental factors that might influence the disease under study. Two further examples may illustrate the universal usefulness of the DSS: It allows studying how the distribution of mosquito populations relates to the geographic pattern of malaria incidence. Molecular markers of malaria host susceptibility or of parasite resistance to antimalarials can be traced within the population across time and space.

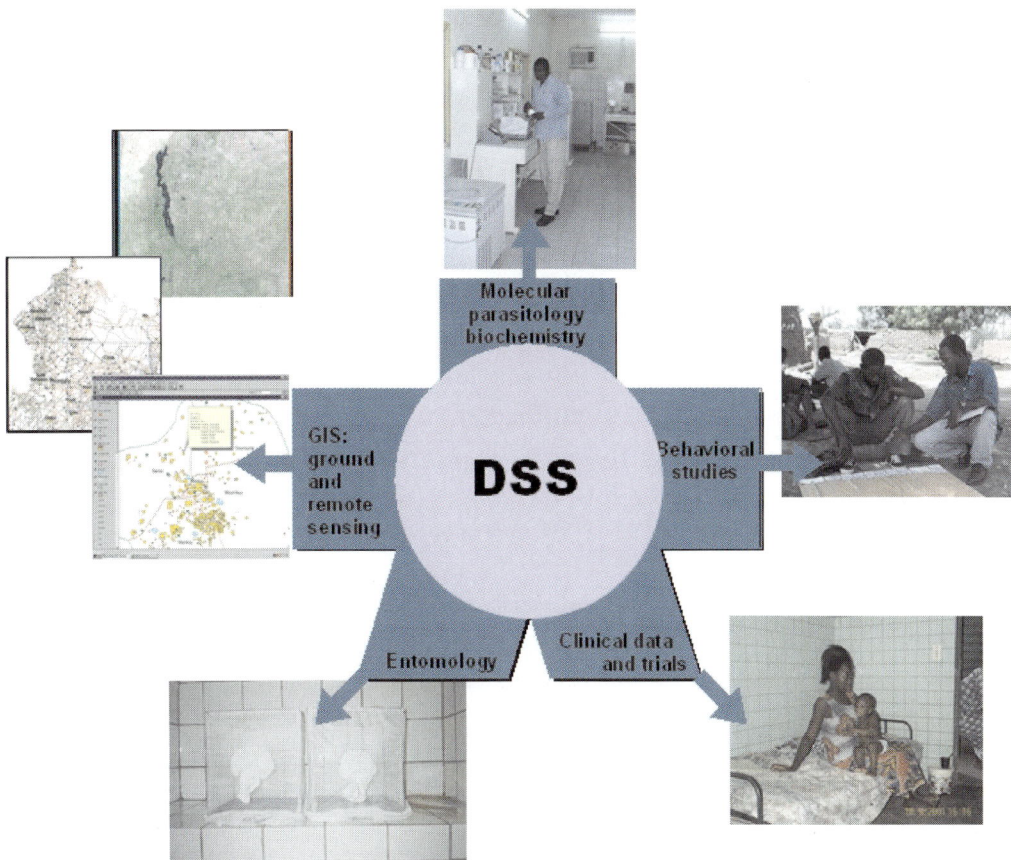

Figure 4: The demographic surveillance system (DSS) as the focal point of different research disciplines

The path towards financial sustainability

Research is costly and funding scarce, particularly in low income countries. On the other hand there are huge amounts of funds available for first-class research proposals. Some funding agencies make particular efforts to build research capacity during the life-time of a project. The art of squaring the circle consists in 1) cooperating with supportive research institutions in the north in joint projects, initially led by them. 2) aiming to be principal investigator if at all possible, in collaborative projects with established partners in the north. This has been increasingly the case in the past three years and reflects increasing skills in proposal writing and competent mastery of research methods on the part of Center staff. 3) Joining hands with other partners in the south in networks whose critical mass enhances the chances of acquiring soft money research grants. The INDEPTH network described in chapter 1.3. is an example for such an endeavor.

Since its creation in 1999, the CRSN has consequently followed this path. It has now a portfolio of more than 15 projects including several large grants where a staff member of the CRSN is principal investigator. Successful acquisition of research funds paves the way to financial sustainability, or doesn't it?

The total revenue of the Center has more than doubled in 4 years, from 230,000 Euro in 1999 to 570,000 in 2003. Figure 5 illustrates the steady increase of self funding, which reached 52 % in 2004. The contribution of the Burkinian Ministry of Health, largely in covering personnel cost, has slightly increased in relative terms from 10% in 1999 to 13.4% in 2003. In absolute terms this means that the amount the Ministry contributes has more than doubled in the last 4 years.

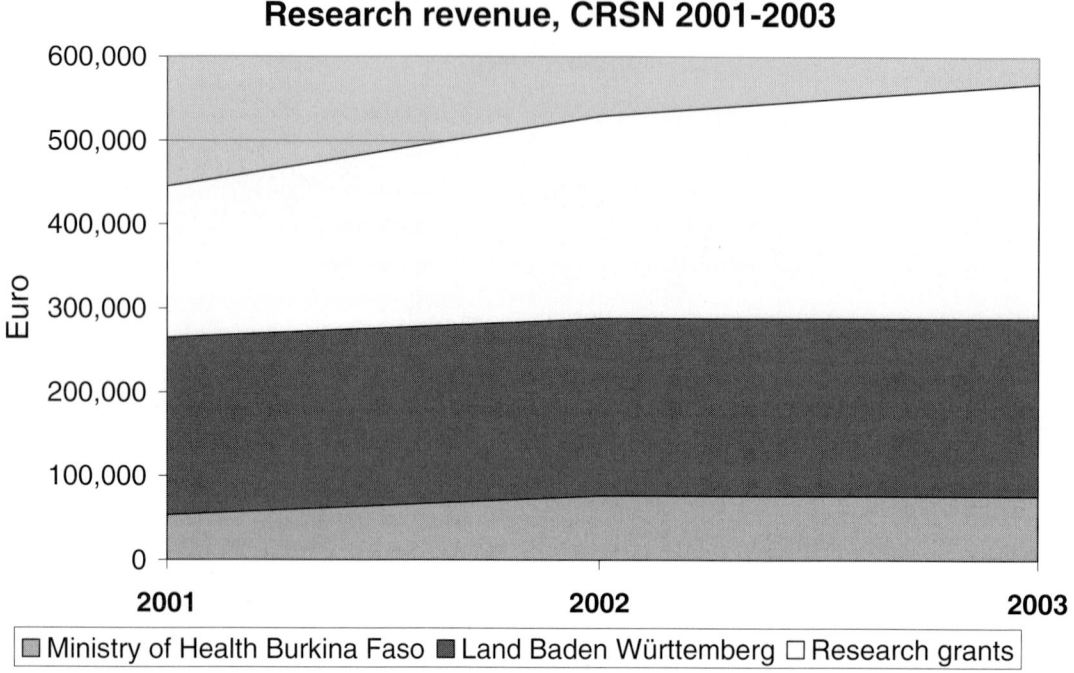

Figure 5: Increasing self-funding of the CRSN which still relies on modest core funding

In contrast the funding of the Land of Baden Wuerttemberg has remained quite stable in absolute terms. Its relative share has considerably fallen from an initial 60% to about 33%, in 2003. While this is a great success for such a young center, it shows that it is very hard to fund such a sophisticated research center exclusively based on soft money. The core funding, in German "Grundausstattung" cannot be borne by the host country. In fact, even a German university enjoys a considerable amount of core funding. The collaborating Department of Tropical Hygiene and Public Health had roughly a similar proportion of core funding through public budgets: 44% versus 56% of acquired research grants. It is inconceivable and unfair to require a research institution from one of the poorest countries to operate without such core support.

There is therefore a need for a modest, but sustained core funding by international solidarity. Of the other 28 similar research institutions, Sweden funds the core expenditures of no fewer than 5 such research centers, the Wellcome trust 3, the Rockefeller foundation 2, the CDC 1 etc.. Given that the majority of such centers are much older and had thus a longer period for capacity building and networking, the success of the CRSN to draw more than 50 % of its revenue from competitive grants is all the more impressive.

The future of the CRSN therefore depends both on continued strengthening of scientific capacity in Nouna, its effective partnerships both with the south and the north. It does, however, also rely on a visionary funding institution in the north who is committed to provide moderate funds (in the order of 200,000 Euro annually) for many years to come.

1.2 Nouna DSS Data structure, data exchange and routine epidemiologic procedures

HEIKO BECHER, GABRIELE STIEGLBAUER, YAZOUME YÉ

University of Heidelberg, Department of Tropical Hygiene and Public Health, Im Neuenheimer Feld 324, 69120 Heidelberg. Germany

Tel.: +49 6221 565031

Email: Heiko.becher@urz.uni-heidelberg.de

Epidemiology is one of the key fields of research in the Nouna-Heidelberg collaboration. The respective research results are outlined in chapter three, whereas in this chapter some of the necessary organisational structures are presented which are the basis for descriptive and analytical studies and which allow an effective collaborative work.

Most of the past epidemiological activities were based on the Nouna DSS population. More recent studies try to put data from this study population into a broader national and international – African – context. The INDEPTH network has played an important role in that respect (see chapter 1.3). In order to allow an effective joint project work between scientists working in Nouna and Heidelberg, well-functioning data management and exchange procedures are necessary. The data exchange between Nouna and Heidelberg has been designed progressively over about the last ten years; however, it was put in writing in October 1999 in Nouna after a meeting with Heidelberg and Nouna team. It is a system which takes the technical conditions in both institutions into account and is well functioning. Some key features are given below:

The Nouna DSS uses a self designed and developed relational database based on Microsoft Access. The database is designed for longitudinal data entry and management and allows first stage systematic consistency and plausibility check. The database structure is comprised of five entities (tables or files) related to each other by one to one and one to many relationships. These entities are: Individual, Membership, Household, Residence and Observation:

- *Individual*. This entity contains invariant records, mainly demographical characteristics (name, sex, date of birth, ethnic and religion) on individuals who reside or have ever resided in the DSS area. Records are uniquely identified by the individual ID. To allow genealogical linkage this entity also includes the ID and name of the mother and father.
- *Household.* The household entity stores information (head of household, geographical location to allow linkage with the Geographical Information System, date of entry of creation of the household) of a particular social group, a household defined as a group of people living together and sharing food and production. The household is composed of one or several members and can be linked to the Membership entity through household unique identification.
- *Membership*. Membership record establishes the link of an individual to a particular household. Data on relationship within household members are stored.

- **Residence**. This entity contains variant information, susceptible to changes over time, like residence, marital, occupation and education status. An individual residence episode within study area or household is defined by the date of entry (birth, in migration) and date of exit (death, out migration). Similarly, marital, occupation and education status can also change with a starting and ending date. Residence can be linked to individual entity by the individual ID.
- **Observation.** Individuals are visited four times a year to update information. The source of observation entity keeps track of the observations that led to any new information; therefore, information of type of observation (census or vital registration survey) and date of observation are stored. Records on the interviewer who did the observation is also included.

The database has been in use for several years with minor modifications and has proved to be effective for the researchers needs. A conversion into other database systems was under discussion but has not taken place. Data entry takes place in Nouna with five well trained data entry clerks. A data-entry supervisor is responsible for data quality security matters. He is supported by a fully trained computer scientist, who is responsible for updating the database programme and developing other database (household survey) links to the DSS.

In regular intervals a copy of the original ACCESS-database with anonymous (according to the national data regulation) individual data is stored and transferred to Heidelberg. Until about the year 2000 this was done with ZIP-discettes, which has now been replaced by CD-ROM. In order to guarantee data security, the sealed CD is brought by visiting scientists from Nouna to Heidelberg. Raw data are not sent by mail or by internet. The DSS database is regularly updated two times a year. Old versions are stored to allow verification of published results at any time in the future.

The database is stored in Heidelberg on a central server with limited access to the core group at the Department of Tropical Hygiene and Public Health. This procedure guarantees that researchers in both institutions have access to an identical database.

For more sophisticated procedures for checking data consistency and for most epidemiologic analyses, we use the statistical software package SAS. The data of relevant ACCESS tables are extracted and imported into this software.

Within SAS a data checking procedure is installed, which checks the imported data for inconsistencies, mainly in date variables (date of birth, date of entry, date of exit). Inaccurate data are corrected and set to new plausible values. Should there be data records with completely lacking information or apparently implausible information which cannot be corrected, these are excluded. A listing with these implausible data is given back to the CRSN for further clarification and correction.

After cleaning the data, a SAS master data file for the routine statistical analysis of the DSS data is generated, including all valid records and relevant variables. The actual data concerning cause of death (Verbal Autopsy database) supplements this file.

On demand or request, data for different research topics from SFB-groups are retrieved, provided in a user-friendly form according to the particular needs.

The SAS master data file is the basis of a statistical routine for a menu-guided analysis of the DSS data (based on a SAS program) und for generating an epidemiological report including basic epidemiological and demographic measures e.g. the annual population size (midyear population, person years), age specific death rates, crude death rates and age standardized death rates and graphical presentations.

The routine analysis modules are currently in a development process and will be established and evaluated in close cooperation with the CRSN Nouna.

As an example of the graphical output, figure 1 shows the age pyramid of the Nouna DSS population as of December 31st, 2001.

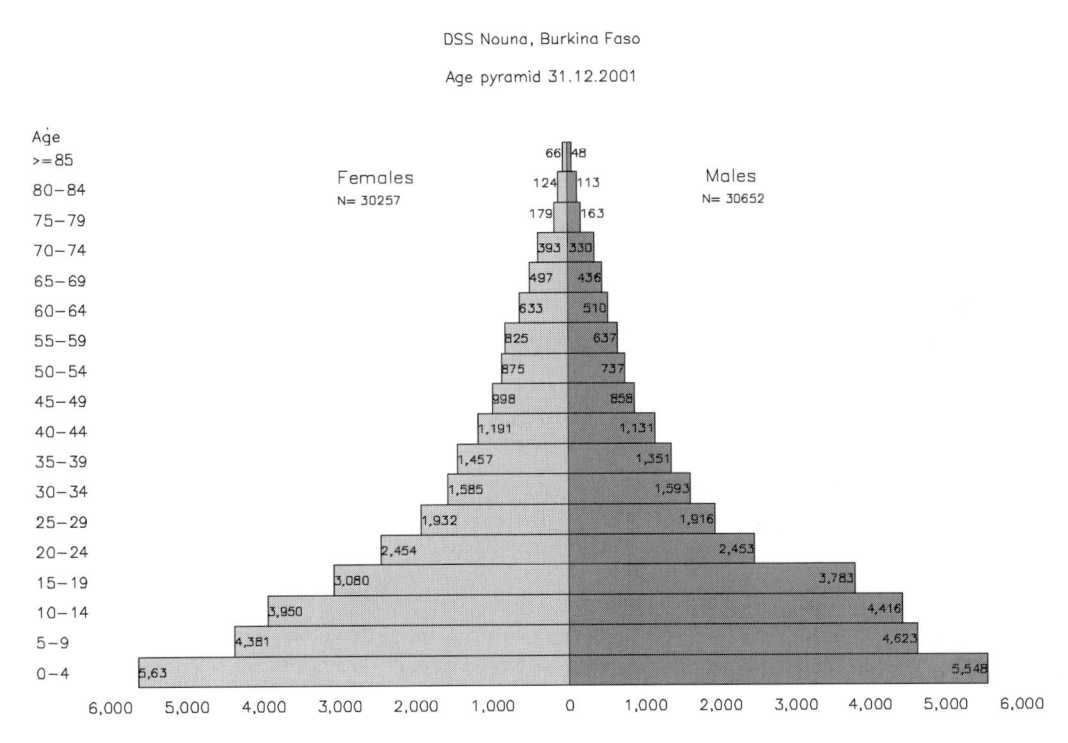

Figure 1: Age pyramid, Nouna DSS, December 31, 2001

1.3 INDEPTH Network: Generating Empirical Population and Health Data in Resource-constrained Countries in the Developing World

OSMAN A. SANKOH AND FRED BINKA

On behalf of the INDEPTH Network

INDEPTH Network Secretariat, P.O. Box KD 213 Kanda, Accra, Ghana
Tel./Fax:+233 21 254752
Email: osman.sankoh@indepth-network.org
         fred.binka@indepth-network.org

Abstract

There is a general lack of a reliable information base to support the longitudinal identification, assessment and monitoring of population health status and of cost-effective interventions for disease and associated socio-economic issues in resource-constrained countries in the developing world. Demographic surveillance systems (DSSs) such as the Nouna DSS in rural Burkina Faso, have been used to generate empirical population and health data at the household level in such settings. In these information systems, geographically-defined populations, mostly in rural areas, first determined by an initial census, form dynamic cohorts associated with residential units and households. Cohort sizes increase by births and in-migration and decreases by deaths and out-migration. Data are collected via survey cycles and verbal autopsies on total and cause-specific mortality, morbidity and disability, pregnancies and fertility, socio-economics, and lifestyle. Demographic surveillance systems are a viable, increasingly affordable but under-used solution to the dearth of empirical population and health data, especially in the poorest countries often without efficient national vital registration systems. Since 1997 efforts started to harness the collective potential of DSS field sites in addressing the void in empirical population and health data in the developing world. These efforts led to the constitution of the INDEPTH Network in 1998 which is currently composed of 36 DSS field sites in 19 countries in Africa, Asia, Oceania and Latin America. This chapter presents the processes for and examples of the generation of empirical population and health data in resource-constrained countries such as Burkina Faso in the developing world. The discussion is anchored on the cross-site activities of the INDEPTH Network in which the Nouna DSS in Burkina Faso is a member.

It is evident today that countries that can monitor mortality and its causes are those that have made substantial progress in health and social security[1]. This ability enables the countries to guide more effectively the performance of their national health systems. On the contrary, in many countries in the developing world such as Burkina Faso, many births, lives and deaths are never officially recorded. With this lack of functioning national vital registration systems, demographic surveillance systems (DSS) established in small sample or sentinel areas, mostly rural but also in urban areas, generate empirical, longitudinal, population-based health information in countries where the burden of disease is high. Among the earliest demographic surveillance system sites that continue today are the Matlab DSS in Bangladesh established in 1960, Niakhar DSS in Senegal established in 1962, Bandafassi DSS in Senegal established in 1970, Ballabgarh DSS in India established in 1972 and the Bandim DSS in Guinea-Bissau established in 1978.

After identifying the potential contribution the DSS could make to understanding population and health dynamics in the developing countries, members of 17 initial field sites from 13 countries in Africa and Asia with continuous demographic evaluation of populations and their health formed the INDEPTH Network (www.indepth-network.net). These countries include Burkina Faso in West Africa. The INDEPTH Network mission focuses on the need to collect and analyze reliable data from resource-poor countries and to support capacity building in these countries. Today, there are 36 field sites in 19 countries. These sites include the Nouna DSS operated by the Nouna Health Research Center in Burkina Faso. Figure 1 shows the distribution of countries with INDEPTH field sites. Table 1 provides a list of INDEPTH member sites as of mid-2004 with the years they were established and the populations under continuous evaluation.

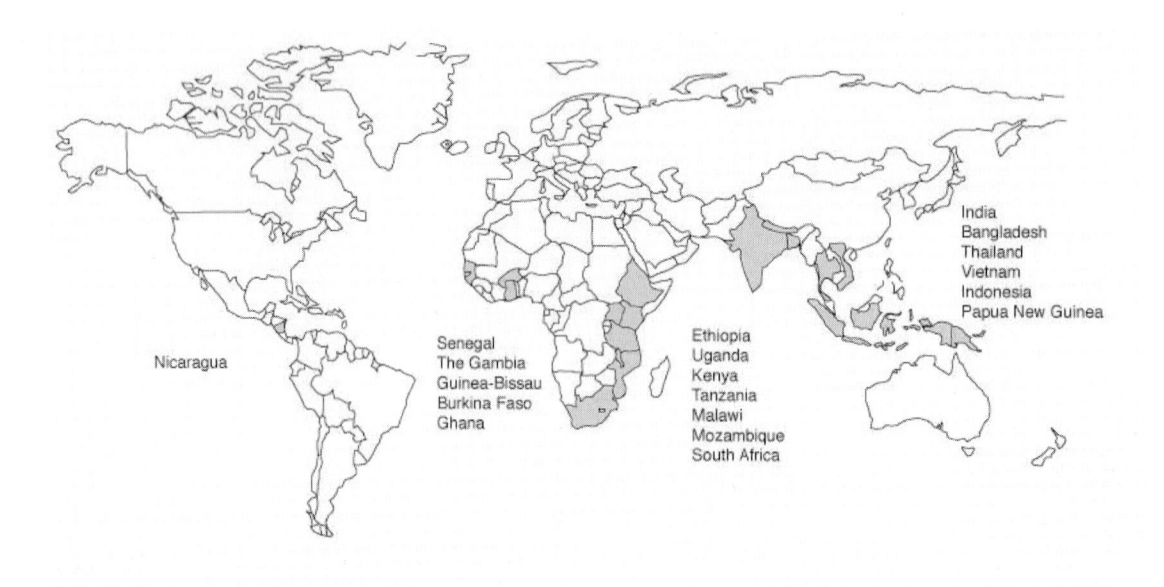

Countries with Demographic Surveillance System (DSS)
Field Sites participating in the INDEPTH Network

Figure 1: Countries with Demographic Surveillance System (DSS) Field Sites participating in the INDEPTH Network

Table 1: List of current INDEPTH DSS member sites

Africa			
Country	**Name of DSS site/host institution**	**Start Year**	**Population**
Burkina Faso	Centre de Recherche en Sante de NOUNA	1992	60,000
Burkina Faso	Centre National de Recherche et de formation sur le Paludisme (OUBRITENGA)	1993	150,000
Burkina Faso	Observatoire de Population de Ouagadougou (Quagadougou Urban Health and Equity Initiative, Burkina Faso)	2002	5,000
Ethiopia	Butajira Rural Health Project	1987	35,000
Gambia	Farafenni Field Station	1981	16,000
Ghana	Navrongo Health Research Centre	1993	139,000
Guinea Bissau	Bandim Project	1978	101,000
Kenya	Kisumu Project	1992	55,000
Kenya	African Population Health Research Centre (Nairobi)	2000	60,000
Mali	Observatoire de Population a Kolondieba	1997	10,000
Mozambizue	Manhica	1996	35,000
Malawi	Karonga Prevention Study	2002	40,000
South Africa	Agincourt Health and Population Programme	1992	63,000
South Africa	Dikgale Demographic and Health Study	1995	8,000
South Africa	Africa Centre Demographic Information System	1999	75,000
Senegal	Niakhar	1962	29,000
Senegal	Bandafassi	1970	11,000
Senegal	Mlomp	1985	8,000
Tanzania	Adult Morbidity and Mortality Project (Dar es Salaam)	1992	70,000
Tanzania	Adult Morbidity and Mortality Project (Hai)	1992	154,000
Tanzania	Adult Morbidity and Mortality Project (Morogoro)	1992	120,000
Tanzania	Ifakara Health Research and Development Centre	1996	55,000
Tanzania	Tanzanian Essential Health Intervention Project (TEHIP) Rufiji Project	1999	90,000
Uganda	Rakai Project	1989	12,000
Asia			
Country	**Name of DSS site / host institution**	**Start Year**	**Population**
Bangladesh	Matlab	1960	212,000
Bangladesh	Health System and Infectious Disease Surveillance (HSID)	1982	127,000
Bangladesh	Watch Project	1996	90,000
India	Ballabgarh DSS (All India Institute of	1972	41,000

	Medical Sciences (AIIMS)		
India	Vadu Rural Health Project, KEM Hospital, Pune District, India (Vadu)	2002	64,000
Indonesia	Community Health Nutrition and Research Laboratories. (Purworejo)	1994	18,000
Thailand	Institute for Population and Social Research, Mahidol University (Kanchanaburi)	2000	43,000
Vietnam	Epidemiological Field Laboratory for Health Research (Filabavi)	1998	50,000
Vietnam	Chililab-Chi Linh District	1998	64 000
Oceania			
Country	**Name of DSS site/ host institution**	**Start Year**	**Population**
Papua new Guinea	Wosera DSS, PNG Institute of Medical Research	2003	140,000
Latin America			
Country	**Name of DSS site/ host institution**	**Start Year**	**Population**
Nicaragua	Center for Demographic and Health Research (CIDS), Leon University	2003	55,000

Source: INDEPTH Network[2]

The field sites such as the Nouna DSS, provide longitudinal, population-based health information including data on all births, deaths, causes of death and migration for sample populations. The generated empirical data enable levels, patterns, causes and trends of mortality to be identified and set the stage for the monitoring and evaluating a wide range of innovations in health care as well as social, economic, behavioral and health interventions and research studies.

Demographic Surveillance Systems in the developing world

A DSS such as the one operated by the Nouna Health Research Center in rural Burkina Faso, is a set of field and computing operations to handle the longitudinal follow-up of well-defined entities or primary subjects (individuals, households, and residential units) and all related demographic and health outcomes within a clearly circumscribed geographic area. Unlike a cohort study, a DSS follows up the entire population of such a geographic area.

In such a system, an initial census defines and registers the target population, usually the total resident population of a geographically bounded area. From the populations shown in Table 1, the average site population is 70,000 people. After the initial census, regular subsequent rounds of data collection at prescribed intervals make it possible to register all new individuals, households, and residential units and to update key variables and attributes of existing subjects. The core system provides for monitoring of population dynamics through routine collection and processing of information on births, deaths, and migrations and is often complemented by various other data sets that provide important social and economic correlates or contexts of population and health dynamics.

A DSS operates in a defined demographic surveillance area (DSA). For example, the Nouna DSS operates in the Kossi Province in Northwest Burkina Faso. This is an area with clear and permanently delineated boundaries, and is recognizable on the ground by physical features. DSSs collect data during rounds or cycles of visits to registered and new residential units in the demographic surveillance area.

Every DSS is required to define the population under surveillance. Thereafter, a set of inclusion criteria must be applied to distinguish eligible from ineligible individuals or subjects (e.g. *de facto* residents) within each subject category. To know the size of the registered resident population at any time, a DSS collects information about three events that alter this size, namely, births, deaths, and migrations. Pregnancies and their outcomes for all women registered in the DSS are recorded regardless of the place of occurrence of such events. Deaths of all registered and eligible individuals are recorded, regardless of the place of death. Some DSSs such as the Nouna DSS, collect more detailed information about deaths to establish the cause of death, generally through verbal autopsies. Deaths are usually identified continuously through community key informants. Update rounds also identify deaths as well as check those already identified by community key informants.

Furthermore, migrations in and out of demographic surveillance areas are important considerations in a DSS because they influence the registration of births and deaths. Meaningful and identifiable segments of time started and ended by events, including births, deaths, migrations, and other events such as nuptiality or marital status are of interest. Most DSSs collect information about events such as marriage and divorce. Other events recorded by DSSs depend on their complexity and research interests but may include the change of a head of household, a household's formation or dissolution, or the construction or destruction of building structures.

Generating DSS indices and measures

Demographic estimates undertaken in the DSS sites employ both indirect and direct methods, using retrospective single-round surveys and prospective multi-round ones[2]. Selection and establishment of the demographic surveillance area are prerequisites of any DSS site. Depending on the nature of a particular research project, which may be hosted in a DSS site, sites employ probability or non-probability sampling methods, or both, in drawing their sample population from within the demographic surveillance area. The INDEPTH Network[2] has described in detail common procedures for DSS data collection.

Typical indices / outcome measures generated by these efforts are total and cause-specific mortality based on empirical data. Further information generated empirically includes morbidity and disability, pregnancies and fertility, socio-economics, and lifestyle. All field workers are made aware of ethical concerns and key respondents, especially household heads sign an informed-consent form at the outset of most research activities, especially those which are based on the DSS.

Table 2 shows an example of data produced by INDEPTH sites including the Nouna DSS, on infant and child mortality for the 1995-99 period. More recent data are being analyzed for new Network publications. A new INDEPTH standard age population[2] that more appropriate reflects the young populations in developing countries was used to standardize the infant and child mortality rates. Hence, the rates have not been compared with others published by other international organizations which often use standard age populations that are based on aging populations in industrialized countries.

Table 2: Infant and child mortality at 19 INDEPTH sites, 1995-99

DSS Site	IMR per 1000	Male (per 1000)				Female (per 1000)			
		$_1q_0$	$_4q_1$	$_5q_0$	$_1q_0/_4q_1$	$_1q_0$	$_4q_1$	$_5q_0$	$_1q_0/_4q_1$
Agincourt, South Africa	16.93	15.06	17.52	32.32	0.86	16.63	17.35	33.69	0.96
Matlab treat.[a], Bangladesh	50.58	47.38	15.92	62.54	2.98	59.88	20.88	79.51	2.87
Matlab comp.[b], Bangladesh	70.05	65.96	23.67	88.08	2.79	80.24	21.64	100.15	3.71
Mlomp, Senegal	45.18	48.24	42.61	88.80	1.13	49.42	51.57	98.60	0.96
Hai, Tanzania	67.13	66.78	26.73	91.73	2.50	56.54	26.68	81.71	2.12
Dar es Salaam, Tanzania	71.13	66.38	50.86	113.86	1.30	67.20	52.49	116.16	1.28
Butajira, Ethiopia	67.82	65.62	57.73	119.56	1.14	71.09	62.20	128.87	1.14
Ifakara, Tanzania	93.22	76.12	52.23	24.37	1.46	86.09	50.27	132.03	1.71
Nouna, Burkina Faso	40.85	34.31	107.53	138.15	0.32	42.71	106.82	144.97	0.40
Manhica, Mozambique	72.65	85.75	68.91	148.75	1.24	59.37	60.41	116.19	0.98
Farafenni, The Gambia	74.65	68.04	110.47	171.00	0.62	66.46	109.12	168.32	0.61
Rufiji, Tanzania	143.00	147.54	37.54	179.55	3.93	175.60	33.10	202.88	5.31
Navrongo, Ghana	109.59	106.58	83.54	181.21	1.28	102.96	73.23	168.65	1.41
Gwembe, Zambia	NA	105.24	87.26	183.32	1.21	111.94	78.78	181.90	1.42
Morogoro, Tanzania	116.73	105.24	87.26	183.32	1.21	111.94	78.78	181.90	1.42
Oubritenga, Burkina Faso	96.49	102.25	95.97	188.41	1.07	91.88	104.84	187.09	0.88
Niakhar, Senegal	NA	89.80	146.84	223.45	0.61	72.16	129.14	191.98	0.56
Bandim, Guinea-Bissau	NA	112.37	129.78	227.57	0.87	101.52	128.31	216.80	0.79
Bandafassi, Senegal	124.88	138.60	134.59	254.54	1.03	116.43	114.29	217.42	1.02

Note: IMR, Infant Mortality Rate (Number of deaths of infants <1 year old per 1000 live births in a given year);

NA, not available;

$_1q_0$, probability that a newborn will die before reaching its first birthday;

$_4q_1$, probability that a child that has reached its 1st birthday will die before its reaching 5th birthday;

$_5q_0$, probability that a newborn child will die before reaching its 5th birthday;

$_1q_0/_4q_1$, ratio of probability of death faced by children before and after their 1st birthday.

[a] Treatment area

[b] Comparison area

The results in Table 2 show a wide range in the level of child mortality, but except at the very low and very highest levels, no geographical clustering is apparent. The probability that a newborn dies before reaching its fifth birthday ranges from 32 to 255 per 1000 for males and from 34 to 217 per 1000 for females. For Nouna DSS in Burkina Faso, the probabilities were 108 per 1000 for males and 107 per 1000 for females. The infant mortality rate for the Nouna DSS was 40.9 per 1000 for the 1995-99 period. The Agincourt site in South Africa recorded a comparatively very low level of child mortality, followed by the cluster comprising Matlab sites in Bangladesh, Mlomp in Senegal, and Hai in Tanzania. The lowest levels are found in South Africa and Asia, and the highest levels are reported from West Africa. Highest levels of infant mortality were recorded by Bandafassi in Senegal, Morogoro in Tanzania, and Navrongo in Ghana.

Processing DSS-generated data

The DSS sites have a generic data system for storage of data that enables data rules and concepts to be standardized across sites. Sites have developed software systems to maintain a consistent record of significant demographic events in their populations. To support field operations and routine cleaning of data, the sites also keep track of where, when, and by whom a particular event was recorded and include fields to designate the place a migrant is moving to or from. The processes involved in developing DSS software are time-consuming, and prone to conceptual and programming errors due to the complex DSS systems. INDEPTH is developing data models that will simplify this process. Some technical details for the Nouna DSS are given in 1.2.

Assessing the quality of DSS-generated Data

Potential errors in data generated by DSS operations may take the form of coverage errors, resulting from omission or repeated counting of persons, or content errors, arising from incorrect reporting of the characteristics of respondents. It is therefore necessary to establish whether the data are of reasonable quality. A variety of quality control procedures are used at the field, data-processing, and analysis stages. Careful, methodological, and conscientious interviewing is required. Trained fieldworkers and supervisors are used to monitor data quality through regular supervisory visits, form checking, and re-interviews.

Statistical procedures are also used to determine the completeness of coverage and reliability of the data. Re-interviews of representative samples are done and individual records are matched case-by-case from two data sources. Also absolute and relative numbers from successive periods of the DSS are compared to identify deviations from expected patterns. In addition, a population pyramid that gives a detailed picture of the age–sex structure of the population is used to assess the quality of age reporting.

Determining Cause of Death

Practical experience working at DSS sites has shown that information on cause of death is only sometimes available from death certificates, since most deaths are neither attended by doctors nor medically certified through post-mortem autopsy. Therefore death registration is frequently incomplete, and even when death certificates are available, diagnoses reported are often non-specific. Consequently, published statistics on both cause-specific and overall rates of mortality in such countries would mostly consist of extrapolations.

The method that is commonly used to measure cause-specific mortality where data on cause of death are lacking or inadequate is the verbal autopsy method[3-4]. There was need to improve the situation regarding the dearth of data on cause-specific mortality in resource-constrained communities where the use of clinical autopsies will not be available or possible. Verbal autopsies are done for deaths to registered members of the demographic surveillance area. Such deaths are notified to the system by community key informants and also at household survey update rounds. Verbal autopsies involve specially trained interviewers who interview relatives about signs and symptoms related to the terminal event using a structured questionnaire. The information from completed questionnaires is then summarized and interpreted to give a likely cause for each death.

The most common method for ascribing causes of death from verbal autopsy questionnaires is when the completed questionnaires are reviewed by one or more physicians who ascribe probable causes of death[3-5]. All parts of the questionnaire, particularly any open-ended sections, are thus incorporated into the diagnosis. For verbal autopsies to be comparable, they need to be based on similar interviews, and the cause of death needs to be arrived at in the same way in all cases. Thus standardization and local validation of the verbal autopsy tool is important since sensitivity and specificity can be affected when there is a bias in the information being collected.[3]

A standardized verbal autopsy instrument has recently been developed by the INDEPTH Network through a series of workshops in which representatives from DSS sites in the developing world and from other external institutions such as WHO participated. This instrument can be downloaded from the INDEPTH website (www.indepth-network.net). Several INDEPTH sites have started using the INDEPTH tool and a few sites are now considering validation and reliability tests of the verbal autopsy tool. DSS sites are finding the method of verbal autopsy as the most viable one for determining the most likely cause of death in especially in rural areas where most deaths take place at home.

Measuring Health Equity in Small Areas

Many recent publications on inequalities and health[6-8] and those which focus on global health equity have indicated renewed commitments and a need for empirical research and evidence-based interventions in these areas. Many policies that are geared towards addressing the needs of the global poor are largely based on indirect estimates and on data from urban centers and health facilities that do not accurately reflect their experience.

The DSS sites located mostly in the rural areas make it possible to explore and engage in the long-term assessment of health equity[9]. Case studies recently completed at DSS sites have shown that in all these areas real differentials exist in social and material wealth, health status, and in the use of health services.[10] Nouna DSS worked on health inequalities in district of Nouna in rural Burkina Faso.[11] The studies show that tools and concepts for measuring health status are far more developed than those for measuring deprivation and disadvantage. Some DSS sites focused on measures of material wealth and poverty through the creation of composite proxies of income/expenditure based on ownership of household assets or individual attributes such as educational attainment and occupation, while others explored well-being in terms of social support and networks. The magnitude of the disparities varies by site and by indicator used, and depending on factors considered. For instance, sites which divided the households or population studied into quintiles, revealed significant inequalities between the bottom and top 20% for almost all health status and service use indicators, with the top 20% being consistently better-off than the bottom 20%. The extent to which these inequality and inequity gradients can be flattened over time will be a measure of how successful pro-poor policies are. The INDEPTH Network is now funding projects that develop intervention studies or manipulate existing interventions to have a pro-poor focus in order to inform policy.

Knowledge from DSS

Numerous publications from DSS sites show the strides by these sites in remote areas to monitor mortality and its causes, and also demonstrate how much knowledge taken for granted that has come from DSS sites. Many of the most important cost-effective health interventions now in use in developing countries were originally tested and proven in DSS sites. A collection of publications from DSS sites is available from the INDEPTH website. The DSS provides a platform for a wide range of health system innovations as well as social, economic, behavioural and health interventions, all closely associated with research activities. Consequently, apart from the core activities involving measuring mortality, many of the DSS sites conduct specific studies in areas including the following, depending on their current priorities: Cause specific mortality; Health equity; Malaria; HIV/AIDS; Migration and urbanisation; Reproductive health; Adult health, chronic disease and aging; Ethics; and applications of research to policy and practice.

DSS sites in Africa and Asia have been contributing to national efforts. For example, since its inception in 1989, Navrongo DSS in northern Ghana has rapidly gained recognition as a world leader in developing-country health research. Its first study, which found that providing Vitamin A supplements to children below the age of five reduced the number of deaths by one fifth, led to the program's adoption throughout Ghana. Its second study found that bed nets soaked in permethrine cut child deaths by 17 per cent. As a result, bed net provision has been incorporated into health policies across Africa. And its third study, which found that moving nurses into communities and mobilising community volunteers to help them reduced overall fertility and mortality, is now part of Ghana's national health care policy and has sparked international interest.

Matlab DSS in Bangladesh, which is part of the Public Health Sciences Division of The International Centre for Diarrhoeal Disease Research, Bangladesh (ICDDR,B) has been developing and promoting realistic solutions to the major health, population and nutrition problems facing the poor people of Bangladesh and other settings. Its work has had major impacts on local, national and international health policy in the realms of diarrhoeal and infectious disease, nutrition, population programmes and child survival strategies. Family planning strategies tested at Matlab have been adopted nationwide and led to Bangladesh's recognition at the 1994 United Nations Conference on Population and Development in Cairo as a family planning success story. Also, the Matlab rural intervention for vaccine trials yielded important findings on the effectiveness of injectable and oral cholera vaccines. The oral cholera vaccine tested by the Centre is now recommended by the World Health Organisation.

As well as influencing policy at local and national levels, several INDEPTH DSS sites have participated in major international efforts to improve health in developing countries. For example, the Ifakara DSS (Tanzania) took part in a multi-country study funded by the Gates Foundation to determine the effect of intermittent preventive anti-malarial drug treatment on children. The study found that intermittent treatment helped control malaria among children under the age of five. The DSS sites at Manhica (Mozambique) and Kisumu (Kenya), along with a site in Mali, are at the forefront of global efforts to develop a malaria vaccine. They are testing the three vaccines that are at the heart of the Malaria Vaccine Initiative's current work. The project is co-funded by USAID.

Conclusion

The core DSS outputs are mortality rates (all-cause and cause-specific), life tables, fertility rates and migration rates. The systems can also produce numerous demographic, health and poverty indicators for understanding trends and determinants for population characteristics, household characteristics, health status and disease burdens, access and use of health services, etc. They can also be used as platforms for analyzing trends in cause-specific mortality, morbidity, fertility and migration, understanding causal and contextual determinants, informing priorities for health research and development, and for measuring impact of interventions and reforms. However, it should be noted that although DSSs generate high quality data, the conditions for data collection in the remote areas have their limitations. These include underreporting of cases or incomplete recording of events. DSS sites strive to ensure that such limitations are addressed over time so that there is no meaningful negative impact on the data produced.

The INDEPTH Network harnesses the collective potential of DSS sites in resource-poor countries in the developing world. INDEPTH cultivates cross-site activities through comparative studies and exchange of experiences on critical common problems. It generates longitudinal data and analysis that can be used to impact ongoing health and social reforms, inform health and social policy and practice and contribute to governmental, NGO, private and community health efforts. The Network broadens the scope of health research by addressing the emerging agenda of non-communicable diseases and aging, accidents, violence and injury, and the problems associated with vulnerable populations. It is important to note that INDEPTH continually improves the methods and technologies used by member sites to ensure all participating groups have access to the most valid and appropriate methodologies available. Finally, INDEPTH generates visibility and recognition for the Network itself and member sites among critical constituencies, including academic, government and international agencies and donors.

Acknowledgements

This paper is written on behalf of the INDEPTH Network. It is based on the INDEPTH monograph volume 1[2] and on ongoing Network research work on Cause of Death and Health Equity. The authors would therefore like to thank editors and all contributing authors to the first volume, research teams in current INDEPTH studies, including site administrators, data managers, field workers and all other staff who continue to collect the data. The authors wish to acknowledge the financial support from current INDEPTH sponsors - the Rockefeller Foundation, the World Bank, Sida/SAREC and the Wellcome Trust. Finally, the authors would like to thank Dr. Don de Savigny whose comments increased the clarity of several sections of the paper.

References

1. Szreter S. Health and human security in an historical perspective. In Global Health Challenges for Human Security. Edited by Chen L, Leaning JN, V. Cambridge. Harvard University Press; 2003.

2. INDEPTH Network. Population and Health in Developing Countries. Volume 1. Population, Health and Survival at INDEPTH Sites. Ottawa, Canada: IDRC; 2002.

3. Kahn K, Tollman SM, Garenne M, Gaer JS. Validation and application of verbal autopsies in a rural area in South Africa. Tropical Medicine and International Health. 2000; 5:824-831.

4. Chandramohan D, Setel P, Quigley M. Effect of misclassification of causes of death in verbal autopsy: can it be adjusted?. *International Journal of Epidemiology*. 2001;30:509-514,

5. Bang AT, Bang RA, and the SEARCH Team. Diagnosis of Causes of Childhood Deaths in Developing countries by Verbal Autopsy: Suggested Criteria. *Bulletin of the World Health Organization.* 1992;70(4):499-507.

6. Kim JY, Millen JV et al., Eds. Dying for Growth. Global Inequality and the Health of the Poor. 2000. Munroe, Maine, Common Courage Press.

7. Evans T, Whitehead M et al., Eds. Challenging Inequities in Health. From Ethics to Action. 2001. New York, Oxford University Press

8. Ngom P, Binka FN, Phillips, JF, Pence, B, Macleod B. Demographic surveillance and health equity in sub-Saharan Africa. *Health Policy and Planning*. 2001;16:337-344.

9. Foege WH. Global public health: targeting inequities. *JAMA*. 1998;279:1931-1932

10. INDEPTH Network. Report from thirteen INDEPTH DSS Sites in Africa and Asia. INDEPTH Network Project Report to the Rockefeller Foundation, 2003, New York.

11. Traore, C and Pale, A. Health Inequalities in the Rural District of Nouna, Burkina Faso. Report from thirteen INDEPTH DSS Sites in Africa and Asia. INDEPTH Network Project Report to the Rockefeller Foundation, New York.

1.4 Ethics of biomedical research in developing countries

OLAF MÜLLER[1] AND BOCAR KOUYATÉ[2]

[1] *University of Heidelberg, Department of Tropical Hygiene and Public Health, Im Neuenheimer Feld 324, 69120 Heidelberg, Germany*

Tel.: +49 6221 565035

E-mail: olaf.mueller@urz.uni-heidelberg.de

[2] *Centre de Recherche en Santé de Nouna, BP 02 Nouna, Burkina Faso*

Tel.: +226-20-537043

Email: bocar.crsn@fasonet.bf

History of ethical codices for biomedical research

Ethical principles with regard to medical interventions in humans have already a long history. The *Hippocratic Letters* have been written some 2.500 years ago, and four of its six stated principles are still fully relevant to modern medicine. However, these principles were rarely applied in the past and the results of unethical experiments on humans have even regularly been published, particularly during the first half of the 20th century.

The *Nürnberg Codex* resulted directly from the Doctors Trial after Second World War. In this trial, 23 persons (mainly German medical doctors), were accused of crimes against humanity during their brutal experiments with prisoners in concentration camps during the National Socialist regimen. The Nürnberg Codex, which was formulated in 1947, was the first internationally recognised codex on the conduct of medical experiments on humans. However, despite the existence of international accepted ethical principles and guidelines there were still a number of unethical studies implemented in the second half of the 20th century. Examples from the USA are the experiments on soldiers with radioactivity in the 1950s and the infamous Tusgegee Study in a population of afro-american men which lasted until the 1970s. The societal changes in the Western World which started in the 1970s finally led to a greater awareness of ethical issues in biomedical research. This resulted in individual questioning of the paternalistic physician-patient relation as well as in more public awareness for human rights issues which were already fixed in the UN Declaration of Universal Human Rights from 1948.

The *Declaration of the World Medical Association from Helsinki* (1964) and its subsequent revisions in Tokyo (1975), Venedig (1983), Hongkong (1989), Somerset West (1996), and Edinburg (2000) is a consequent development from the Nürnberg Codex. The Declaration of Helsinki with its currently thirty-two paragraphs remains the best known and accepted international ethical codex in the field of biomedical research on human subjects, despite the fact that its latest version has only been approved by 44 of 195 UN member states and that it is legally not binding (WMA 2002).

Today, the Declaration of Helsinki is no longer the only internationally relevant ethical codex. Of particular importance are:

- The *International Ethical Guidelines for Biomedical research Involving Human Subjects of the Council for International Organisations of Medical Sciences (CIOMS)*, with its particular goal to translate the Declaration of Helsinki into guidelines which are practicable in developing countries (1982, 1993, 2002) (CIOMS/WHO 2002)

- The *International Ethical Guidelines for Epidemiological Research* Involving Human Subjects of the Council for International Organisations of Medical Sciences (1991)

- The *Guidelines on Good Clinical Practice of the World Health Organisation,* which are of relevance to drug registration in the EU, USA and Japan (1995)

- The *Guidelines of the International Conference of Harmonising* the Technical Prerequisites for the Registration of Pharmaceuticals for Use in Humans, which are also of relevance to drug registration in the EU, USA and Japan (1996)

- The *Guidelines of the Nuffield Council on Bioethics* (Medical Research Council UK, Nuffield Foundation, Wellcome Trust) on The Ethics of Clinical Research in Developing Countries (1999)

- The *Guidelines of UNAIDS* on Ethical Aspects during the Conduct of HIV Vaccine Trials (2000)

- The *Convention of Human Rights of the European Council,* which is legally binding for member states (2004)

- The *European Guidelines for Adaptation of Legislation and Administration regarding Implementation of Good Clinical Practice* during the Conduct of Clinical Studies on Pharmaceuticals in Humans, which are also legally binding for member states (2004)

Definition of biomedical research (CIOMS)

Progress in the prevention and treatment of human disease depends on different kinds of studies in the field of physiology and pathophysiology, epidemiology, anthropology, and clinical medicine. Research involving human subjects may employ either observation or physical, chemical or psychological intervention.

Biomedical research involving human subjects thus includes:

- Studies of a physiological, biochemical or pathological process or of the response to a specific intervention – whether physical, chemical or psychological – in healthy subjects or patients.

- Controlled trials of diagnostic, preventive or therapeutic measures in larger groups of persons, designed to demonstrate a specific generalizable response to these measures against a background of individual biological variation.

- Studies designed to determine the consequences for individuals and communities of specific preventive or therapeutic measures.

- Studies concerning human health-related behaviour in a variety of circumstances and environments.

Biomedical research is principally different from routine medical practice, although clinical studies may frequently become integrated into health service delivery. However, in the treatment of diseases where no standard of care exists, no clear differentiation can be made between experiments and published case series (CIOMS/WHO 2002).

General ethical principles (CIOMS)

All research involving human subjects should be conducted in accordance with three basic ethical principles, namely respect for persons, beneficence and justice.

Respect for persons incorporates at least two fundamental ethical considerations:

- respect for autonomy, which requires that those who are capable of deliberation about their personal choices should be treated with respect for their capacity for self-determination, and

- protection of persons with impaired or diminished autonomy, which requires that those who are dependent or vulnerable be afforded security against harm or abuse.

Beneficence refers to the ethical obligation to maximize benefits and to minimize harms. This principle gives rise to norms requiring that the risks of research be reasonable in the light of expected benefits, that the research design be sound, and that the investigators be competent both to conduct the research and to safeguard the welfare of the research subjects. Beneficence further proscribes the deliberate infliction of harm on persons. This aspect is sometimes expressed as a separate principle – nonmaleficence (do not harm).

Justice refers to the ethical obligation to treat each person in accordance with what is morally right and proper. In biomedical research the principle refers primarily to distributive justice, which requires the equitable distribution of both the burdens and the benefits of participation in research. Special provision must be made to the rights and welfare of vulnerable persons.

Sponsors of research or investigators cannot be held accountable for unjust conditions where the research is conducted, but they must refrain from practices that are likely to worsen unjust conditions. Neither should they take advantage of the relative inability of developing countries or vulnerable populations to protect their own interests, by conducting research inexpensively and avoiding complex regulatory systems of industrialized countries in order to develop products for lucrative markets. In general, the research project should leave communities in developing countries better off than previously, and should be responsive to their health needs in that any product developed is made reasonably available to them (CIOMS/WHO 2002).

Ethical guidelines in biomedical research (CIOMS)

1. **Ethical justification and scientific validity of biomedical research involving human beings**
The ethical justification of biomedical research is the prospect of discovering new ways of benefiting people`s health. Such research can be ethically justifiable only if it is carried out in ways that respect and protect the subjects of that research and are morally acceptable within the communities in which the research is carried out. Moreover, because scientific invalid research is unethical in that it exposes research subjects to risks without possible benefit, investigators and sponsors must ensure that proposed studies conform to generally accepted scientific principles and are based on adequate knowledge of the pertinent scientific literature.

2. **Ethical review committees**
All proposals to conduct research involving human subjects must be submitted for review of their scientific merit and ethical acceptability to one or more scientific review and ethical review committees. The review committees must be independent of the research team, and any direct financial or other material benefit they may derive from the research should not be contingent on the outcome of the review. The investigators must obtain their approval before undertaking the research. The ethical review committee should conduct further reviews as necessary in the course of the research, including monitoring of the progress of the study.

3. **Ethical review of externally sponsored research**
An external sponsoring organisation and individual investigators should submit the research protocol for ethical and scientific review in the country of the sponsoring organisation, and the ethical standards applied should be no less stringent than they would be for research carried out in that country. The health authorities of the host country, as well as a national or local ethical review committee, should ensure that the proposed research is responsive to the health needs and priorities of the host country and meets requisite ethical standards.

4. **Individual informed consent**
For all biomedical research involving humans the investigator must obtain the voluntary informed consent of the prospective subject or, in the case of an individual who is not capable of giving informed consent, the permission of a legally authorised representative in accordance with applicable law. Waiver of informed consent is regarded uncommon and exceptional, and must in all cases be approved by an ethical committee.

5. **Obtaining informed consent: essential information for prospective research subjects**
Before requesting an individual`s consent to participate in research, the investigator must always provide the following informations: that participation is voluntary, withdrawl will be possible without penalty, design and details of the study, risks and benefits to individuals and respective communities, right to data access, availability of safe and effective products after the study, existence of alternative interventions, privacy and confidentiality, provision of medical care, and compensation for harm.

6. **Obtaining informed consent: obligations of sponsors and investigators**
Sponsors and investigators have a duty to refrain from unjustified deception, undue influence, or intimidation, to seek consent only after ascertaining that the prospective subject has adequate understanding of the relevant facts and of the consequences of participation, to obtain from each subject a

signed form as evidence of informed consent, and to renew the informed consent if new information becomes available.

7. Inducement to participate
Subjects may be reimbursed for lost earnings, travel costs and other expenses incurred in taking part in a study, and they may also receive free medical services. Subjects, particularly those who receive no direct benefit from research, may also be paid or otherwise compensated. The payments should not be so large, however, or the medical services so extensive as to induce prospective subjects to consent to participate in the research against their better judgement. All payments, reimbursements and medical services provided must have been approved by an ethical review committee.

8. Benefits and risks of study participation
The investigators must ensure that potential benefits and risks are reasonably balanced and risks are minimised. Interventions or procedures that hold out the prospect of direct diagnostic, therapeutic or preventive benefit must be justified by the expectation that they will be at least as advantageous in the light of foreseeable risks and benefits as any available alternative. Risks of interventions that do not hold out the prospect of direct benefit must be justified in relation to the expected benefits to society. The risks presented by such interventions must be reasonable in relation to the importance of the knowledge to be gained.

9. Special limitations on risk when research involves individuals who are not capable of giving informed consent
When there is ethical and scientific justification to conduct research with individuals incapable of giving informed consent, the risk from research interventions that do not hold out the prospect of direct benefit for the subject should be not greater than the risk attached to routine examination. Slight increases above such risk may be permitted when there is an overriding scientific rationale and when an ethical review committee has approved them.

10. Research in populations and communities with limited resources
The sponsor and the investigator must make every effort to ensure that the research is responsive to the health needs and the priorities of the population or community in which it is to be carried out, and that any intervention or product developed, or knowledge generated, will be made reasonably available for the benefit of that population or community.

11. Choice of control in clinical trials
Research subjects in the control group of a trial of a diagnostic, therapeutic or preventive intervention should receive an established effective intervention. In some circumstances it may be ethically acceptable to use an alternative comparator, such as placebo or no treatment. Placebo may be used when there is no established effective intervention, when withholding an established effective intervention would expose subjects to, at most, temporary discomfort, or when use of an established effective intervention as comparator would not yield scientifically reliable results and use of placebo would not add any risk of serious and irreversible harm.

12. Equitable distribution of burdens and benefits in the selection of groups of subjects in research

Groups or communities to be invited to be subjects of research should be selected in such a way that the burdens and benefits will be equitably distributed. The exclusion of groups or communities that might benefit from study participation must be justified.

13. Research involving vulnerable persons

Special justification is required for inviting vulnerable individuals to serve as research subjects and, if they are selected, the means of protecting their rights and welfare must be strictly applied.

14. Research involving children

Before undertaking research in children, the investigator must ensure that the research might not equally well be carried out with adults, the purpose of the research is to obtain knowledge relevant to the health needs of children, a parent or legal representative has given permission, the agreement of each child has been obtained to the extent of the child's capabilities, and a child's refusal to participate or continue in the research will be respected.

15. Research involving individuals who by reason of mental or behavioural disorders are not capable of giving adequately informed consent

The investigator must ensure that such persons will not be subject of research that might equally well be carried out on normal persons, the purpose of the research is to obtain knowledge relevant to the health needs of this group, the individual consent has been obtained to the extend of that person's capabilities, and permission is obtained from a responsible family member or legal representative.

16. Women as research subjects

Investigators, sponsors or ethical review committees should not exclude women of reproductive age from biomedical research. However, a thorough discussion of risks to the pregnant woman and to her foetus is a prerequisite for the woman's ability to make a rational decision. If participation might be hazardous to a foetus or a woman if she becomes pregnant, a pregnancy test and access to effective contraceptive methods has to be guaranteed.

17. Pregnant women as research participants

Investigators and ethical review committees should ensure that pregnant women are adequately informed about the risks and benefits to themselves, their pregnancies, the foetus and their subsequent offspring, and to their fertility. Research should only be performed if it is relevant to the particular health needs of pregnant women or her foetus, or to the health needs of pregnant women in general, and, when appropriate, if it is supported by reliable evidence from animal experiments, particularly as to risks of teratogenicity and mutagenicity.

18. Safeguarding confidentiality

The investigator must establish secure safeguards of the confidentiality of subjects' research data. Subjects should be told the limits, legal or other, to the investigators' ability to safeguard confidentiality and the possible consequences of breaches of confidentiality.

19. Right of injured subjects to treatment and compensation

Investigators should ensure that research subjects who suffer injury as a result of their participation are entitled to free medical treatment for such injury and to such financial or other assistance as would compensate them equitable for any resultant impairment, disability or handicap. In case of death as a result of their participation, their dependants are entitled to compensation. Subjects must not be asked to waive the right to compensation.

20. Strengthening capacity for ethical and scientific review and biomedical research
Many countries lack the capacity to assess or ensure the scientific quality or ethical acceptability of biomedical research proposed or carried out in their jurisdiction. In externally sponsored collaborative research, sponsors and investigators have an ethical obligation to ensure that biomedical research projects for which they are responsible in such countries contribute effectively to national or local capacity to design and conduct biomedical research, and to provide scientific and ethical review and monitoring of such research.

21. Ethical obligation of external sponsors to provide health-care services
External sponsors are ethically obliged to ensure the availability of health care services that are essential to the safe conduct of the research, treatment for subjects who suffer injury as a consequence of research interventions, and services that are a necessary part of the commitment of a sponsor to make a beneficial intervention or product developed as a result of the research reasonably available to the population or community concerned (CIOMS/WHO 2002).

HIV/AIDS and research ethics

The international discussion on ethical aspects of biomedical research in developing countries was and still is very much influenced by the development and the consequences of the HIV/AIDS pandemic. A paper which was published in The New England Journal of Medicine in September 1997 and two accompanying editorials in The New England Journal and in The Lancet sharply critized a group of externally financed placebo-controlled trials on the prevention of perinatal HIV transmission carried out in eleven developing countries of Africa, Asia and America (Lurie and Wolfe 1997; Angell 1997; Anonymous 1997a). They argued that using placebo would be unethical, as a study which was published in The New England Journal three years before had clearly shown a major reduction of perinatal HIV transmission associated with a complex antiretroviral drug regimen in industrialised countries and has thus to be considered the international standard. If this standard would not be systematically implemented in HIV/AIDS research, they argued, exploitation of poor countries by rich countries would be guaranteed. During the major controversial discussion over the following years, many experienced scientists from both industrialised and developing countries argued against such a view which was considered totally unrealistic and should even be judged as ethical imperialism (Varmus and Satcher 1997; DeCock et al. 1997; Anonymous 1997b, Anonymous 1997c; Aaby et al. 1997;Phanuphak 1998; Merson 1998; Lallemant et al. 1998; Gambia Government/MRC Joint Ethical Committee 1998; . Their main argument was that if always the highest international standard has to be implemented for the comparator group in poor developing countries, many trials of importance to the health of populations in such countries would be made impossible. Thus low-cost technologically appropriate solutions for HIV/AIDS and other major public health problems could no longer be developed for the populations who most urgently need them.

The international discussion on this ethical conflict finally resulted in a Note of Clarification on Paragraph 29 of the Declaration of Helsinki, which for the first time authorised the use of placebo even if an effective international standard exists provided that there are overriding scientific arguments to do so (WMA 2002). These aspects were also appropriately included into the adaptation of the CIOMS Guidelines in 2002, although here the conflicting views could not be totally reconciled (CIOMS/WHO 2002).

The ethical complexities associated with HIV/AIDS research will continue to fuel the international discussion on ethical aspects of biomedical research in developing countries (Cleaton-Jones 1997; Barry 1998; Angell 1998; Angell 2000; Richards 2002; Tusker and Slack 2003; Mukherjee 2003; Fitzgerald et al 2003; Berkley 2003). In particular the internationally funded large studies on HIV/AIDS vaccines which are currently starting will again be accompanied by a critical discussion. Some questions of importance to the ethics of such studies concern the right to lifelong treatment of research subjects being found to be HIV infected or having become infected during studies, the stigma associated to vaccine-induced HIV seroconversion, the conflict between the right to treatment and prevention and the scientific interest to measure endpoints such as virus load and seroconversion, and the right of study communities to be provided with an affordable vaccine in case of success.

Summary and outlook

The application of ethical principles does not principally differ between industrialized and developing countries. However, cultural differences and in particular the huge differences in income and in the availability and quality of medical services can produce conflicts when implementing externally supported biomedical research on human subjects in developing countries. Ethical conflict mainly concerns the following four areas:

Individual informed consent
In many communities of developing countries individual consent can only be asked after permission of community leaders has been obtained. Moreover, the concepts of biomedical research are usually not easy to explain to the often uneducated study subjects which is likely to impair the validity of individual informed consents (Préziosi et al. 1997).

Comparator in clinical trials and respecting local research priorities
Here the main aspect remains the exceptional use of a comparator other than an established effective intervention (international standard) in controlled clinical trials. This concerns situations in which an established effective intervention is not available and unlikely in the foreseeable future to become available, usually for economic or logistic reasons. The scientific and ethical review committees must be satisfied that the established effective intervention cannot be used as comparator because it would not yield scientifically reliable results that would be relevant to the health needs of the study population (Varmus and Satcher 1997).

Ethical review committees
Local, institutional or national committees which are capable to undertake scientific and ethical review of research proposals do not always exist in developing countries or do not have a sufficient capacity for their tasks. Thus, the sponsors and investigators of externally supported studies often have a strong obligation to support capacity building for scientific and ethical review in developing countries.

Obligation of external sponsors to provide health-care services

Although sponsors are, in general, not obliged to provide health-care services beyond that which is necessary for the conduct of the research, there is a moral obligation to do so particularly in countries where the standard of care for many diseases in practice is no treatment. The extent of services always needs to be negotiated beforehand and should be clearly stated in the research protocol. It also has to be clarified beforehand how an effective intervention will be made available to the study population and community after the end of the study. This is particularly challenging in the increasing number of studies on chronic diseases, which often require lifelong treatment (Cleaton-Jones 1997).

Beside the already mentioned ongoing ethical conflicts in the area of HIV/AIDS, there are a number other reasons why we can expect an even intensified discussion in the field of ethics of biomedical research in developing countries in the near future. As a result of the rapid progress in biotechnology, the number of health products (drugs, vaccines, etc.) available for testing in humans will continue to increase. This development is accompanied by recent major improvements in supporting biomedical research in developing countries through private foundations (e.g. Bill and Melinda Gates Foundation, Clinton Foundation) and international partnerships (e.g. European and Developing Countries Clinical Trial Partnership, Global Fund against AIDS, tuberculosis and malaria). Finally, the increasing international emphasis on the importance of evidence-based decisions in health will further accelerate the implementation of biomedical research in human subjects in developing countries. Future ethical conflicts during conduct of such studies can only be solved through mutually respectful partnerships between scientists from industrialised countries and their colleagues from developing countries.

References

Aaby P, Badiker A, Darbyshire J, et al. (1997) Ethics of HIV trials. The Lancet 350, 1546

Angell M (1997) Editorial: The ethics of clinical research in the third world. The New England Journal of Medicine 337, 847-49

Angell M (1998) Editorial: Ethical imperialism? Ethics in international collaborative clinical research. The New England Journal of Medicine 339, 1081-83

Angell M (2000) Editorial: Investigators responsibilities for human subjects in developing countries. The New England Journal of Medicine 342, 967-69

Anonymous (1997a) Editorial: The ethics industry. The Lancet 350, 897

Anonymous (1997b) Editorial: Scientific imperialism. BMJ 314, 840-42

Anonymous (1997c) Editorial: Ethics and international research. BMJ 315, 965-66

Barry M (1998) Ethical considerations of human investigation in developing countries – the AIDS dilemma. The New England Journal of Medicine 339, 1083-85

Berkley S (2003) Thorny issues in the ethics of AIDS vaccine trials. The Lancet 326, 992

CIOMS/WHO (2002) International Ethical Guidelines for Biomedical Research involving Human Subjects. Council for International Organisations of Medical Sciences (CIOMS), WHO, Geneva (www.cioms.ch)

Cleaton-Jones PE (1997) An ethical dilemma: availability of antiretroviral therapy after clinical trials with HIV infected patients are ended. BMJ 314, 887-89

DeCock K, Shaffer N, Wiktor S, Simonds RJ, Rogers M (1997) Ethics of HIV trials. The Lancet 350, 1546-47

Fitzgerald DW, Pape JW, Wasserheit JN, Counts GW, Corey L (2003) Provision of treatment in HIV-1 vaccine trials in developing countries. The Lancet 362, 993-94

Gambia Government/Medical Research Council Joint Ethical Committee (1998) Ethical issues facing medical research in developing countries. The Lancet 351, 286-87

Lallemant M, McIntosh K, Jourdain G, et al. (1998) Ethics of placebo-controlled trials of zidovudine to prevent the perinatal transmission of HIV in the third world. The New England Journal of Medicine 338, 839-40

Lurie P, Wolfe SM (1997) Unethical trials of interventions to reduce perinatal transmission of the human immunodeficiency virus in developing countries. The New England Journal of Medicine 337, 853-56

Merson M (1998) Ethics of placebo-controlled trials of zidovudine to prevent the perinatal transmission of HIV in the third world. The New England Journal of Medicine 338, 836

Mukherjee JS (2003) HIV-1 care in resource-poor settings: a view from Haiti. The Lancet 362, 994-95

Phanuphak P (1998) Ethical issues in studies in Thailand of the vertical transmission of HIV. The New England Journal of Medicine 338, 834-35

Préziosi MP, Yam A, Ndiaye M, Simaga A, Simondon F (1997) Practical experiences in obtaining informed consent for a vaccine trail in rural Africa. The New England Journal of Medicine 33, 370-73

Richards T (2002) Developed countries should not impose ethics on other countries. BMJ 325, 796

Tucker T, Slack C (2003) Not if but how? Caring for HIV vaccine trail participants in South Africa. The Lancet 362, 995

Varmus H, Satcher D (1997) Ethical complexities of conducting research in developing countries. The New England Journal of Medicine 337, 1003-05

WMA (2002) World Medical Association Declaration of Helsinki: Ethical principles for medical research involving human subjects. WMA General Assembly, Washington (www.wma.net)

1.5 Health Information Systems

KLAUS KRICKEBERG

Le Châtelet, 63270 Manglieu, France

and

Grosser Kamp 4, 33619 Bielefeld, Germany

Tel.: +33 4 73 69 20 46 and +49 521 100 760

Email: krik@ideenwelt.de

Abstract

We describe the functions of health information systems in developing countries and sketch the principles to be followed when designing such a system or reforming an existing one.

1.5.1 Sources of health information

Obtaining, and rationally using, information on all aspects of health is vital for the well-being of people in developing countries. In economically rich countries the lack of a coherent overall structure for collecting and exploiting health-related information renders many parts of the health services less efficient but the ensuing waste usually remains bearable. In poor countries, it becomes disastrous. In many developing countries including Burkina Faso health planners have therefore started very early to think about health information and attempted to build mechanisms for obtaining and handling it. They have almost always hurt themselves at obstacles like lack of material resources, scarcity of trained manpower, and insufficient administrative services. In some countries, overly bureaucratic health administrations have presented an additional difficulty. However, these difficulties have overshadowed the main problem: the absence of clear ideas about the objectives and functions of the various mechanisms for dealing with health information, and the lack of rigorous structural principles and technical rules for designing, implementing, and operating them. It is in fact these conceptual elements that allow us to overcome many of the afore-mentioned material hurdles.

When talking about health information we will be taking a global view from the beginning, i.e. look at the health services as a whole. Thus we are dealing with clinical, epidemiologic, economic, and administrative information. Most information of relevance can be represented numerically, i.e. in the form of data or indicators, if necessary upon previous coding.

Health information in developing countries flows from three sources, well distinguished in principle although overlapping and interacting in practice. The first one consists of *sample surveys* where a sample of people, families, communities, or institutions like rural health centres is taken and information in the form of data about these "sampling units" is recorded. The data may concern the moment of selecting the sample only, or some or all units sampled may be followed over a certain period to give rise to a *longitudinal study.* In particular, the sample may be fixed once for all. For instance, faced with the problem of obtaining reliable information regularly from all communal health centres of a given country, health planners have sometimes selected so-called *sentinel centres* whose capabilities were enhanced by furnishing some laboratory equipment, paying additional trained staff, and ensuring better communications. Sentinel centres may, however, furnish biased information because the measures taken to upgrade the selected centres alter the health situation there. More people may indeed be attracted to use these facilities, better treatment can influence the dynamics of the transmission of infectious diseases, and additional health education will reduce the incidence of many ailments including injuries. Recently, the concept of a sentinel centre was extended by installing Demographic Surveillance Systems (DSSs) in various "field sites", i.e. in geographically defined populations, in order to monitor their health and demographic status. Finally, since 1998, an "International Network of field sites with continuous Demographic Evaluation of Populations and Their Health in developing countries" (INDEPTH) is being built up in order to link existing field sites, to strengthen them, and to enhance their visibility and use. This is described in chapter 1.3 of the present volume.

The second source of health information is composed of *research studies,* in particular epidemiologic ones. In contrast to normal sample surveys, they focus on relations between variables of a different nature like exposure and disease outcome, and they are designed with a view of one or several specific questions. A large part of the present volume (chapter five) is devoted to them. There is, of course, an inherent relation between this and the aforementioned source of information since the epidemiological studies reported in chapter five are based on the population of the Nouna DSS or a sample taken from it.

The third source of health information, which is the subject of the present chapter, is the *daily work of the health services* themselves, be it clinical or preventive, accounting or managing. The underlying idea is to exploit to a maximum the information that arises more or less automatically during the normal activities of the health worker, and to do it with a minimum of additional work and structures. A mechanism to this end is called a Health Information System (HIS). Its functions are to collect, transmit, and analyze information from the health care system in a routine fashion. It is based on registers and reports within the network of health institutions. The funding of HIS is thus not based on research grants, as a DSS often is, but on the national health budget.

In line with the principle of being rooted in normal health care activities, a HIS ought to cover the whole country and all health facilities. It should serve all users of health information and all essential objectives of health care. It needs to be closely coordinated with the other two sources of health information regarding definition of concepts, notations, choice of topics. In particular, for obvious but unfortunately often forgotten reasons of efficiency, sample surveys and special research studies should not be undertaken if the results can just as well be obtained from the HIS.

In the following section we shall have a closer look at the users and objectives of a HIS, and in the final one we shall deal with its design and structure.

1.5.2 Objectives of a health information system

Different users have different ideas about the objectives of a HIS. Hence let us describe the various users first. In most existing HISs, health authorities like district and provincial health departments and the Ministry of Health have been considered the main beneficiaries. In many countries, institutes and networks devoted to special tasks like hygiene and prevention, controlling tuberculosis or malaria, and mother and child health, exist and use partial HISs that are separated from the one of the Ministry of Health. In addition, a plethora of so-called *vertical programmes* have appeared in order to handle particular health problems. An early example was Control of Diarrhoeal Diseases (CDD), a recent one the eradication of poliomyelitis. They were mostly planned by WHO but implemented by other international or national, governmental or non-governmental organizations. Each programme is run vertically, from its top administration down to the basic providers of health care, and its managers have usually felt the need for a partial HIS of their own.

Some functions of a HIS are quite classical. Health authorities including managers of vertical programmes use it for obtaining indicators like incidence or prevalence of the main diseases, mortalities and case fatalities and information on health facilities and staff including their activities, on logistics of drugs and vaccines, and on expenses. One objective in doing this is to publish health statistics and health yearbooks, another one is yearly budgeting, and a third one is general management of the health services. In fact, sometimes the term "Health Management Information System" is being employed instead of HIS, which is misleading because a comprehensive HIS needs to include information that is remote from management, especially information of an epidemiologic nature. Building a separate information system devoted to management only will necessarily result in redundancies and inefficiencies.

In addition to these *general* classical tasks there is a more specific, and equally classical, one, namely epidemic surveillance of infectious diseases. Most developing countries do not have an extended health insurance system, but when building one, a general HIS could certainly provide the information needed for operating it. A separate information system for health insurance is superfluous.

A potentially very important but still little considered objective of a HIS is the planning and implementation of *health strategies* along the lines of vertical programmes, but more adapted to the situation of a specific country. The main issue at hand is to regard several health problems and several options at a time in order to attack them in a global way and to set priorities given the existing means and the expected benefits. Another one is to plan strategies for handling new problems not yet covered by specialized institutions or vertical programmes like the nicotine addiction pandemic.

The functions of a HIS described up to here are *global* in the sense that they concern the whole country. The users are health authorities at the top of the hierarchy, and information reaches them via reports. Remember, however, that the source of information in the system is the routine work within the basic health facilities that are in direct contact with the population for curative and preventive activities. These basic facilities are also themselves *users* of information. Clinical work, i.e. case-management in the largest sense, can profit tremendously from recording and exploiting data on a consultation or a case. In addition, there is what WHO once called "epidemiology at the basis", which concerns a smaller geographic or administrative entity, usually a commune. For example, knowing and interpreting indicators on the frequencies of the various diseases including traumata that present themselves at a communal health centre not only has a practical value for guiding the centre but also an educative one; it can be a motivation for the health worker as well. There may even be simple but illuminating epidemiologic studies based on the registers of the HIS only that link an incidence to a social or geographic risk factor. Data on expenses, sale of drugs and the like allow the local management of a health centre or hospital. Finally, the totality of data that have been registered in a health facility makes it possible to monitor and evaluate its overall performance as well as that of some of its components or procedures, for instance the quality of diagnostic rules that are not based on laboratory tests but only on clinical symptoms.

For an example of a HIS, or rather of all partial HISs, in a developing country that possesses a well-structured network of communal health centres, see the report on Vietnam by Krickeberg (1999).

1.5.3 Design of a health information system

In spite of a long history of attempts to design HISs for specific purposes, it is only recently that the underlying principles have been investigated in a systematic way (Krickeberg 1994, 2003; Lippeveld et al. 2000).

We have mentioned in the beginning several obstacles of a general nature to building a good HIS. Having described the typical users, we are now in a position to talk about a more specific, and formidable, one, namely the egoism of the various players in the health sector. As said above, some specialized institutes and many vertical programmes insist on operating their own partial HIS and these partial systems are little coordinated. This represents an intolerable burden on the health worker in basic health facilities who has to keep many registers, usually in the form of heavy books, and to file a large number of reports of varying structure and layout in many directions to the detriment of her or his medical activities. This problem plays a key role in the structural principles on which a HIS should rest, and in the technical rules to be followed in order to satisfy all essential requirements. Once it is solved, many of the other difficulties can be overcome much more easily.

Most basic principles have already appeared in the preceding discussions. Thus the HIS needs of course to have been designed in view of its *objectives*. It must contain rules for analyzing and exploiting the information gathered. It has to be *integrated* which means that the same system serves all users and all uses, be it curative clinical work, prevention, management, etc. Given its objectives, it should be *minimal*, should not contain redundant information, registers or reports, should not produce superfluous information, and should function at minimal cost. This has, in particular, an implication regarding the flow of information. Routine reports must be filed only from and to institutions as really needed, following operational priorities and not hierarchical dictates.

The HIS ought to be *simple* and practical and have a clear and transparent structure so it can easily be handled and perhaps even liked by health workers at all levels, from those in communal health centres to those in the Ministry of Health. This is indeed the best way to motivate the health staff to handle the system correctly, which in turn is indispensable for getting closer to another basic though unattainable desideratum, *reliability*. Moreover, only a well-structured HIS can be computerized although there have been quite a few attempts, always futile, at saving a badly designed system be the use of computers. The information system must also be *flexible* so it can easily be adapted to changes of all kind: changes of the epidemiological situation, changes of the structure of the health system or of health strategies and medical knowledge and techniques, economic and sociologic changes of the country, and changes in information technology.

There have to be clearly defined rules that tell health officials what to do about wrong or missing information, i.e. there have to exist *error-correcting* procedures.

The design of a HIS with a view of these principles and requirements needs to be based on a few technical concepts and rules, all of them fairly elementary and often evident. We will have to recall them here, though, because there is no general agreement on the definition of the basic concepts, and the importance of rigorous rules is largely underestimated. For details, see Krickeberg (1994, 2003, 2004).

Information as it is being registered and treated in the form of data may concern anything: people, institutions, objects, actions etc; these are the underlying *units*. In any concrete situation, the first thing to do is to specify well the so-called *target population,* which consists of all units in question. For instance, a unit may be a child under 5 living at a given moment in a given village, and the target population is composed of all these children; or the target population may consist of all consultations done during a certain month in a certain health centre. Data are the values of one or several *variables.* A variable is, mathematically speaking, a function defined on a target population. For example, for the first target population mentioned before, the variable "age" assigns, to each child, his or her own age. All the values together, indexed by the respective children, form the data. For the second target population, the variable "diagnosis" attributes, to every consultation, the diagnosis made, properly coded. A *register* is a concrete, explicit, and usable representation of the data of one or several variables, usually on paper or on a computer disk. We will not enter into technical details like sub-registers or linked registers.

An *indicator,* in contrast to data, concerns a target population as a whole, but not individual units. It depends on one or several variables defined on the same target population. Two examples, concerning our first and second example of a variable, respectively: the mean age of these children, and the number of "diarrhoea" cases recorded. In practice, an indicator is a summary statistic, computed from all the values of the underlying variables as recorded in a register.

Registers are *the* fundamental, and often neglected, components of a HIS. They need to obey the following "golden" rule: in any basic institution, there is *only one register for a given target population,* i.e. for a given type of unit. For example, it is mandatory that there exist, in a health centre or a ward of a hospital, only one register of consultations, not a "general" one for the Ministry, and one more for each vertical programme and for other special purposes.
Well-designed registers are in particular the main tools for the local use of the HIS sketched above. Their multiple functions demand a clear definition of the variables involved.

The second function of a register, namely to serve as the basis of the routine reports to be filed, should also follow rigorous structural rules. This applies both to paper-based and computer-based HISs. We note first that most information contained in routine reports is in the form of *indicators*, be they epidemiologic, economic, or others. The transmission of *data* on individual units, e.g. on cases, from one institution to another one is indeed rare and mainly restricted to epidemic surveillance and registers of special diseases. For indicators resulting from clinical activities which are the most prominent ones, the structural rule in question looks like this: the clinical act giving rise to the data, the immediate use of these data in the act itself, their recording in the relevant register, and the drawing up of the reports based on these data, have to be *integrated* conceptually and technically. In particular, the *layout* of the register and that of the reporting forms need to be closely coordinated so as to allow calculating the indicators and writing the report in a single, transparent, and almost automatic operation.

In this way, many indicators of quite a different nature can be easily computed and transmitted to various institutions and according to needs that may change, all based on the *same* registers and on the *same* variables. However, on no account should there exist a register that is not tied operationally to some function within the health system and whose only purpose is to calculate and report indicators.

There have been attempts at designing HISs by starting with a list of the indicators to be covered in view of the goals of the system. This idea may be tempting at first sight but is in fact naïve. Such lists have always been long and very much subject to debate, they leave no room for flexibility, and they are at variance with the basic structural principles as outlined above. What we have to fix in the beginning are the *variables* needed; doing this well is crucial. The second step will then be the design of the *registers.*

Reliability of information is a particularly difficult problem in the context of a developing country. Statistical standard procedures to assure quality of data and indicators can only be applied to a rather limited extent. Motivation of the health worker is a somewhat more efficient measure but gaps and errors will remain. The topic of what to do when confronted with them has many facets. The available theory concerns errors and missing data in a *single* statistical, in particular epidemiologic study. In the realm of HISs, however, we have to handle them *routinely,* e.g. for every monthly report of a district health administration to its superiors. To this end, simple rules and algorithms need to be developed which can function under the specific conditions. This is the subject of ongoing research.

The manifold practical and organizational problems that arise when one starts to implement a HIS have been very well described in detail by Lippeveld et al. (2000). They should on no account be underestimated. They are not the subject of the present article, though.

References

Krickeberg K (1994) Health information in developing countries. In: Frontiers in Mathematical Biology, Lecture Notes in Biomathematics 100:550-568

Krickeberg K (1999) The health information system in Vietnam in 1999. Joint Health Systems Development Programme Vietnam-EU (Unpublished report, available from the author: krik@ideenwelt.de)

Krickeberg K (2003) Health information systems in developing countries. Bull International Statistical Institute 54th Session Proceedings, Invited Paper Meeting 54. ISI, Den Hague

Krickeberg K (2004) Epidemiology in developing countries. In: Handbook of Epidemiology, Springer, Heidelberg-New York

Lippeveld Th, Sauerborn R, Bodart C (eds) (2000) Design and implementation of health information systems. World Health Organization, Geneva

Further reading:

Azubuike MC, Ehiri JE. (1999) Health information systems in developing countries: benefits, problems, and prospects J R Soc Health 119:180-4

Cibulskis RE, Hiawalyer G (2002) Information systems for health sector monitoring in Papua New Guinea. Bull World Health Organ 80:752-8.

Pappaioanou M, Malison M, Wilkins K, Otto B, Goodman RA, Churchill RE, White M, Thacker SB. (2003) Strengthening capacity in developing countries for evidence-based public health: the data for decision-making project. Soc Sci Med. 57:1925-37

Rotich JK, Hannan TJ, Smith FE, Bii J, Odero WW, Vu N, Mamlin BW, Mamlin JJ, Einterz RM, Tierney WM(2003) Installing and implementing a computer-based patient record system in sub-Saharan Africa: the Mosoriot Medical Record System. J Am Med Inform Assoc. 10:295-303

Williamson L, Stoops N, Heywood A (2001) Developing a District Health Information System in South Africa: a social process or technical solution? Medinfo 10:773-7

2 Clinical Research

2.1 Overview

2.1.1 Malaria studies in Nouna, Burkina Faso

OLAF MÜLLER

University of Heidelberg, Department of Tropical Hygiene and Public Health, Im Neuenheimer Feld 324, 69120 Heidelberg, Germany

Tel.: +49 6221 565035

Email: olaf.mueller@urz.uni-heidelberg.de

Introduction

Malaria is the most frequent vector-borne disease in the world. The absolute number of individuals at risk for malaria has increased up to three billion in 2002 worldwide (Hay et al., 2004). Sub-Saharan Africa, including Burkina Faso, is the most severely affected region in the world.

Malaria is holoendemic but seasonal in the Nouna study area. Transmission of malaria is intense in the villages surrounding Nouna town, with an Entomological Inoculation Rate ranging from 100 to 1000 infective bites per person per year (Traoré 2004). *Plasmodium falciparum* is the dominating malaria parasite, but *P. ovale* and *P. vivax* also occur mainly as a mixed infection with *P. falciparum* (Müller et al. 2001, chapter 2.2). Malaria tropica is consequently a major cause of morbidity and mortality in young children of this region, and most clinical malaria episodes occur during or shortly after the rainy season which usually lasts from June until October (Müller et al. 2001, chapter 2.2; Müller et al. 2003a, chapter 3.6 Traoré 2004).

Soumaya, the local illness concept closest to the biomedical term malaria, covers a broad range of signs and symptoms (Okrah et al. 2002, chapter 3.3). *Djokadjo* and *Kono* are local terms for the more severe disease manifestations associated with jaundice and convulsions respectively. While *Soumaya* is known by most of the population to be caused by mosquitoes, the more severe manifestations of malaria are often thought to be caused by supernatural forces. As a consequence, such atypical manifestations are often first seen by a traditional healer. We are currently analysing the data from an anthropological study, which has been carried out in 2003/2004, on the role of traditional healers in the treatment of atypical malaria presentations in the study area.

Malaria treatment seeking behaviour in the Nouna area depends on a number of factors such as perceived cause and severity of the disease, income, and accessibility of health services (Müller et al. 2003a, chapter 3.6). Most treatment thus takes place in the households, and only a small proportion of febrile illness episodes are seen in local health centres. Chloroquine and paracetamol, which are often bought in shops and through local drug sellers, are the most frequent western drugs used against uncomplicated malaria in this rural area of Burkina Faso. However, traditional treatment is still used alternatively or in addition to western treatment in a substantial proportion of malaria cases (Okrah et al. 2002, chapter 3.3; Müller et al. 2003a, chapter 3.6).

Anaemia is highly prevalent in young children of the study area, but surprisingly malaria was not identified as the main risk factor for severe anaemia in a longitudinal study over the main malaria transmission season in 1999 (Müller et al. 2003, chapter 2.4). Instead of malaria, malnutrition was significantly associated with severe anaemia development in this large prospective study (Müller et al. 2001, chapter 2.2; Müller et al. 2003b, chapter 2.4). Moreover, there was some evidence from analysing verbal autopsy data that cerebral malaria and not severe anaemia causes most of the malaria-deaths in young children of the study area (Müller et al. 2003a, chapter 3.6; Traoré 2004).

The association between protein-energy malnutrition (PEM) and malaria has been discussed controversially for a long time. A large cohort of preschool children has been followed in the Nouna area for a six months period over the main malaria transmission period. There was no association between PEM and malaria morbidity, but malnourished children had a more than two-fold higher risk of dying than non-malnourished children (Müller et al. 2003c, chapter 2.6). Moreover, a randomised double-blind placebo-controlled trial on zinc supplementation in young children of this area with a high prevalence of malnutrition showed no effect of the intervention on malaria morbidity (Müller et al. 2001, chapter 2.2).

Chloroquine resistance and the development of alternative malaria drugs

The increasing resistance development against the well-known malaria drug chloroquine is considered a major public health disaster in Sub-Saharan Africa (SSA). While in most of the southern and eastern African countries chloroquine failure rates had reached already a level which required a change in the malaria first-line treatment during recent years, chloroquine has remained the official first-line drug in many western African countries including Burkina Faso until today. However, chloroquine resistance is also increasing in Burkina Faso and it is only a question of time until a change in policy will be required. The chloroquine treatment failure rate in young children followed over a period of 14 days has been shown to be 10 percent and thus still acceptable in 2001 in the villages surrounding Nouna town (Müller et al. 2003d, chapter 2.5). This finding of a failure rate around 10 percent in the rural CRSN study area has been confirmed by a chloroquine efficacy study carried out in the frame of a multi-centre study on the effects of malaria home treatment in 2003 (unpublished observations). However, a clinical study carried out on young children of Nouna town in 2003 demonstrated a very high failure rate of around 30 percent (unpublished observations). Although the other affordable malaria drug pyrimethamine-sulfadoxine (which is the current official second-line malaria drug) has not been used much in Burkina Faso and thus been shown to be still highly effective, resistance to this drug is expected to develop rapidly in case of widespread monotherapy (Müller et al. 2004, chapter 2.8).

Combination therapy has now become the new paradigm in malaria control, and artemisinin-based combination therapy (ACT) is widely recommended because of the rapid action of the artemisinin component against the parasites and the lower probability of resistance development when using two effective drugs together. However, the costs of ACT are still 10-20 times higher compared to chloroquine or pyrimethamine-sulfadoxine monotherapy, supply is currently not sufficient for the huge amount of malaria cases particularly in SSA, potential partner drugs which are both synergistic and have a comparable short half-life are currently not available, and considerably cheaper pragmatic non-ACT have been shown to be even more effective in a number of African countries. Moreover, external support of systematic ACT through the Global Fund may not be sustainable for all of SSA. Against this background, the Ruprecht-Karls-University Heidelberg in collaboration with the CRSN has started the development of an affordable alternative malaria drug combination called BlueCQ (Schirmer et al. 2003, chapter 5.2). This combination consists of chloroquine and the old malaria drug methylene blue. Animal experiments and *in vitro* tests were promising and three subsequent safety studies conducted in 2003 in healthy volunteers in Heidelberg, in G6PD deficient adult men in Burkina Faso, and in young children with uncomplicated falciparum malaria in Burkina Faso have shown no relevant side effects of BlueCQ (Müller et al. submitted). A BlueCQ dose-finding study has now been started at the beginning of the rainy season of 2004 in Nouna town. If a likely effective BlueCQ dose regimen will be identified, a phase III efficacy trial comparing chloroquine with BlueCQ and other potential alternative drug combinations will follow.

The role of insecticide-treated mosquito nets in malaria control

In five large randomised and controlled field studies carried out in African countries with very different malaria transmission intensity, insecticide-treated mosquito nets (ITN) have consistently been shown to reduce all-cause child mortality by around 20 percent and malaria morbidity by around 50 percent. However, as all these studies have only followed children over short periods of time and as there was some evidence from ecological studies on higher malaria mortality in hypo/mesoendemic as compared to hyper/holoendemic areas, there remained a considerable concern that the interference of ITN protection with the development of immunity could even lead to harmful effects of the intervention in high-transmission areas. Against this background we had designed and implemented a large controlled ITN trial in young children of the whole rural CRSN study area since June 2000. A total of 3.400 newborns were individually randomised to ITN protection from birth until their 5th birthday versus ITN protection from months 6 until their 5th birthday. Preliminary data analysis points to no differences in mortality between groups and a significant morbidity advantage in protecting children since birth. Moreover, we were one of the first research groups who tested the efficacy of a prototype of a promising long-lasting ITN in Africa (Müller et al. 2002, chapter 2.3).

The challenge of the coming years thus lies in achieving a high coverage with ITN protection of young children and pregnant women in rural SSA. There is currently an ongoing and highly controversial discussion about two different models: The first one is on providing ITN free of charge to all African households of malaria endemic areas, while the second one is on distributing ITN through a social marketing system. Both are supported through limited evidence from a few pilot projects. We consider these two approaches as not mutually exclusive and are planning from 2005 onwards to study the effectiveness of distributing long-lasting ITN free of charge to pregnant women attending antenatal care services in half of the peripheral health centres of Nouna Health District, compared to a distribution system based on social marketing.

Conclusions and outlook

Like most of the other SSA countries, Burkina Faso will have to live with malaria for the years to come. However, although the disease cannot be eradicated with current technology in the highly endemic areas, a number of effective interventions are now available. These are first of all the provision of early diagnosis and prompt treatment of malaria episodes with an effective first-line drug, and secondly the prevention of a significant proportion of malaria episodes through protection with ITN. As access to modern health facilities will remain limited in the rural areas of SSA in the near future, home treatment of febrile episodes in children is considered a promising supplementary measure and needs to be further evaluated. Although nutritional interventions have unfortunately not been shown to have a direct impact in malaria control, long-term strategies to reduce the high prevalence of childhood malnutrition are urgently needed for Burkina Faso and other SSA countries. For malaria control, scaling up the implementation of effective malaria combination therapies, ITN and home treatment should be considered the primary goal of national programmes in all of the malaria endemic areas of SSA. The CRSN in collaboration with the Heidelberg University will continue to contribute with relevant clinical and epidemiological research to such a development.

References

Traoré C. The epidemiology of malaria in rural north-western Burkina Faso. Dissertation, Medical Faculty, Ruprecht-Karls-University Heidelberg, 2004

Hay SI, Guerra CA, Tatem AJ, Noor AM, Snow RW. The global distribution and population at risk of malaria: past, present, and future Lancet Infect Dis. 2004; 4(6):327-36

2.1.2 Introduction of a program for prevention of transmission of human immunodeficiency virus from mother to infant in rural Burkina Faso: first operative results

[1]Böhler Thomas, [2]Sarker, Malabika, [3]Ganamé, Jean, [3]Coulibaly, Boubacar, [1]Hofmann, Jennifer, [3]Nagabila, Youssouf, [3]Boncoungou, Justine, [1]Tebit, Denis Manga, [2]Snow, Rachel C., [1]Kräusslich Hans-Georg

[1] University of Heidelberg, Departments of Virology and of [2]Tropical Hygiene and Public Health, Im Neuenheimer Feld 324, 69120 Heidelberg, Germany

Tel. :   +49 6221 565001

Email : hans-georg.kraeusslich@med.uni-heidelberg.de

[3]Centre de Recherche en Santé de Nouna, BP 02 Nouna, Burkina Faso

Tel.: 00226-20-537043

Email: bocar.crsn@fasonet.bf

Abstract

As an extension of the ongoing collaboration between the Centre de la Recherche en Santé de Nouna (CRSN) and the University of Heidelberg, a newly designed service for HIV voluntary counseling and testing (VCT) and prevention of mother-to-child-transmission (PMTCT) was introduced at the Centre Médical avec Antenne Chirurgical (CMA) in Nouna, rural Burkina Faso. In order to increase field acceptability of the PMTCT program, trained collaborators of the CRSN and the CMA conducted a community sensitisation program as well as individual interviews and focus group discussions (FGDs) with different population groups in Nouna town. Information on knowledge, attitudes, and operational preferences regarding HIV/AIDS, VCT, PMTCT and related health services allowed us to adapt the design of the PMTCT program in order to minimise the risk of stigmatisation for the participants. The program, which is based on national guidelines for VCT and PMTCT services in Burkina Faso, was launched in July 2003 and attracted an increasing number of female users during the first months of its activity. Data from an anthropologic field study on breast feeding and breast pathologies in lactating women together with information on the uptake of the service (including HIV prevalence in pregnant women and the frequency of MTCT in Nouna) as well as results of forthcoming community surveys will be used for continuous adaptation of the program to the needs of the population.

Approximately half of the world's 38 million HIV-infected persons are women, and 700,000 infants were infected last year through mother to child transmission (UNAIDS 2004). A woman infected by HIV can transmit the virus to her child during pregnancy, during delivery or while breastfeeding (Newell 1998). Mechanisms of breast-milk transmission, however, are not yet fully understood. HIV has been detected in breast milk (Nduati 1995) and a meta-analysis of studies of mother-to-child transmission (MTCT) via breast-milk illustrated a cumulative probability of postnatal MTCT of at least 9.3% at 18 months of age (BHITS 2004). Preventing mother-to-child transmission (PMTCT) has become a major focus of HIV control programs (DeCock 2000). Short course regimens for PMTCT are being disseminated in high prevalence settings and new treatments are under investigation (Bulterys 2004). While numerous studies demonstrate the "proof of concept" for VCT and PMTCT, sufficient experience has not yet evolved to allow delineation of best practice for either intervention, and there is evidence of substantial variation in the public acceptance of these services in different settings (Rutenberg 2003).

Social factors such as differences in local perception of risk, cultural independence of women, social security, ethnicity, or religion may all impact the acceptance of VCT and PMTCT, and better understanding of such associations will influence program design and implementation. In Western Europe and North America health care authorities have increasingly encouraged patients to contribute to the planning and development of health services (Crawford et al. 2002). Underlying these incentives is the belief that involving patients leads to more accessible and acceptable services and improves the health and quality of life of patients. A report from Preston Hall Hospital, Maidstone, U.K., decribed a doubling of the number of clients accepting HIV testing simply by introducing a more "user-friendly" HIV testing protocol after consultation with client groups (Read and Wincelaus 2003). Similar strategies may be applied in developing countries in order to increase field acceptability of VCT and PMTCT services (Rutenberg 2003).

In collaboration with the Ministry of Health of Burkina Faso, the National Program for PMTCT of HIV was extended to Nouna in 2002. In the research project A6 of the collaborative research grant "Control of tropical infectious diseases" we tried to identify local awareness of HIV, local perceptions of risk, public demand for services, and perceived obstacles to accessing VCT and PMTCT interventions.

Women's knowledge, attitudes and risk perception regarding HIV/AIDS

In spring 2002, a random household survey was conducted among 300 women aged 15 to 29 years and living in Nouna town to investigate knowledge, attitudes and risk perception regarding HIV/AIDS (Sarker, in press). Using the Nouna DSS (see chapter one for details) a weighted random sample from the census list of 3,026 (15-29 year old) women residing in one of the seven sectors of Nouna town was drawn from a total population of 21,430. Five local interviewers were recruited and trained in the use of the study questionnaire which was translated into the local language Djula. Risk perception on HIV/AIDS and disease related knowledge was assessed in personal interviews. The nature of the study and questionnaire was explained to all participants; they were assured about confidentiality and had to provide verbal consent.

Women living in Nouna had a high level of HIV/AIDS related knowledge, with few incorrect beliefs about virus transmission (Table 1). In contrast to this relatively good knowledge, nearly two-thirds of the study population was unaware that a person can be HIV positive without showing any symptoms. Accordingly, the understanding that a person infected with HIV can be asymptomatic but nevertheless infective needs to be addressed more agressively. Women currently living in Nouna had far more knowledge (77%) about MTCT compared to a study conducted in Bobo-Dioulasso, Burkina Faso six years ago (8%), consistent with a general increase in awareness about HIV vertical transmission world-wide. However, 38% of women did not know any means of PMTCT prior to the presentation about short-course therapy provided within the context of the study. 'Avoiding breast-feeding' as a means to avoid infecting the baby with HIV was listed by just under two-thirds of women. However, there is no charitable service offering infant formula in Nouna, and given the high rates of infant malnutrition and death in Burkina Faso, national recommendations for HIV-infected women to continue breastfeeding for 4 months and start weaning after that appear appropriate.

Table 1: Answers of women who had heard of HIV/AIDS (n=275) to questions regarding HIV testing, PMTCT services and HIV positive status disclosure in Nouna town (DSS-based survey in spring 2002).

	Yes (%)
If a woman feels at risk of having AIDS, do you think she would like to do a test ?	190 (69%)
If a woman is HIV+, could she convince her partner to have an HIV test?	237 (86%)
Would a woman take her baby for HIV testing?	228 (83%)
If a woman is pregnant, do you think that she would like to have an HIV test?	253 (92%)
If a woman is pregnant and learns that she has HIV, what do you think she would prefer to do thereafter?:	
• Take medication (to reduce the chances that the baby has HIV)	207 (75%)
• Undergo an abortion	5 (2%)
• Trust in God	56 (20%)
• Does not know	7 (3%)
Perceptions about women's ability to disclose HIV positive status (multiple answers possible):	
If a woman knows that she is HIV positive, could she share that with her partner ?	171 (62%)
If a woman knows that she is HIV positive, could she share that with her family ?	148 (55%)
If a woman knows that she is HIV positive, could she share that with her friends?	75 (27%)

Willingness to undergo HIV testing if a woman feels at risk was high (69%) and increased to 92% after a short presentation of the planned PMTCT program. Regarding maternity care, women demanded an improved staff performance and reduced service and medicine cost. In summary, this young female population possessed a high level of HIV/AIDS knowledge, while condom prevention knowledge was quite low. Willingness to participate in a HIV testing program was very high as seemed the expressed demand for a PMTCT program.

Men's knowledge, attitudes and risk perception regarding HIV/AIDS

In summer 2002, a regional focus-group study was undertaken in 4 sectors of Nouna town among married men, aged 25 to 50 years, and living as heads of a court or household. Following a pre-test in a mixed ethnic group, additional participants were recruited from five ethnic groups living in town (Mossi, Peulh, Samo, Marka, Bwaba; n=74). Alternatively, participants were required to hold an occupation as civil servants ("fonctionnaire"; n=8), these participants met as a separate group. Trained collaborators of the CRSN identified and recruited participants for the study. The promoters followed strictly the selection criteria for recruitment. The size of the seven discussion groups ranged from 6 to 22 participants.

Participants generally knew that HIV/AIDS can be transmitted by heterosexual relationships, dirty objects (e.g. knives), and contact with blood and used syringes. Transmission from mother to child during birth was also mentioned. Less frequently, transmission of HIV/AIDS was attributed to mosquito bites, sharing food with people suffering from AIDS, and circumcision. It was known that prophylaxis of HIV/AIDS is possible by the use of preservatives during sexual intercourse. Other ways of prevention mentioned include fidelity between partners, sexual abstinence, strict observation of religious rules, HIV-testing before marriage and good education and socialisation. The fight against poverty may also help to prevent AIDS. Most of the discutants stated that there is currently no African drug available for the treatment of HIV/AIDS.

People talk about AIDS only on special occasions (e.g., a neighbor or a family member suffering or dying from AIDS). In families there is communication about modes of prevention both between husbands and wives and between parents and adolescent children. In married couples a positive test result in one of the partners may be followed by divorce. Overall, men are in favor of the organisation of a VCT service in the community and the use of antiretroviral prophylaxis for PMTCT. However, several individuals raised the question how to deal with the enormous social problems which may potentially arise. It is generally perceived that women cannot freely talk about a positive test result with their husbands or other family members. Disclosing the serostatus in a couple, especially if it is discordant, may cause severe conflicts and may have a deep impact on the perception of the VCT and PMTCT service.

Most but not all discussions concluded that husbands and wives should be tested together. Nearly unanimously it was stated that the test results should be available immediately, i.e. the same day. People should be prepared psychologically before receiving a positive test result. The counseling staff must be able to keep secrets and respect confidentiality. Men preferred to be counseled by men, women should be counseled either by male or by female counselors.

Women's attitudes and risk perception regarding breastfeeding

In order to obtain detailed information regarding knowledge, attitudes, beliefs and practice of breastfeeding of women in Nouna, qualitative data were collected through in-depth interviews with 37 women who had experienced problems during previous periods of breastfeeding, participant observation in households of lactating women and focus group discussions using questionnaires, tape recordings, photo documentation and a diary. An ethnologist (J.H.) recruited study participatants during announced meetings with women living in randomly chosen neighborhoods in Nouna town from January to March 2003. The study showed that women perceived breast milk as the best and cheapest way to nourish an infant. Breast milk gives "strength" and identity to the child and establishes the emotional bond between mother and infant. Breast milk also has a dangerous potential of causing diarrhea and transmitting disease, e.g. HIV. However, the inability to breastfeed an infant was perceived as the most serious threat to the infant's life since poverty does not allow the mother to buy artificial food if breastfeeding is not possible. Perceived causes for breast pathologies which may challenge the women's ability to breastfeed are listed in table 2.

Table 2: Reasons for breast problems during lactation given by women in Nouna town (n=37; multiple answers were possible)

Causes for breast pathologies mentioned	Number of women
Lateral sucking of the child (pulling of nipple) / wrong practices of breastfeeding	9
Parasites (entry of worms)	7
Coughing/belching of the child during breastfeeding (Although this is known to cause swelling but not abscess)	4
"balls" which are not exploded during process of "l'ecrasement"	4
Sorcery, enemy who sends illness (maladie surnaturelle)	4
God (Dieu)	4
Large breasts	2
Plugging in coins inside the bra	2
The infant didn't drink enough maternal milk	2
Non-compliance with prohibitions (protect the breast, wearing of shoes and fula), biting of the nipple, hygiene, small white crumbs ("choses") are not to remove from the mammary gland, eating of pieces of the broom (not hygienic meals), drinking of sour water, being left by the infant's father, war (Ivory Coast) etc.	Each 1
No reason reported (« Je ne peux pas connaître la cause »)	12

It was concluded from this ethnological field study that interventions for the prevention of mother-to-child transmission of HIV in rural Burkina Faso should (a) promote exclusive breastfeeding, (b) aim at prevention and appropriate treatment of breast pathologies during lactation in collaboration with indigenous healers, (c) help women to establish a relationship of trust towards the PMTCT service and (d) address health education programs on PMTCT and infant feeding issues not only to women in reproductive age, but also to other family members involved in decision making on the use of economic resources of the household.

Community sensitization in Nouna town and introduction of the service

Activities for community sensitisation and social mobilisation regarding VCT and PMTCT were undertaken from April to December 2003 by the team in Nouna. These activities consisted in organised meetings with the complete staff of the CMA, the ethics committee at the CRSN, numerous women's and patient's organisations, religious leaders, veterans' associations, local administative authorities, workers' unions, trade unions, staff and pupils of colleges and high schools. A total of 1752 persons were thus contacted and informed about VCT and the PMTCT service in Nouna. In general, these persons appreciated the launching of the program and expressed their willingness to take the responsibility for further social mobilisation and expanding information regarding the service in the community.

The PMTCT program started in July 2003. After 6 months of regular activities the staff at Nouna had performed group counseling on HIV, testing and PMTCT for 532 attendees of antenatal care at the CMA (393 pregnant women). In the same period a total of 1197 pregnant women had attended antenatal care. Thus, group counseling had reached approximately one third of all pregnant women in antenatal care. Individual counseling was requested by 563 pregnant women (47% of all women in antenatal care), 429 (76%) of these women agreed to HIV testing. Thus, 36% of all pregnant women in antenatal care accepted an HIV test. An algorithm describing the sample flow for laboratory testing is shown in figure 1.

> **Hb concentration, blood group, VDRL (all pregnant women)**

> **HIV serology (all women who accept VCT)**
▼
2 different rapid screening tests (*Determine, Genie II*)
▼
quality control by *ELISA* (Behring und Murex)
▼
Western Blot *INNO-LIA*: confirmation & distinction between HIV-1 and HIV-2
▼
CD4 counts, viral load, *PCR* and *molecular analysis* (gag-pol-env)

Figure 1: Flow chart showing the sample flow of laboratory testing in the Nouna PMTCT program

A positive HIV test result was obtained in 21 women (5% of tested), 408 blood samples were seronegative for HIV. In 345 cases post-test counseling was performed (80% of those tested; 19 seropositive and 305 seronegative women). 25 male partners were tested as well. In 24 cases post-test counseling was performed (1 seropositive and 23 seronegative male partners). One seropositive partner did not return for communication of the test result and post-test counseling.

As of April 2004, ten of the HIV positive women had delivered and seven of them had completed the nevirapine protocol and are currently being followed up. Blood and breast milk samples were collected from mothers and blood spot samples from newborns at specified time points post delivery. Analysis by PCR and sequencing revealed that CRF02.AG and CRF6.cpx are the two major strains circulating in Nouna, similar to a previous study in Burkina Faso. Furthermore, PCR analysis of early samples from children indicated that one of them was infected. Infection probably occurred before delivery since the sample on the first day after delivery was already positive. This transmission was associated with a low CD4 T cell number (<200 cells /mm^3) in the mother.

Discussion

The newly launched joint PMTCT service of the CMA and the CRSN is highly accepted by the population in Nouna and has immediately reached and maintained a high level of acceptance among pregnant women attending antenatal care at the CMA. Nearly half of the women requested individual counseling on HIV/AIDS, its transmission and prevention. More than three quarters of women who received individual counseling accepted an HIV test and nearly two thirds wanted to know the test result and returned for post-test counseling (80% of women who were tested). Thus, the strategy of voluntary group counseling, followed by individual counseling and testing on demand of the client (even at a later time point) and individual post-test counseling (all services offered to pregnant women and their male partners) seems to be successful among antenatal care attendees in Nouna. However, only 6% of the male partners of women who accepted VCT agreed to be tested together with their wives. This is in sharp contrast to the declarations of men in Nouna during the focus group discussions in the year before.

The Centre Médical St. Camille in Ouagadougou, the capital of Burkina Faso, also offers a comprehensive PMTCT service in collaboration with the national PMTCT program. After 9 months of regular activities, the Centre reports an acceptance rate for VCT (pre-test counseling) of approximately 22% (Centre Médical St. Camille 2003). However, nearly all of these women have undergone HIV testing and have received their test results during post-test counseling. As observed in Nouna, only approximately 7% of sexual partners accepted VCT. It may be speculated that the low rate of male partners tested may be largely due to lack of general antiretroviral therapy. Accordingly, there is little perceived benefit to male partners. In many PMTCT sites, expansion of the program to include combination antiretroviral therapy to HIV-positive women with low CD4-counts and their male partners is currently being implemented (PMTCTplus) and this is also planned for Nouna. It may be anticipated that availability of PMTCTplus will significantly increase the rate of male partners tested and it will be important to monitor this closely.

In a publication on field acceptability and effectiveness of services to reduce MTCT of HIV in West Africa, Meda et al. (DITRAME-ARNS 049 Study Group 2002) described a high acceptance of HIV pre-test counseling and testing in pregnant women (ca. 90%). However, only approximately 30% of these women did return for post-test counseling and recruitment into a clinical trial of PMTCT. In contrast, in St. Camille only 22% of women participated in VCT, but >90% of these agreed to be tested and returned for their test results. The current numbers in Nouna are between these two figures. It appears likely that there are multiple reasons for the observed differences in acceptance rates of VCT and in participation in the PMTCT program (see below). One important aspect may be how vigorously participation is recommended at a specific site. In some cases, all women attending antenatal care are strongly encouraged to participate in VCT, while in other sites (e.g. St. Camille), women are informed about the service but have to actively choose VCT ("opt-in" versus "opt-out" strategy). It appears likely that "opt-out" programs have a significantly higher rate of VCT participation with a relatively lower return rate, while "opt-in" programs – e.g. St. Camille – have a lower rate of VCT-participation with a very high return rate. In the case of Nouna, participation in the VCT program is recommended by the counselor, but not vigorously advocated and this may explain why the relative numbers in Nouna are in between those observed in the DITRAME study and in St. Camille, respectively.

Despite the fact that efficacy of antiretroviral prophylaxis of MTCT was proven and the entire process of care was free of charge, a significant part of women who had agreed to be tested for HIV did not want to know their test results in all studies. In the DITRAME study, the authors suggested that this may be due to a long delay in the availability of test results, a bad quality of staff-client interactions, lack of treatment for HIV-infected mothers, and the fear of negative social consequences as potential reasons for this refusal. They suggested that women's partners should be involved in decision making regarding HIV testing and treatment in order to increase the uptake of pregnant women in a MTCT reduction programme.

In summary, information obtained during our study and from the review of published literature may help in the continuous process of updating the Nouna PMTCT service and its adaptation to the expressed needs of the population. Current plans include the enlargement of the capture area to the surrounding villages as well as the availability of antiretroviral combination therapy for HIV-infected women and their partners who participate in the research project. Immunologic and virologic research aiming at identifying protective factors for HIV-transmission during breast-feeding will address the important question of how seropositive mothers can safely feed their uninfected infants.

Acknowledgements:

This work was supported by a grant from the DFG within SFB544 "Control of tropical infectious diseases" and by a grant from the ministry of research of the state of Baden-Württemberg and the medical faculty Heidelberg.

We are strongly indebted to B. Kouyaté, the director of CRSN, who made implementation of the program possible. We also thank the Nouna District Medical Officer M. Yé, as well as A. Palé, and N. Dembele for help in various parts of the project.

References

BHITS (Breastfeeding and HIV International Transmission Study Group): Late postnatal transmission of HIV-1 in breast-fed children: an individual patient data meta-analysis. J Infect Dis 2004; 189:2154-2166

Bulterys M, Fowler MG, van Rompay KK, Kourtis AP: Prevention of mother-to-child transmission of HIV-1 through breast-feeding: past, present, and future. J Infect Dis 2004; 189:2149-2153

Cartoux M, Msellati P, Meda N et al.: Attitude of pregnant women towards HIV testing in Abidjan, Côte d'Ivoire and Bobo-Dioulasso, Burkina Faso. AIDS 1998; 12:2337-2344

Centre Medical St. Camille de Ouagadougou: Prevention de la transmission mere-enfant du VIH/SIDA (PTME) - Rapport technique N° 2, february 2003

Crawford MJ, Rutter D, Manley C et al.: Systematic review of involving patients in the planning and development of health care. Br Med J 2002; 325:1263-1268

Dabis F, Newell ML, Fransen L, Cartoux M, Meda N, Whynes DK et al. Prevention of mother to child transmission of HIV in developing countries: recommendations for practice. Health Policy Planning 2000;15:34-42

De Cock KM, Fowler MG, Mercier E, de Vincenzi I, Saba J, Hoff E et al. Preventing mother to child transmission of HIV in resource poor countries: translating research into policy and practice. JAMA 2000;283:1175-1182

Guzman-Garcia S, Snow R, Aitken I: Preferences for contraceptive attributes: voices of women in Ciudad Juárez, Mexico. International Family Planning Perspectives 1997; 23:52-58

Meda N, Leroy V, Viho I et al.: Field acceptability and effectiveness of the routine utilization of zidovudine to reduce mother-to-child transmission of HIV-1 in West Africa. AIDS 2002; 16:2323-2328

Nduati RW, John GC, Richardson BA, Overbaugh J, Welch M, Ndinya-Achola J, Moses S, Holmes K, Onyango F, Kreiss JK. Human immunodeficiency virus type 1-infected cells in breast milk: association with immunosuppression and vitamin A deficiency. J Infect Dis. 1995 Dec;172(6):1461-8.

Newell ML: Mechanisms and timing of mother-to-child transmission of HIV-1. AIDS 1998; 12: 831-837

Read J, Wincelaus SJ: New strategies for increasing the detection of HIV: analysis of routine data. Br Med J 2003; 326:1066-1067

Rutenberg N, Baek C, Kalibala S, Rosen J: Evaluation of United Nations-supported pilot projects for the prevention of mother-to-child transmission of HIV. UNICEF, New York, 2003

Sarker M, Milkowski A, Slanger T, Gondos A, Sanou A, Kouyate B, Snow R. HIV risk perception among rural women in Burkina Faso: the importance of knowledge of asymptomatic nature of HIV and ethnicity. AIDS Behavior (in press)

UNAIDS 2004. Report of Global AIDS epidemic, UNAIDS/04.16E June 2004).
(http://www.unaids.org/bangkok2004/GAR2004_pdf/GAR2004_Execsumm_en.pdef)

2.2 Effect of zinc supplementation on malaria and other causes of morbidity in west African children: randomised double blind placebo controlled trial

Müller O, Becher H, van Zweeden AB, Ye Y, Diallo DA, Konate AT, Gbangou A, Kouyaté B, Garenne M

British Medical Journal. 2001 Jun 30;322(7302):1567.

Reprinted with permission from the BMJ Publishing group.

Papers

Effect of zinc supplementation on malaria and other causes of morbidity in west African children: randomised double blind placebo controlled trial

Olaf Müller, Heiko Becher, Anneke Baltussen van Zweeden, Yazoume Ye, Diadier A Diallo, Amadou T Konate, Adjima Gbangou, Bocar Kouyate, Michel Garenne

Abstract

Objective To study the effects of zinc supplementation on malaria and other causes of morbidity in young children living in an area holoendemic for malaria in west Africa.

Design Randomised, double blind, placebo controlled efficacy trial.

Setting 18 villages in rural northwestern Burkina Faso.

Participants 709 children were enrolled; 685 completed the trial.

Intervention Supplementation with zinc (12.5 mg zinc sulphate) or placebo daily for six days a week for six months.

Main outcome measures The primary outcome was the incidence of symptomatic falciparum malaria. Secondary outcomes were the severity of malaria episodes, prevalence of malaria parasite, mean parasite densities, mean packed cell volume, prevalence of other morbidity, and all cause mortality.

Results The mean number of malaria episodes per child (defined as a temperature ≥37.5°C with ≥5000 parasites/µl) was 1.7, 99.7% due to infection with *Plasmodium falciparum*. No difference was found between the zinc and placebo groups in the incidence of falciparum malaria (relative risk 0.98, 95% confidence interval 0.86 to 1.11), mean temperature, and mean parasite densities during malaria episodes, nor in malaria parasite rates, mean parasite densities, and mean packed cell volume during cross sectional surveys. Zinc supplementation was significantly associated with a reduced prevalence of diarrhoea (0.87, 0.79 to 0.95). All cause mortality was non-significantly lower in children given zinc compared with those given placebo (5 v 12, P = 0.1).

Conclusions Zinc supplementation has no effect on morbidity from falciparum malaria in children in rural west Africa, but it does reduce morbidity associated with diarrhoea.

Introduction

The annual incidence of malaria is about 300-500 million cases, causing between 1.5 and 2.7 million deaths.[1] Tropical Africa accounts for 90% of the morbidity and mortality attributed to malaria; severe disease and death mainly occur among infants in remote rural areas.[2][3] Prevailing poverty, lack of functioning health services, climatic and environmental change, and the rapid spread of chloroquine resistance contribute to a deteriorating malaria situation in Africa.[1-6]

Zinc deficiency is common in children in developing countries.[7] It has been associated with an increased susceptibility to a variety of infections because of its effects on the immune system.[8] In several studies, mainly from Asia and Latin America, zinc supplementation has been shown to have therapeutic and preventive effects on acute and chronic diarrhoea, dysentery, and pneumonia.[9-22] Only two studies have provided data on the possible efficacy of zinc supplementation in reducing morbidity from malaria.[23][24] We aimed to test the hypothesis that zinc supplementation reduces morbidity from falciparum malaria in African children.

Participants and methods

Study area

Our study took place between June and December 1999 in the Nouna district of northwestern Burkina Faso. This area is a dry orchard savanna, populated mainly by subsistence farmers of different ethnic groups. Malaria is a major cause of morbidity and mortality in children in this region, with most transmission occurring during and shortly after the rainy season from June to October.

The main staple food is millet, so children usually receive a diet with little protein. Food intake is particularly low during the rainy season, when workload and disease incidence are high.[25] As in most of sub-Saharan Africa, zinc supplementation for the control of diarrhoea is not available in Nouna.

Study design

Our study was designed as a randomised, placebo controlled, double blind efficacy trial. We identified eligible children from the demographic surveillance system of the Centre de Recherche en Santé de Nouna.[26] Eligible children were aged between 6 and 31 months at enrolment and were permanent residents in 18 of the 39 villages of the study area. We recruited children by lot-

Department of Tropical Hygiene and Public Health, Ruprecht Karls University, 69120 Heidelberg, INF 324, Germany
Olaf Müller
clinical epidemiologist
Heiko Becher
professor of epidemiology and biostatistics

Centre de Recherche en Santé de Nouna, Nouna, Burkina Faso
Anneke Baltussen van Zweeden
general practitioner
Yazoume Ye
data manager
Adjima Gbangou
research officer
Bocar Kouyate
director of research

Centre National de Recherche et de Formation sur le Paludisme, Ouagadougou, Burkina Faso
Diadier A Diallo
epidemiologist
Amadou T Konate
general practitioner

Centre Français sur la Population et le Dévelopement, 75270 Paris, Cedex 06, France
Michel Garenne
director of research

Correspondence to: O Müller
olaf.mueller@urz.uni-heidelberg.de

BMJ 2001;322:1-6

tery (names were drawn blindly at random from a box); 30 from 12 small villages and 60 from six larger villages. Children were allocated zinc or placebo in blocks of 30 (15 zinc, 15 placebo) by computer generated randomly permutated codes (prepared by the World Health Organization). We excluded children with serious underlying illness, and we excluded from the final analysis those who were absent from the study area for more than 14 consecutive days. Assuming a mean of one malaria episode per child per season and allowing for 20% loss to follow up, we used a sample size of 720 children to detect a 20% reduction in episodes of falciparum malaria with 90% power ($\alpha = 0.05$).

The children were given 12.5 mg (half a 25 mg tablet) zinc sulphate (Biolectra Zinc, Hermes Arzneimittel, Munich) or placebo daily (except Sundays) for six months. This dose has been recommended by the WHO and has been used successfully in randomised controlled trials in children in developing countries.[9-23] The tablets were identical in appearance and taste. They were stored in waterproof plastic tubes labelled with the child's identification number. Fieldworkers based in the villages provided the tablets and were also trained to take finger prick blood samples and to prepare blood films. They were visited twice weekly by supervisors who checked their work, collected completed forms and blood slides, and regularly reported to the study physician based in Nouna (AB). The study supervisors performed random checks of the fieldwork.

The children were seen daily, except for Sundays, by their fieldworker, who took their axillary temperature with an electronic thermometer (Digital Classic, Hartmann, Germany) and filled in a structured questionnaire based on the parents' reported morbidity symptoms of their child, visits to the healthcare providers, and any Western or traditional treatments received. If temperatures were 37.5°C or higher, blood samples were taken and thick and thin blood films prepared. If children were sick during the visits the parents were advised to take them to the local health centre.

Three cross sectional surveys were undertaken at baseline (June), mid-study (September), and the end of the study (December). The children were examined by the same physician (OM) during visits. Data on personal characteristics and risk factors (age, sex, ethnicity, use of mosquito nets), clinical data (history, symptoms, temperature, spleen size by Hackett grade, weight, height or length, mid-arm circumference), and parasitological data (thin and thick blood films) were collected from all the children, whereas packed cell volumes and serum zinc concentrations were measured only in random subsamples of 100 children.

Laboratory procedures
Blood was usually taken by finger prick, and the packed cell volume was measured in the field with a portable microhaematocrit centrifuge (Compur Microspin, Bayer Diagnostics, Germany). Blood films were kept in closed slide boxes until transportation to Nouna (two or three times a week during longitudinal follow up and daily during cross sectional surveys). They were stained with Giemsa at the Nouna hospital laboratory and transported to the Centre National de Recherche et de Formation sur le Paludisme in Ouagadougou for reading. The films were examined by two laboratory technicians and checked by a third investigator in cases of discrepancy. Blood films were analysed for the species specific parasite density per microlitre by counting against 500 white blood cells and multiplying by 16 (assuming 8000 white blood cells per microlitre of blood). If no parasites were seen in 400 fields on the thick film a negative result was declared. A 10% random sample of blood films was re-examined at the laboratory of the Heidelberg School of Tropical Medicine, showing an overall 97% concordance for *Plasmodium falciparum* parasitaemia. Venous blood was kept in a cold box until centrifugation on the same day in Nouna. Serum samples were stored at −20°C until zinc determination at the Heidelberg University laboratory by flame atomic absorption spectrometry (Perkin-Elmer 1100 B, Germany).

Statistical analysis
Data forms were checked by supervisors before computer entry (version 97, Microsoft Access) at the Centre de Recherche en Santé de Nouna. Parasitological data were entered into EpiInfo (version 6.0) at the Centre National de Recherche et de Formation sur le Paludisme, and the data were transferred to the Centre de Recherche en Santé de Nouna. All data were checked for range and consistency, and all parasitological data and data from cross sectional surveys were double entered. Any differences were resolved by checking against the original case record forms. The randomisation code was broken after the database was closed. Analysis was by intention to treat.

The primary outcome was the incidence of clinical episodes of falciparum malaria (in the presence or absence of *P malariae* or *P ovale*). An episode was defined as an axillary temperature of 37.5°C or higher with at least 5000 parasites/µl and no other obvious causes for the fever. This is similar to the case definition used in studies from the Gambia.[27] Additional definitions of fever and any parasite count and a parasite count of 100 000/µl or more were also applied as they represent traditional case definitions for mild and heavy infections.

Secondary outcomes were the duration and severity of falciparum malaria episodes, the prevalence of other causes of morbidity, and all cause mortality. Diarrhoea, fever, and cough were calculated by the number of child days of the respective disease divided by the total number of days of observation. We also investigated the mean species specific prevalences and densities of malaria parasites, mean packed cell volume, mean spleen grade, and mean values for anthropometric measurements during follow up visits for the cross sectional surveys.

The relative risk of falciparum malaria in children supplemented with zinc was calculated as the ratio of incidence densities between the zinc and placebo groups. We defined incidence densities as the number of *P falciparum* episodes divided by the number of days of observation. Relative risks, 95% confidence intervals, and P values were calculated. To exclude recrudescent malaria episodes, the individual observation time was defined as the time interval from the first to last day of observation minus 20 days for each defined episode. In a Poisson regression model we modelled the individual number of malaria episodes as a function of treatment with and without adjustment for covariates (age, weight, and height at start of study; sex; ethnic group). In addition, we analysed the effect of treatment on mortality with a proportional hazards regression model both with and without adjustment for covariates. We performed χ^2 analysis to test differences in distributions and t tests to compare arithmetic means. All analyses were done with SAS (version 6.12).

Ethical aspects

We received ethical approval for our study from the ethical committee of the Heidelberg University Medical School and the Ministry of Health in Burkina Faso. The trial was explained to the Nouna health district authorities, the villagers, and the head of each participating compound. Oral consent was obtained from the parents and carers of the children before enrolment. Sick children seen during surveys or visits by the supervisors were treated in the village or referred to Nouna hospital free of charge.

Results

Of 713 eligible children (one village had only 23 children of the required age group), 709 were enrolled and randomised to either zinc (n=356) or placebo (n=353). The children were not treated for 4349 days in total owing to absence, an average of 6.3 days per child (2163 zinc, 2186 placebo). Overall, 661 of 685 children (96%) were examined during the cross sectional surveys (figure).

Table 1 shows the characteristics of the children at baseline in June. The two groups were similar, except for the children being slightly older in the zinc group (18.7 v 17.5 months, P=0.03). At baseline 26% of the children were aged 6-12 months, 27% were 13-18 months, 26% were 19-24 months, and 21% were 25-31 months.

The prevalence of malnutrition was high at baseline (table 2), with 36.3% of children below −2 z score for height for age (stunting) and 24.6% below the −2 z score for weight for height (wasting). The effects of zinc on anthropometric measurements will be published elsewhere.

Serum zinc values paired for June and September were available for 81 children (41 zinc, 40 placebo; table 2). Mean zinc concentrations at baseline were 11.7 µmol/l, with no differences between the two groups, and 72% of the children were zinc deficient according to the reference laboratory's threshold of 13.0 µmol/l. After three months (mid-study survey), children in the zinc group had significantly higher serum zinc concentrations than children in the placebo group (15.3 v 12.4 µmol/l, P=0.005), and the proportion of zinc deficient children significantly declined in the zinc group but not in the placebo group (11/41 v 28/40, P=0.0001).

Spleen enlargement (Hackett score >1) was common at baseline and increased significantly until the end of the study (87% in zinc group v 98% in placebo group, P=0.001; table 2). At the height of the rainy season (September) a quarter of the children reportedly slept under an untreated mosquito net the night before their visit, with no significant differences between the zinc and placebo groups (24% v 27%). Parasitological results were available for 511 of 661

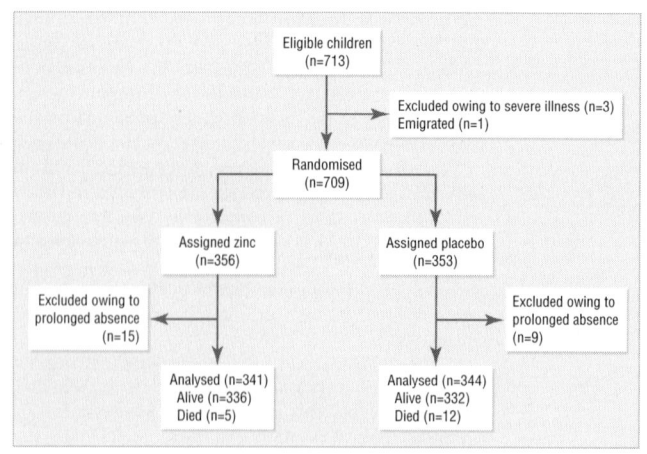

Trial profile

(77%) and 615 of 661 (93%) children at baseline and at the end of the study, respectively (table 2). Overall, P falciparum was the most common parasite (99%), and most of the children who had P malariae (6%) and P ovale (10%) also had P falciparum. The prevalence of falciparum malaria (1.4% in zinc group v 6.2% in placebo group, P=0.001) and of P falciparum, P malariae, and P ovale parasitaemia (62.8% v 89.6%, P=0.001; 4.2% v 13.2%, P=0.001; 0.6% v 20.2%, P=0.001), and the mean density of P falciparum (2909 v 7954, P=0.001) increased significantly over the study. Mean packed cell volume values, measured in 70 children (39 zinc, 31 placebo) at baseline and at follow up, significantly decreased from 32.0 to 29.1 over the study period (P=0.001). No differences were found in clinical or parasitological characteristics between the two groups, either at mid-study (data not shown) or at the end of the study.

Table 3 shows the results for morbidity at follow up in the longitudinal study. Parasitological results were available for 2065 of 2324 (89%) febrile episodes. Over the six months of the study, the mean number of episodes of falciparum malaria a month was 0.38 (parasite density ≥1/µl), 0.28 (≥5.000/µl), and 0.02 (≥100 000/µl), with no differences between the zinc and placebo groups at any of the respective three parasite thresholds (relative risk 0.99, 95% confidence interval 0.89 to 1.11, P=0.94; 0.98, 0.86 to 1.11, P=0.77; 1.00, 0.64 to 1.60, P=0.91). This finding remained the same after analysis of the effects of zinc on the incidence of P falciparum by age group (data not shown). No difference was found between the two

Table 1 Characteristics of participants at baseline. Values are numbers (percentages) unless stated otherwise

	Baseline	
	Zinc group (n=332)	Placebo group (n=329)
Mean (range) age (months)	18.7 (6-31)	17.5 (6-31)
Boys	165 (50)	160 (49)
Ethnic group:		
Marka	155 (47)	149 (45)
Mossi	63 (19)	66 (20)
Bwaba	66 (20)	64 (20)
Peulh	35 (11)	42 (13)
Others	13 (4)	8 (2)

Papers

Table 2 Clinical and parasitological data at baseline and end of study for cross sectional survey. Values are means (ranges) unless stated otherwise

	Baseline		End of study	
	Zinc group (n=332)	Placebo group (n=329)	Zinc group (n=334)	Placebo group (n=327)
Clinical characteristics				
Weight (kg)	8.8 (4.9-15.0)	8.6 (3.4-15.0)	9.9 (5.9-16.1)	9.6 (3.9-16.1)
Height (cm)	76.1 (62-94)	75.4 (56-99)	81.0 (65-97)	80.2 (58-99)
No (%) with enlarged spleen*	272 (87)	275 (87)	300 (97)	288 (98)
No (%) with temperature ≥37.5°C*	27 (8.1)	16 (4.9)	30 (9.0)	32 (9.8)
No (%) with clinical malaria†	4 (1.6)	3 (1.2)	18 (5.7)	20 (6.7)
Packed cell volume (%)‡	32.6 (26-44)	31.7 (24-38)	28.6 (18-38)	29.7 (22-36)
Parasitological characteristics				
No (%) with *Plasmodium falciparum* density:				
≥1/µl	154 (60.1)	169 (65.5)	287 (90.3)	264 (88.9)
≥5000/µl	20 (7.9)	31 (12.0)	128 (40.3)	122 (41.1)
≥100 000/µl	0 (0)	0 (0)	1 (0.3)	3 (1.0)
Mean *P falciparum* density/µl	2754	3090	7602	8333
No (%) with *P malariae* density ≥1/µl	10 (4.0)	11 (4.3)	46 (14.5)	35 (11.8)
Mean *P malariae* density/µl	914	219	674	907
No (%) with *P ovale* density ≥1/µl	1 (0.4)	2 (0.8)	68 (21.4)	57 (19.2)
Mean *P ovale* density/µl	16	345	348	498
Zinc measurement§				
Serum zinc (mmol/l)	11.5 (5.2-27.2)	11.9 (5.6-20.5)	15.3 (4.8-30.2)	12.4 (5.0-27.4)

*Individuals with missing data were excluded from denominator.
†Temperature ≥ 37.5°C, ≥5000 parasites/µl.
‡In paired subsample of 70 children (39 zinc, 31 placebo) at baseline and end of study.
§In paired subsample of 81 children (41 zinc, 40 placebo) at baseline and mid-study.

groups for mean temperature (38.3°C in zinc group v 38.3°C in placebo group) and mean parasite density (44 529 v 44 316) during episodes of falciparum malaria (≥37.5°C with ≥5000 parasites/µl).

Table 3 also shows the effects of zinc supplementation on the number of reported days with other morbidity outcomes. No differences were found in the number of days with fever (relative risk 1.01, 0.95 to 1.07, P=0.62) and the number of days with cough (1.05, 0.97 to 1.15, P=0.22) between the two groups, but the number of days with diarrhoea was significantly lower in the zinc group (0.87, 0.79 to 0.95, P=0.002).

More children in the placebo group than zinc group died during the study (12 v 5), but this difference did not reach significance. The estimated relative risk in the survival analysis with a proportional hazards model was 0.41 (0.15 to 1.19, P=0.1). The relative risk did not change appreciably (0.47) when covariates were adjusted for.

Discussion

We found no evidence for zinc supplementation being effective against falciparum malaria in a population of west African children with a high prevalence of malnutrition and zinc deficiency. Recipients of zinc were no different for number of episodes of falciparum malaria or any other malariometric measurement than the recipients of placebo. This was so for all age groups and was consistently seen during both the longitudinal study and the cross sectional surveys.

Our study was a large randomised controlled trial, which had reasonable power to detect a moderate efficacy of the intervention. Case detection was intense and sustained, loss to follow up was small, and individual randomisation made systematic errors unlikely. Dilution of the intervention through fieldworkers mixing up the allocation of zinc or placebo also seems unlikely owing to training and supervision. Moreover, the intervention was followed by a significant increase in serum zinc concentration in the zinc group, whereas zinc concentration remained unchanged in the placebo group.

Our results do not confirm the findings of two community based studies on zinc supplementation and malaria.[23][24] One study, on children aged 7-28 months in the Gambia, showed 32% fewer clinical epi-

Table 3 Effect of zinc supplementation on febrile episodes of falciparum malaria and other causes of morbidity

Morbidity	Zinc group	Placebo group	Relative risk (95% CI)†
Febrile episodes*	(No of children)		
No of episodes with parasite density ≥1/µl:			
0	26	44	
1	116	98	
2	128	115	0.99 (0.89 to 1.11)
3	51	69	
4	19	17	
5	1	1	
No of episodes with parasite density ≥5000/µl:			
0	69	78	
1	138	133	
2	104	92	0.98 (0.86 to 1.11)
3	24	30	
4	5	11	
5	1	0	
No of episodes with parasite density ≥100 000/µl:			
0	306	310	
1	34	33	1.0 (0.64 to 1.6)
2	1	1	
Reported symptoms	(child days)		
Fever	2133	2095	1.01 (0.95 to 1.07)
Cough	1006	949	1.05 (0.97 to 1.15)
Diarrhoea	869	997	0.87 (0.79 to 0.95)‡

Observation time was 49 086 child days for zinc group and 49 021 child days for placebo group; for analysis of incidence of falciparum malaria, children were removed from numerator and denominator for 20 days after malaria episode.
*Temperature ≥37.5°C and specified parasite density.
†Based on Poisson regression model.
‡P=0.002.

> **What is already known on this topic**
>
> Zinc deficiency is common in infants in developing countries
>
> Zinc supplementation has been shown to reduce morbidity from infectious disease in such populations, particularly through reductions in morbidity from diarrhoea and respiratory infections
>
> Limited evidence exists for zinc supplementation being effective in reducing morbidity from malaria
>
> **What this study adds**
>
> Zinc supplementation has no effect on falciparum malaria in children in rural west Africa
>
> It is effective in reducing morbidity from diarrhoea and may help to reduce mortality from all causes

sodes of malaria in children given zinc compared with those given placebo after follow up over 15 months.[23] This was, however, a small study on 110 children matched for age and sex, zinc supplementation was given only twice weekly, no information was provided on the methods for diagnosis of malaria, and the effects on malaria were only of borderline significance. The other study looked at the effects of zinc supplementation on morbidity from malaria in 274 children aged 6-60 months in Papua New Guinea.[24] The children were randomly assigned to 10 mg zinc gluconate or placebo for six days a week for 10 months. The trial reported a 30-35% reduction in attendances to a health centre due to malaria in those children receiving zinc compared with those receiving placebo.

Even mild zinc deficiency can impair multiple mediators of host immunity.[8] Some evidence shows that zinc deficiency predominantly affects the cell mediated immune system.[28-32] In this context, our inability to show an effect of zinc supplementation on morbidity from malaria may provide evidence for cell mediated immunity being less important in malaria in humans. Furthermore, such a hypothesis would be supported by the overwhelming evidence for malaria not behaving as an opportunistic infection in African children with HIV or AIDS.[33-35]

Overall, 17 of the 709 (2.4%) children died during the study, which confirms the unacceptably high level of childhood mortality from malaria in rural African regions.[1-3] We found a tendency for zinc to be protective against all cause mortality, which could be a real finding given the known effects of zinc on gastro-intestinal and respiratory infections.[9-22] This is supported by our finding of a significantly lower prevalence of diarrhoea in children given zinc rather than placebo. Our study was not designed to look in detail at the effects of zinc on other causes of morbidity, and such findings must be interpreted with caution.

We thank Walter Fiehn of Heidelberg Medical School for determining the serum zinc values, the team of the Heidelberg Tropical Institute for quality control of the malaria slides, Brian Greenwood for his advice during the design and implementation of the study, the staff of the Centre de Recherche en Santé de Nouna, and the children and their parents.

Contributors: OM was responsible for the overall coordination of the study and contributed to the study design, enrolment and examination of the children, field supervision, and data analysis; he will act as guarantor for the paper. HB was responsible for data analysis and contributed to the study coordination. ABvZ was responsible for the coordination and supervision of the fieldwork and contributed to the analysis and interpretation of the data. YY was responsible for the management of the data in Nouna and contributed to the design of the study. DAD contributed to the design, field supervision, and laboratory supervision of the study. ATK contributed to the coordination, field supervision, and analysis and interpretation of the data. AG and BK contributed to the design and coordination of the study. MG contributed to the study design and coordination and data analysis. All authors contributed to the writing of the paper.

Funding: The World Health Organization and the Deutsche Forschungsgemeinschaft (SFB 544, control of tropical infectious diseases).

Competing interests: None declared.

1. World Health Organization. World malaria situation in 1994. *Wkly Epidemiol Rec* 1997;72:269-92.
2. Greenwood B, Bradley A, Greenwood A, Byass P, Jammeh K, Marsh K, et al. Mortality and morbidity from malaria among children in a rural area of the Gambia, West Africa. *Trans R Soc Trop Med Hyg* 1987;81:478-86.
3. Snow RW, Craig M, Deichmann U, Marsh K. Estimating mortality, morbidity and disability due to malaria among Africa's non-pregnant population. *Bull WHO* 1999;77:624-40.
4. Kilian A, Langi P, Talisuna A, Kabagambe G. Rainfall pattern, El Nino and malaria in Uganda. *Trans R Soc Trop Med Hyg* 1999;93:22-3.
5. Marsh K. Malaria disaster in Africa. *Lancet* 1998;352:924.
6. Müller O, Garenne M. Childhood mortality in Africa. *Lancet* 1999;353:673.
7. Gibson RS, Ferguson EL. Assessment of dietary zinc in a population. *Am J Clin Nutr* 1998;68:S430-4.
8. Shankar AH, Prasad AS. Zinc and immune function: the biological basis of altered resistance to infection. *Am J Clin Nutr* 1998;68:S447-63.
9. Sachdev HPS, Mittal NK, Mittal SK, Yadav HS. A controlled trial on utility of oral zinc supplementation in acute dehydrating diarrhea in infants. *J Pediatr Gastroenterol Nutr* 1988;7:877-81.
10. Sachdev HPS, Mittal NK, Yadav HS. Oral zinc supplementation in persistent diarrhea in infants. *Ann Trop Paediatr* 1990;10:63-9.
11. Sazawal S, Black R, Bhan MK, Bhandari N, Sinha A, Jalla S. Zinc supplementation in young children with acute diarrhea in India. *N Engl J Med* 1995;333:839-44.
12. Sazawal S, Black R, Bhan MK, Jalla S, Bhandari N, Sinha A, et al. Zinc supplementation reduces the incidence of persistent diarrhea and dysentery among low socioeconomic children in India. *J Nutr* 1996;126:443-50.
13. Sazawal S, Black R, Bahn MK, Jalla S, Sinha A, Bhandari N. Efficacy of zinc supplementation in reducing the incidence and prevalence of acute diarrhea—a community based, double blind, controlled trial. *Am J Clin Nutr* 1997;66:413-8.
14. Ruel MT, Rivera JA, Santiazo MC, Lönnerdal B, Brown KH. Impact of zinc supplementation on morbidity from diarrhea and respiratory infections among Guatemalan children. *Pediatrics* 1997;99:808-13.
15. Penny ME, Peerson JM, Marin RM, Duran A, Lanata CF, Lönnerdal B, et al. Randomized, community based trial of the effect of zinc supplementation, with and without other micronutrients, on the duration of persistent childhood diarrhea in Lima, Peru. *J Pediatr* 1999;135:208-17.
16. Faruque ASG, Mahalanabis D, Haque SS, Fuchs GJ, Habte D. Double-blind, randomized, controlled trial of zinc or vitamin A supplementation in young children with acute diarrhea. *Acta Paediatr* 1999;88:154-60.
17. Roy SK, Tomkins AM, Haider R, Akramuzzaman SM, Behrens RH, Mahalanabis D. Impact of zinc supplementation on subsequent growth and morbidity in Bangladeshi children with acute diarrhea. *Eur J Clin Nutr* 1999;53:529-34.
18. Sazawal S, Black RE, Jalla S, Mazumdar S, Sinha A, Bhan MK. Zinc supplementation reduces the incidence of acute lower respiratory infections in infants and preschool children: a double-blind, controlled trial. *Pediatrics* 1998;102:1-5.
19. Ninh NX, Thissen JP, Collette L, Gerard GG, Khoi HH, Ketelslegers JM. Zinc supplementation increases growth and circulating insulin-like growth factor I in growth-retarded Vietnamese children. *Am J Clin Nutr* 1996;63:514-9.
20. Rosado JL, Lopez P, Munoz E, Martinez H, Allen LH. Zinc supplementation reduced morbidity, but neither zinc nor iron supplementation affected growth or body composition of Mexican preschoolers. *Am J Clin Nutr* 1997;65:13-9.
21. Umeta M, West CE, Haidar J, Deurenberg P, Hautvast JGAJ. Zinc supplementation and stunted infants in Ethiopia: a randomised controlled trial. *Lancet* 2000;355:2021-6.
22. Bhurta ZA, Black RE, Brown KH, Gardner JM, Gore S, Hidayat A, et al of the Zinc Investigators' Collaborative Group. Prevention of diarrhea and pneumonia by zinc supplementation in children in developing countries: pooled analysis of randomized controlled trials. *J Pediatr* 1999;135:689-97.
23. Bates CJ, Evans PH, Dardenne M, Prentice A, Lunn PG, Northrop-Clewes CA, et al. A trial of zinc supplementation in young rural Gambian children. *Br J Nutr* 1993;69:243-55.

24 Shankar AH, Genton B, Tamja S, Arnold S, Wu L, Baisor M, et al. Zinc supplementation can reduce malaria-related morbidity in preschool children [abstract]. *Am J Trop Med Hyg* 1997;57:249.
25 Sauerborn R, Nougtara A, Diesfeld HJ, eds. *Les couts economiques de la maladie pour les menages au milieu rural du Burkina Faso*. Frankfurt: Peter Lang Verlag, 1996.
26 Benzler J, Sauerborn R. Rapid risk household screening by neonatal arm circumference: results from a cohort study in rural Burkina Faso. *Trop Med Int Health* 1999;3:962-74.
27 D'Alessandro U, Olaleye BO, McGuire W, Langerock P, Bennett S, Aikins MK, et al. Mortality and morbidity from malaria in Gambian children after introduction of an impregnated bednet programme. *Lancet* 1995;345:479-83.
28 Pekareh RS, Sandstead HH, Jacob RA, Barcome DF. Abnormal cellular immune responses during acquired zinc deficiency. *Am J Clin Nutr* 1979;32:1466-71.
29 Chandra RK, Au B. Single nutrient deficiency and cell-mediated immune responses, I. Zinc. *Am J Clin Nutr* 1980;33:736-8.
30 Beisel WR. Single nutritients and immunity. *Am J Clin Nutr* 1982;35:S417-68.
31 Chandra RK. 1990 McCollum award lecture. Nutrition and immunity: lessons from the past and new insights into the future. *Am J Clin Nutr* 1991;53:1087-101.
32 Beck FWJ, Prasad AS, Kaplan J, Fitzgerald JT, Brewer GJ. Changes in cytokine production and T cell subpopulations in experimentally induced zinc-deficient humans. *Am J Physiol* 1997;272:E1002-7.
33 Müller O, Moser R. The clinical and parasitological presentation of falciparum malaria in Uganda is unaffected by HIV infection. *Trans R Soc Trop Med Hyg* 1990;84:336-8.
34 Butcher GA. HIV and malaria: a lesson in immunology? *Parasitol Today* 1992;8:307-11.
35 Chandramohan D, Greenwood BM. Is there an interaction between human immunodeficiency virus and Plasmodium falciparum? *Int J Epidemiol* 1998;27:296-301.

(Accepted 22 March 2001)

2.3 Evaluation of a prototype long-lasting insecticide-treated mosquito net under field conditions in rural Burkina Faso

MÜLLER O, IDO K, TRAORÉ C

Trans R Soc Trop Med Hyg. 2002; 96 (5): 483-4

Reprinted with permission from the Royal Society of Tropical Medicine and Hygiene, London

Short Report

Evaluation of a prototype long-lasting insecticide-treated mosquito net under field conditions in rural Burkina Faso

O. Müller[1]*, K. Ido[2] and C. Traoré[2] [1]*Department of Tropical Hygiene and Public Health, Ruprecht-Karls-University, INF 324, 69120 Heidelberg, Germany;* [2]*Centre de Recherche en Santé de Nouna, Burkina Faso*

Abstract
Insecticide measurements and standard World Health Organization bioassays on random samples of new unwashed, traditionally washed and up to 18 months field-used 'long-lasting' deltamethrin treated mosquito nets demonstrated a rapid reduction of efficacy under field conditions. The technology of 'long-lasting' insecticide-treatment needs much improvement.

Keywords: malaria, insecticide-treated mosquito nets, Burkina Faso

Introduction
The efficacy of insecticide-treated mosquito nets (ITNs) in reducing malaria morbidity and mortality has been repeatedly demonstrated in sub-Saharan Africa (LENGELER, 1998). However, beside the obvious problems with achieving good ITN coverage and compliance, regular re-treatment remains a major challenge to community effectiveness when householders are asked to pay for the insecticide (LINES, 1996; ARMSTRONG-SCHELLENBERG et al., 1999).

Long-lasting insecticide-treatment, ideally lasting the entire lifetime of a mosquito net, is considered a possible solution to this problem. PermaNet™, a product of the Vestergaard Frandsen Group (Kolding, Denmark), is marketed as a prototype of a long-lasting ITN. Deltamethrin (target dose 56 mg/m²) is bound to the fibre of this mosquito net in a way which is claimed to delay the loss of the insecticide over time. According to the manufacturer, the product has been tested by an independent reference laboratory in Europe, where it remained effective even after being washed 21 times (www.vestergaard-frandsen.dk). We report our results from an 18-months field evaluation of PermaNets™ in Burkina Faso.

Methods
This study forms part of a large ITN intervention trial in the study area of the Nouna Health Research Centre (CRSN) in north-western Burkina Faso, an area highly endemic for malaria (MÜLLER et al., 2001). PermaNets™ (family size, rectangular, green, 100 denier) are used for protection of the study children.

The PermaNet™ evaluation was undertaken in December 2001. Deltamethrin concentration was measured on random samples of new unwashed nets, nets which had been washed once or twice by traditional methods and nets used in villages and collected after up to 18 months. Deltamethrin was determined using xylene extraction and capillary gas chromatography with [63]Ni electron capture detection (Department de Phytopharmacie, Ministère des Classes Moyennes et de l'Agriculture, Belgium). ITN efficacy was measured by standard bioassays with World Health Organization

*Author for correspondence; phone +49 6221 565035, fax +49 6221 565039, e-mail olaf.mueller@urz.uni-heidelberg.de

Table. Deltamethrin concentration and mosquito mortality (24 h after 3 min exposure) on new and field-used PermaNets™, evaluated in December 2001 in rural Burkina Faso

	New mosquito nets			Field-used mosquito nets		
	Not washed	1 wash	2 washes	6 months	12 months	18 months
Number of nets	6	3	3	8	11	5
Mean deltamethrin concentration on net (mg/m²)[a]	47.1 (22.5–88.2)	38.6 (20.4–49.2)	20.1 (13.9–25.4)	24.1 (2.4–103.6)	3.7 (0.4–12.2)	1.6 (0.7–3.5)
Mean number of washes[a]	0	1	2	0.9 (0–2)	2.1 (0–4)	5.8 (2–10)
Number of nets	10			7	9	2
Mosquito mortality	261/269			133/158	96/177	2/28
Percentage[a]	97 (88–100)			84 (41–100)	54 (0–93)	7 (7–8)
Mean number of washes[a]	0			1.1 (0–3)	1.9 (0–4)	3.0 (2–4)

[a]Range in parentheses.

cones, using progeny *Anopheles gambiae s.l.* collected from villages with the endpoint of mortality 24 h after 3 min exposure to the net. Wash frequency and perceived efficacy against mosquitoes were continuously evaluated in the study population through 2-weekly questionnaire surveys from mid-2000 onwards.

Results

Mean deltamethrin concentration was already much reduced after 2 washes of the PermaNet™. Deltamethrin concentration and mosquito mortality steadily declined over time during field use, and had reached unacceptably low levels after 12 months (Table).

Conclusions

PermaNets™, a prototype long-lasting ITN, do not provide sufficient long-term efficacy under field conditions. Possible explanations are specific environmental conditions (heat, dust, dirt), factors associated with traditional washing techniques, or the poor quality control of the manufacturing process.

Acknowledgements

The study was funded by the Deutsche Forschungsgemeinschaft (SFB 544, Control of Tropical Infectious Diseases).

References

Armstrong-Schellenberg, J., Abdulla, S., Minja, H., Nathan, R., Mukasa, O., Marchant, T., Mponda, H., Kikumbih, N., Lyimo, E., Manchester, T., Tanner, M. & Lengeler, C. (1999). KINET: a social marketing programme of treated nets and net treatment for malaria control in Tanzania, with evaluation of child health and long-term survival. *Transactions of the Royal Society of Tropical Medicine and Hygiene*, **93**, 225–231.

Lengeler, C. (1998). Insecticide treated bednets and curtains for malaria control (a Cochrane Review). In: *The Cochrane Library*, Issue 3. Oxford: Update Software (CD-ROM version).

Lines, J. (1996). Mosquito nets and insecticides for net treatment: a discussion of existing and potential distribution systems in Africa. *Tropical Medicine and International Health*, **1**, 616–632.

Müller, O., Becher, H., Baltussen van Zweeden, A., Ye, Y., Diallo, D. A., Konate, A. T., Gbangou, A., Kouyaté, B. & Garenne, M. (2001). Effect of zinc supplementation on malaria and other causes of morbidity among West African children: randomized double-blind placebo-controlled trial. *British Medical Journal*, **322**, 1567–1572.

Received 1 February 2002; revised 3 April 2002; accepted for publication 5 April 2002

2.4 Severe anaemia in west African children: malaria or malnutrition?

Müller O, Traoré C, Jahn A, Becher H

The Lancet. 2003; 361(9351): 86-7

Reprinted with permission from Elsevier.

Severe anaemia in west African children: malaria or malnutrition?

Sir—H Verhoef and colleagues (Sept 21, p 908)[1] show that intermittent administration of iron has a more pronounced effect on the haemoglobin status of Kenyan children than sulfadoxine-pyrimethamine.

We have done an analysis of risk factors for severe anaemia in a cohort of young children in rural Burkina Faso. The cohort consisted of 709 children aged 6–31 months, who were recruited for a randomised placebo-controlled trial on the effects of zinc supplementation on malaria morbidity.[2] Village-based morbidity surveillance took place over the main malaria transmission period in 1999 (June to December), supplemented by two cross-sectional clinical surveys which included anthropometric measurements. Malaria is holoendemic but highly seasonal in the area.

Anaemia status, defined by packed cell volume measurements (Compur Microspin, Bayer Diagnostics, Germany) during the December survey, was available for 544 (79%) of the 685 children successfully followed up. The mean packed cell volume was 29·2% (range 18–38), and 77 (14%) were defined as being severely anaemic (packed cell volume ≤24%). The mean SD scores for height-for-age (HAZ), weight-for-age (WAZ), and weight-for-height (WHZ) were −1·6, −2·0, and −1·2, respectively, in June; and −1·5, −2·0, and −1·3, respectively, in December.

We compared children with and without severe anaemia for the number of falciparum malaria episodes (fever plus ≥5·000 *Plasmodium falciparum* per μL) over the 6-month observation period, for the prevalence of falciparum malaria within 10 days before the December survey, and for their mean HAZ/WAZ/WHZ SD scores. In logistic regression analyses (adjusted for age and sex), anaemia was not associated with the frequency of malaria episodes, nor with malaria prevalence. However, it was significantly associated with malnutrition, defined as HAZ, WAZ, and WHZ of −2 or less (table).

These data contribute to the growing evidence for the importance of malnutrition in the development of anaemia in young children living in malaria-endemic areas.[3] Given the well known grave implications of malnutrition on morbidity and mortality, programmes with the aim of improving the health of young children in developing countries need to put much more emphasis on improving the overall nutritional situation of young children.[4,5] Finally, these findings also have implications for use of anaemia as an outcome in malaria control trials.

*Olaf Müller, Corneille Traoré, Albrecht Jahn, Heiko Becher

*Department of Tropical Hygiene and Public Health, Ruprecht-Karls-University, INF 324, 69124 Heidelberg, Germany (OM, AJ, HB); and Centre de Recherche en Santé de Nouna, Burkina Faso (CT)
(e-mail: Olaf.Mueller@urz.uni-heidelberg.de)

1 Verhoef H, West CE, Nzyuko SM, et al. Intermittent administration of iron and sulfadoxine-pyrimethamine to control anaemia in Kenyan children: a randomised controlled trial. *Lancet* 2002; **360:** 908–14.
2 Müller O, Becher H, Baltussen van Zweeden A, et al. Effect of zinc supplementation on malaria and other morbidity in west African children: randomised double blind placebo controlled trial. *BMJ* 2001; **322:** 1567–72.
3 Nussenblatt V, Semba RD. Micronutrient malnutrition and the pathogenesis of malarial anaemia. *Acta Tropica* 2002; **82:** 321–37.
4 Rice AL, Sacco L, Hyder A, Black RE. Malnutrition as an underlying cause of childhood deaths associated with infectious diseases in developing countries. *Bull World Health Organ* 2000; **78:** 1207–21.
5 Müller O, Jahn A, von Braun J. Micronutrient supplementation for malaria control—hype or hope? *Trop Med Int Health* 2002; **7:** 1–3.

	Children with severe anaemia (n=77)	Children without severe anaemia (n=467)	Odds ratio (95% CI)
Height-for-age	−1·99 (1·40)	−1·39 (1·36)	0·72* (0·60–0·86)
Weight-for-age	−2·44 (1·13)	−1·76 (1·12)	0·58* (0·46–0·73)
Weight-for-height	−1·62 (0·79)	−1·21 (0·89)	0·58* (0·43–0·78)
Number of falciparum malaria episodes in previous 6 months	1·29 (1·04)	1·31 (0·97)	0·92† (0·71–1·18)
Falciparum malaria ≤10 days before haemoglobin measurement (yes/no)	2/75	32/435	0·32† (0·07–1·39)

Data are mean (SD) unless otherwise stated. *For continuous anthropometric score, odds ratio refers to increase of 1, adjusted for sex and age. †Adjusted for sex, age, and weight-for-age.

Association between severe anaemia, falciparum malaria, and malnutrition in young west African children

2.5 Clinical efficacy of chloroquine in young children with uncomplicated falciparum malaria – a community-based study in rural Burkina Faso

Müller O, Traoré C, Kouyaté B

Trop Med Int Health. 2003 Mar; 8(3): 202-3

Reprinted with permission from Blackwell Publishers Ltd.

Short communication: Clinical efficacy of chloroquine in young children with uncomplicated falciparum malaria – a community-based study in rural Burkina Faso

Olaf Müller[1], Corneille Traoré[2] and Bocar Kouyaté[2]

1 Department of Tropical Hygiene and Public Health of the Ruprecht-Karls-University Heidelberg, Heidelberg, Germany
2 Centre de Recherche en Santé de Nouna, Nouna, Burkina Faso

Summary We report on a 14-day study on the efficacy of chloroquine for treating uncomplicated falciparum malaria in young children of a malaria holoendemic area in rural Burkina Faso. In this community-based study, the overall treatment failure rate was 12/120 (10%), with no differences between villages. This supports the evidence for a still sufficient efficacy of chloroquine in north-western Burkina Faso.

keywords malaria, chloroquine, resistance, Africa, Burkina Faso

Introduction

Chloroquine has been the mainstay for malaria control in sub-Saharan Africa (SSA), but the emergence of chloroquine-resistant *Plasmodium falciparum* has put into question the efficacy of this well-known drug (Trape 2001). In fact, increasing resistance has already convinced several SSA countries to replace chloroquine as first line drug for treatment and prophylaxis (Nuwaha 2001). It has been suggested to change to a new first-line drug when the prevalence of RIII parasitological resistance has reached the range of 14–31%, or when the mean duration of clinical response decreases to <14 days (Sudre *et al.* 1992; Bloland *et al.* 1993). We report data on the efficacy of chloroquine treatment in young children of a rural area of Burkina Faso with high *P. falciparum* transmission intensity.

Methods

The study was nested into an ongoing cohort study on the long-term effects of insecticide-treated mosquito nets (ITN) in young children from six villages of Nouna Health District in north-western Burkina Faso. These villages belong to the research zone of the Centre de Recherche en Santé de Nouna (CRSN), consisting of Nouna town and 41 of the surrounding villages. They were purposely selected to represent the rural study population in its sociocultural, demographic and geographical diversity. The Nouna area is a dry orchard savanna, populated mainly by subsistence farmers of different ethnic groups.

Cohort children were visited daily by village-based field staff for temperature measurement and recording of relevant data during illness episodes. In case of fever, blood films were taken and the films were examined by two experienced microscopists of the Nouna Health Research Centre. Malaria is holoendemic but highly seasonal in the area (Müller *et al.* 2001). Approval for the study was granted by the Ethical Committee of the Heidelberg University Medical School and the Ministry of Health in Burkina Faso.

Cohort children were consecutively enrolled from July until October 2001 if they fulfilled the following inclusion criteria: age ≥6 months, falciparum malaria (≥37.5 °C axillary temperature + ≥5.000 *P. falciparum* parasites per microlitre in the absence of another obvious fever cause), absence of antimalarial treatment during past 2 weeks, informed oral consent. All study children received fully supervised treatment with 25 mg/kg bodyweight of chloroquine (drugs taken from the essential drug stock of Nouna Health District) over 3 days. Enrolled children were followed clinically over a 14-day period, and a systematic blood slide was taken on days 7–10. For the evaluation of treatment outcome, we used a modified definition of the WHO protocol for assessment of therapeutic efficacy of antimalarial drugs in areas with intense transmission (WHO 1996). We defined early treatment failure (ETF) as development of severe malaria on days 1–3 or axillary temperature ≥ 37.5 °C on day 3 in the presence of parasitaemia on days 7–10, and late treatment failure (LTF) as development of severe malaria and/or axillary temperature ≥37.5 °C on days 4–14 in the presence of parasitaemia on days 7–10 without previously meeting the criteria of ETF.

Table 1 Parasitological and clinical failure rates of chloroquine treatment in young children with uncomplicated falciparum malaria (fever + ≥5000 parasites/µl) in six villages of rural Burkina Faso, July–October 2001

Village	Parasitological failure	Clinical failure
Koro*	8/25	5/25
Seriba	4/16	2/16
Dionkongo	7/18	2/18
Bourasso*	5/27	1/27
Sikoro	7/27	2/27
Kodougou	1/7	0/7
Total	32/120 (27%)	12/120 (10%)

* Village with a health centre.

Results

A total of 120 children were recruited and there was no loss to follow-up. The mean age was 10.4 months (range 6–15), and the male/female ratio was 0.71. Mean temperature on day 0 was 38.7 (range 37.5–40.7), and mean *P. falciparum* density was 38 400 (range 5500–287 000).

On days 7–10, 32/120 (27%, 95% confidence interval 19–35%) children were still parasitaemic (mean *P. falciparum* density 3620, range 50–23 000). The overall treatment failure rate was 12 of 120 (10%, 95% confidence interval 5–15%), with six of 120 (5%) being ETF and six of 120 (5%) being LTF. None of the children developed severe malaria, and there were no differences in parasitological and clinical failure rates between villages (Table 1).

Discussion

After standard treatment with chloroquine, we found a parasitological failure rate of 27% and a clinical failure rate of 10% in children aged 6–15 months. This significant discrepancy supports the evidence for a rapid development of immunity in young children exposed to intense malaria transmission (WHO 1996).

The first cases of *in vitro* and *in vivo* chloroquine resistance in Burkina Faso were seen in 1983 and 1988, respectively, and reported clinical failure rates after use of chloroquine for treatment of uncomplicated malaria in children were around 5% in the early 1990s (Guigemdé *et al.* 1994). Our finding of a low chloroquine clinical failure rate in a representative group of young children from rural Burkina Faso provides further evidence for chloroquine remaining sufficiently effective after many years of resistance occurence in parts of West Africa (Guigemdé *et al.* 1994; Brasseur *et al.* 1999; Plowe *et al.* 2001).

Acknowledgements

The study was funded by the Deutsche Forschungsgemeinschaft (SFB 544, Control of Tropical Infectious Diseases).

References

Bloland P, Lackritz E, Kazembe P, Were JBO, Steketee R & Campbell CC (1993) Beyond chloroquine: implications of drug resistance for evaluating malaria therapy efficacy and treatment policy in Africa. *Journal of Infectious Diseases* 167, 932–937.

Brasseur P, Guigemdé R, Diallo S *et al.* (1999) Amodiaquine remains effective for treating malaria in West and Central Africa. *Transactions of the Royal Society of Tropical Medicine and Hygiene* 93, 645–650.

Guigemdé TR, Aoba A, Ouedraogo JB & Lamizana L (1994) Ten-year surveillance of drug-resistant malaria in Burkina Faso (1982–1991). *American Journal of Tropical Medicine and Hygiene* 50, 699–704.

Müller O, Becher H, Baltussen A *et al.* (2001) Effect of zinc supplementation on malaria morbidity among West African children: a randomized double-blind placebo-controlled trial. *British Medical Journal* 322, 1567–1572.

Nuwaha F (2001) The challenge of chloroquine resistant malaria in sub-Saharan Africa. *Health Policy and Planning* 16, 1–12.

Plowe CV, Doumbo OK, Djimde A *et al.* (2001) Chloroquine treatment of uncomplicated *Plasmodium falciparum* malaria in Mali: parasitologic resistance versus therapeutic efficacy. *American Journal of Tropical Medicine and Hygiene* 64, 242–246.

Sudre P, Breman JG, McFarland D, Koplan JP (1992) Treatment of chloroquine-resistant malaria in African children: a cost-effectiveness analysis. *International Journal of Epidemiology*, 21, 146–154.

Trape J (2001) The public health impact of chloroquine resistance in Africa. *American Journal of Tropical Medicine and Hygiene* 64 (Suppl.), 12–17.

WHO (1996) *Assessment of Therapeutic Efficacy of Antimalarial Drugs for Uncomplicated Falciparum Malaria in Areas with Intense Transmission.* World Health Organization, Geneva, WHO/MAL/96.1077.

Authors

Dr Bocar Kouyaté, Centre de Recherche en Santé de Nouna, BP34, Nouna, Burkina Faso. E-mail: bocar.crsn@fasonet.bf

Dr Olaf Müller, Department of Tropical Hygiene and Public Health, Ruprecht-Karls-University, INF 324, 69120 Heidelberg, Germany. E-mail: olaf.mueller@urz.uni-heidelberg.de (corresponding author).

Dr Corneille Traoré, Centre de Recherche en Santé de Nouna, BP34, Nouna, Burkina Faso. E-mail: corneille@fasonet.bf

2.6 The association between protein-energy malnutrition, malaria morbidity and all-cause mortality in West African children

MÜLLER O, GARENNE M, KOUYATÉ B, BECHER H

Trop Med Int Health. 2003 Jun; 8(6): 507-11

Reprinted with permission from Blackwell Publishers Ltd.

The association between protein–energy malnutrition, malaria morbidity and all-cause mortality in West African children

Olaf Müller[1], Michel Garenne[2], Bocar Kouyaté[3] and Heiko Becher[1]

1 Department of Tropical Hygiene and Public Health, Ruprecht-Karls-University, Heidelberg, Germany
2 Institut Pasteur, Paris, France
3 Centre de Recherche en Santé de Nouna, Burkina

Summary Both malaria and protein–energy malnutrition (PEM) are highly prevalent in young children of sub-Saharan Africa, and the association between PEM and malaria continues to be discussed controversially. We analysed the association between PEM, malaria morbidity and all-cause mortality in a cohort of 709 children aged 6–30 months in a malaria holoendemic rural area of Burkina Faso. Study children were followed over the main malaria transmission period (June–December) in 1999 through longitudinal malaria surveillance complemented by three cross-sectional clinical surveys. There was no association between PEM and malaria morbidity, but malnourished children had a more than two-fold higher risk of dying than non-malnourished children.

keywords Africa, Burkina Faso, malaria, malnutrition, mortality

Introduction

Nutritional status is considered to be one of the major determinants of host resistance to infection (Keusch 1979; Gershwin et al . 1985). Malnutrition is estimated to cause about half of the world's 12 million annual deaths in children less than 5 years of age as well as substantial proportions of infectious disease morbidity (Pinstrup-Andersen et al. 1993; Rice et al. 2000). The relation between nutritional status and mortality is well documented, with decreasing nutritional status being associated with increasing risk ratios of mortality (Van den Broek et al. 1993; Garenne et al . 2000; Rice et al. 2000). More than half of the global burden of childhood deaths is caused by diarrhoea, acute respiratory illness (ARI), malaria and measles, conditions which can easily be prevented or treated (Tulloch 1999). In sub-Saharan Africa (SSA), malaria alone is estimated to kill around one million children every year (Snow et al. 1999).

Young children of SSA are the group most affected by both poor nutrition and malaria, and the relation between both conditions continues to be discussed very controversially. While a number of studies provided substantial evidence for protein–energy malnutrition (PEM) being associated with reduced malaria morbidity, others have not seen such associations or even demonstrated that PEM is associated with more severe manifestations of malaria (McGregor 1988; Shankar 2000). Against this background we studied the association between PEM, malaria morbidity and all-cause mortality in a cohort of West African pre-school children.

Subjects and methods

Study area

The study was conducted in Nouna Health District in northwestern Burkina Faso. Nouna is a dry orchard savannah, populated almost exclusively by subsistence farmers of different ethnic groups. There is a short rainy season, which usually lasts from June to October. Malnutrition is highly prevalent in the study area and malaria is holoendemic, with most transmission occurring during or shortly after the rainy season. HIV/AIDS is still a rare disease in this rural area of Nouna Health District.

Patients

In 1999, we had undertaken a randomized double-blind placebo-controlled trial on the effects of zinc supplementation on malaria morbidity. The main finding was that zinc supplementation had no effect on malaria morbidity (Müller et al. 2001). During this trial, 709 children aged 6–30 months were recruited from 18 villages of the Nouna Health Research Centre (CRSN) study area in Nouna Health District. Anthropometric and malariometric data were systematically collected during three cross-sectional surveys (6 of 99, 9 of 99, 12 of 99), and

685 children were successfully followed up over the 6-month study period.

To survey malaria morbidity, children were seen daily except on Sundays by village-based fieldworkers who took the axillary temperature with an electronic thermometer (Digital Classic, Hartmann, Germany) and filled in a structured questionnaire on further parent-reported information. If a temperature of 37.5 °C or higher was measured, a finger prick blood sample was taken and a thick and thin blood film were prepared. The parents of children found to be sick during daily visits were advised to take them to the nearest local health centre for diagnosis and treatment. During cross-sectional surveys, children were seen and examined by the same physician during all visits. Children found sick during surveys were treated appropriately or referred to Nouna Hospital free of charge. Mothers of malnourished children received intensive advice on feeding practice, and were offered admission to the Nouna Hospital Feeding Centre in case of severe malnutrition. Demographic and risk factor data (age, sex, ethnicity, mosquito net protection in September, socio-economic status defined through possession of radio/bicycle/motorbike), clinical data (history, symptoms, temperature, spleen size by Hackett grade, weight, height/length, mid-arm circumference), and parasitological data (thin and thick blood films) were collected from all children. Demographic and socio-economic baseline variables are shown in Table 1.

Table 1 Distribution of demographic and socio-economic baseline variables

	n	%
Sex		
Male	335	48.9
Female	350	51.1
Age (months) (6/1999)		
6–12	174	25.4
13–18	185	27.0
19–24	181	26.4
>24	145	21.2
Ethnic group		
Dafing	311	45.4
Bwaba	141	20.6
Mossi	132	19.3
Peulh	79	11.5
Samo	12	1.8
Others	10	1.5
Bednet use (9/1999)		
No	489	71.4
Yes	168	24.5
Missings	28	4.1
Socio-economic status		
Low	67	9.8
Middle	229	33.4
High	299	43.7
Missing	90	13.1
Total	685	100.0

Laboratory procedures

Blood films were Giemsa-stained at Nouna Hospital Laboratory and then transported to the Centre National de Recherche et de Formation sur le Paludisme in Ouagadougou for reading. All films were examined by two experienced laboratory technicians using a × 100 oil immersion lens and × 10 eyepieces. In case of significant discrepancy between the results of the two technicians, blood slides were read by a third investigator. Blood films were analysed for the species-specific parasite density per microlitre by counting against 500 white blood cells and multiplying by 16 (assuming 8000 white blood cells per microlitre of blood). Slides were declared negative if no parasites were seen in 400 fields on the thick film.

Anthropometric measurements

Weight was measured during each of the three surveys, while height/length was measured only during the baseline and the end-of-study survey. Weight was measured with one Salter hanging spring scale with 100-g gradations, which was calibrated and checked daily before and after use. Children were allowed to wear a minimum of light clothes. Recumbent length and standing height were measured with a locally produced length board with an upright wooden base and a movable headpiece and a simple anthropometer, respectively. Measures included weight to 0.1 kg and height/length to 1.0 cm. Anthropometric measurements were usually performed by the same fieldworker following standard techniques. The SD scores for height-for-age (HAZ), weight-for-age (WAZ), and weight-for-height (WHZ) were calculated in comparison with the NCHS reference population, using Epi Info, version 6.0. Stunting, underweight and wasting were defined as HAZ ≤ -2, WAZ ≤ -2, and WHZ ≤ -2, respectively (WHO Working Group 1986).

Mortality follow-up

Mortality follow-up took place through the existing Demographic Surveillance System (DSS) of the CRSN (Sankoh et al. 2001). The routine activities of the DSS include three-monthly visits to all households in the CRSN study area, with registration of all births, deaths and migrations.

Statistical analysis

Malaria incidence was calculated by dividing the number of falciparum malaria episodes by the number of days of observation. A falciparum malaria episode was defined as an axillary temperature of 37.5 °C or higher with at least 5000 parasites per microlitre and no other obvious causes for the fever. Additional definitions of fever and parasite counts of ≥1 and ≥100 000/μl were also applied. To exclude recrudescent malaria episodes, the individual observation time was defined as the time interval from the first to last day of observation minus 20 days for each defined episode.

We compared children with malnutrition (mean HAZ/WAZ/WHZ ≤ −2) and without malnutrition (mean HAZ/WAZ/WHZ > −2) for falciparum malaria incidence over the 6-month study period using Poisson regression and all-cause mortality (over a 1-year follow-up period) using logistic regression; children with no anthropometric measurements to calculate the HAZ/WAZ/WHZ scores at the first survey were excluded from the respective analyses. Possible confounding factors (age, sex, ethnicity, village, mosquito net use, and socio-economic status) were taken into account. Relative risks, 95% confidence intervals, and P-values were calculated using the statistical software package SAS and using PROC GENMOD for Poisson Regression, PROC LOGISTIC for logistic regression and PROC CORR SPEARMAN for assessing the relation between age and number of malaria episodes.

Ethical aspects

Approval was granted by the Ethical Committee of Heidelberg University Medical School, the Ethical Committee of the World Health Organization and the Ministry of Health in Burkina Faso. Prior to study participants' recruitment, the trial was explained in detail to all district authorities and village meetings were held to explain the purpose, methods, benefits and risks of the study to the population. The trial was also explained to the respective head of each participating compound and oral consent was sought from the parents and caretakers of study children before enrolment.

Results

Of 685 children followed up for malaria incidence over the 6-month observation period, 232 (36%), were stunted, 314 (48%) underweight and 132 (20%) wasted based on the respective mean HAZ, WAZ and WHZ values. The median number of falciparum malaria episodes over the observation period according to the three case definitions (≥37.5 °C + ≥1 *P. falciparum* parasites/microlitre; ≥37.5 °C + ≥5000 *P. falciparum* parasites/microlitre; ≥37.5 °C + ≥100 000 *P. falciparum* parasites/microlitre) were 2 (range 0–5), 1 (0–5) and 0 (0–2) respectively. The mean SD scores for HAZ, WAZ, and WHZ were −1.6, −2.0, and −1.2 at baseline, respectively; and −1.5, −2.0, and −1.3 after 6-month follow-up, respectively (Table 2). There were no differences in falciparum malaria incidence between malnourished and non-malnourished children after adjustment for possible confounding variables (Table 3).

During the 6 months of the randomized controlled trial 17 of 685 (2.5%) study children died; after 12 months of observation, 28 of 685 (4.1%) of the study children had died. After adjustment for possible confounding variables, malnourished children had a more than two-fold higher risk of dying than non-malnourished children, with a

Table 2 Distribution of anthropometric variables by sex and survey

	Male			Female		
	n	mean	SD	n	mean	SD
First survey (6/1999)						
HAZ	322	−1.69	1.49	326	−1.42	1.39
WAZ	321	−2.03	1.29	332	−1.87	1.15
WHZ	320	−1.28	1.09	325	−1.20	0.95
Second survey (9/1999)						
HAZ						
WAZ	292	−1.89	1.26	307	−1.73	1.12
WHZ						
Third survey (12/1999)						
HAZ	309	−1.60	1.43	307	−1.45	1.34
WAZ	307	−1.99	1.18	319	−1.93	1.13
WHZ	305	−1.30	0.95	306	−1.33	0.83

SD = standard deviation; HAZ = height for age; WAZ = weight for age; WHZ = weight for height.

Table 3 Association between protein–energy malnutrition, falciparum malaria and all-cause mortality

		Malaria defined as												Total mortality		
		≥37.5 °C ≥1 parasite/microlitre				≥37.5 °C ≥5000 parasites/microlitre				≥37.5 °C ≥100 000 parasites/microlitre						
	n	RR*	ME	PDO	95% CI	RR*	ME	PDO	95% CI	RR*	ME	PDO	95% CI	Deaths n (%)	RR**	95% CI
HAZ																
>−2	416	1.0	753	55 901		1.0	545	60 061		1.0	48	70 001		12 (2.9)	1.0	
≤−2	232	1.0	406	30 791	0.9–1.1	1.0	300	32 911	0.9–1.2	0.8	20	38 511	0.5–1.4	15 (6.5)	2.4	1.0–5.7
P-value					0.87				0.59				0.44			0.05
WAZ																
>−2	339	1.0	620	45 616		1.0	448	49 056		1.0	38	57 256		6 (1.8)	1.0	
≤−2	314	1.0	553	41 643	0.9–1.1	1.0	407	44 563	0.9–1.2	0.8	29	52 123	0.5–1.4	21 (6.7)	2.7	1.0–7.3
P-value					0.98				0.68				0.49			0.05
WHZ																
>−2	513	1.0	926	68 911		1.0	669	74 051		1.0	53	86 371		14 (2.7)	1.0	
≤−2	132	1.0	228	17 365	0.9–1.2	1.0	172	18 485	0.9–1.2	1.0	14	21 645	0.5–1.8	13 (9.8)	2.8	1.1–6.7
P-value					0.99				0.58				0.94			0.02

* RR based on Poisson regression model adjusted for age, sex, ethnicity, village (region), mosquito net use, socio-economic status.
** RR based on logistic regression model adjusted for age, sex, ethnicity, village (region), mosquito net use, socio-economic status.
ME = number of malaria episodes; PDO = person days of observation; HAZ = height for age; WAZ = weight for age; WHZ = weight for height.

relative risk of 2.4 [confidence interval (CI) 1.0–5.7, $P = 0.05$] for stunted children, 2.7 (CI 1.0–7.3, $P = 0.05$) for underweight children, and 2.8 (CI 1.1–6.7, $P = 0.02$) for wasted children (Table 3).

Discussion

We measured the association between PEM and malaria morbidity in a well-defined population of young children exposed to high *P. falciparum* transmission intensity. There was no association between PEM and the incidence of falciparum malaria, using the case definition of fever plus at least 5000 *P. falciparum* parasites per microlitre, and after controlling for possible confounding factors. Additional comparisons using traditional case definitions for mild and heavy infections did not change this result. As zinc supplementation assigned randomly to study children was not found related with malaria, it is unlikely to be a confounder (Müller et al. 2001). These findings are in contrast with a number of older studies, which claimed that PEM is associated with decreased malaria morbidity, as well as with some more recent studies providing evidence for PEM being associated with increased malaria morbidity (McGregor 1988; Shankar 2000). A variety of designs have been used in such studies, ranging from hospital-based case–control studies on malaria morbidity and mortality to community-based cohort studies on malaria incidence, and from experimental studies in animals to famine interventions in human populations. Most of these studies have obvious methodological limitations, and are thus difficult to interpret (Shankar 2000). However, in our study we also have to take into account that parasitaemia is not a very good measure of malaria morbidity.

Protein–energy malnutrition is considered to be one of the most important risk factors for overall morbidity and mortality in childhood, particularly in SSA (Murray & Lopez 1997). The strongest evidence for this association comes from observational community-based cohort studies (Rice et al. 2000). As even in cohort studies the direction of the effect can be confused through intermittent illnesses resulting in nutritional deterioration, we chose a PEM definition likely to avoid such bias.

In our study, mortality was significantly associated with a low HAZ, WAZ and WHZ. This supports the evidence for both acute malnutrition (wasting) and chronic malnutrition (stunting) being associated with mortality (Pinstrup-Andersen et al. 1993; Rice et al. 2000). Our findings on the high prevalence of malnutrition and the association between PEM and all-cause mortality in a typical population of young West African children thus confirms the major impact of this risk factor on overall childhood mortality in SSA (Murray & Lopez 1997).

Evidence points to diarrhoea and ARI being the most important causes of deaths related to malnutrition in childhood, while the association between PEM and malaria mortality continues to be discussed controversially (Rice et al. 2000; Shankar 2000). As the majority of young children's deaths in SSA occur at home, verbal autopsy is the only method to estimate cause-specific mortality rates. Unfortunately, it is not very reliable for determining deaths caused by the major diseases in SSA children, and particularly not for malaria (Snow et al. 1992; Todd et al. 1994). Verbal autopsy is likely to become even more unreliable with the emergence of HIV/AIDS as a major determinant of childhood deaths in SSA (Müller & Garenne 1999).

Our results confirm PEM being a major risk factor for all-cause mortality in West African children but provide no evidence for PEM being associated with malaria morbidity.

Acknowledgements

We thank Ms Gabriele Stieglbauer at the University of Heidelberg for her assistance in data management and statistical analysis. The work was supported by a grant from the World Health Organization, and by the Deutsche Forschungsgemeinschaft (SFB 544, Control of Tropical Infectious Diseases).

References

Garenne M, Maire B, Fontaine O, Dieng K & Briend A (2000) *Risques de décès associés à différents états nutritionnels chez l'enfant d'âge préscolaire*. Etudes du CEPED, no 17. CEPED, Paris.

Gershwin ME, Beach RS & Hurley LS (1985) *Nutrition and Immunity*. Academic Press, New York.

Keusch GT (1979) Nutrition as a determinant of host response to infection and the metabolic sequelae of infectious disease. *Seminar of Infectious Diseases* 2, 265–303.

McGregor IA (1988) Malaria and nutrition. In: *Malaria – Principles and Practice of Malariology*. (eds WH Wernsdorfer & I McGregor), Churchill Livingstone, London, pp. 753–768.

Müller O & Garenne M (1999) Childhood mortality in sub-Saharan Africa. *Lancet* 353, 673.

Müller O, Becher H, Baltussen van Zweeden A et al. (2001) Effect of zinc supplementation on malaria and other causes of morbidity in west African children: randomized double blind placebo controlled trial. *British Medical Journal* 322, 1–6.

Murray CJL & Lopez AD (1997) Global mortality, disability, and the contribution of risk factors: global burden of disease study. *Lancet* 349, 1436–1442.

Pinstrup-Andersen P, Burger S, Habicht JP & Peterson K (1993) Protein-energy malnutrition. In: *Disease Control Priorities in Developing Countries*. (eds DT Jamison, WH Mosley, AR Measham & JL Bobadilla) Oxford University Press, Oxford, pp. 391–420.

Rice AL, Sacco L, Hyder A & Black RE (2000) Malnutrition as an underlying cause of childhood deaths associated with infectious diseases in developing countries. *Bulletin of the World Health Organization* 78, 1207–1221.

Sankoh OA, Ye Y, Sauerborn R, Müller O & Becher H (2001) Clustering of childhood mortality in rural Burkina Faso. *International Journal of Epidemiology* 30, 485–492.

Shankar A (2000) Nutritional modulation of malaria morbidity and mortality. *Journal of Infectious Diseases* 182 (Suppl. 1), 37–53.

Snow RW, Armstrong JRM, Forster D et al. (1992) Childhood deaths in Africa: uses and limitations of verbal autopsies. *Lancet* 340, 351–355.

Snow RW, Craig M, Deichmann U & Marsh K (1999) Estimating mortality, morbidity and disability due to malaria among Africa's non-pregnant population. *Bulletin of the World Health Organization* 77, 624–640.

Todd JE, de Francisco A, O'Dempsey TJD & Greenwood BM (1994) The limitations of verbal autopsy in a malaria-endemic region. *Annals of Tropical Paediatrics* 14, 31–36.

Tulloch J (1999) Integrated approach to child health in developing countries. *Lancet* 354, 16–20.

Van den Broek J, Eeckels R & Vuylstek J (1993) Influence of nutritional status on child mortality in rural Zaire. *Lancet* 341, 1491–1495.

WHO Working Group (1986) Use and interpretation of anthropometric indicators of nutritional status. *Bulletin of the World Health Organization* 64, 929–941.

Authors

Olaf Müller (corresponding author) and **Prof. Heiko Becher**, Department of Tropical Hygiene and Public Health, Ruprecht-Karls-University Heidelberg, Im Neuenheimer Feld 324, 69120 Heidelberg, Germany. E-mail: olaf.muller@urz.uni-heidelberg.de; heiko.becher@urz.uni-heidelberg.de
Michel Garenne, Institut Pasteur, 28 rue du Docteur Roux, 75724 Paris Cedex 15, France. E-mail: mgarenne@bhdc.jussien.fr
Bocar Kouyaté, Centre de Recherche en Santé de Nouna, B.P. 34, Nouna, Burkinu Faso E-mail: bocar.crsn@fasonet.bf

2.7 Effect of zinc supplementation on growth in West African children: a randomized double-blind placebo-controlled trial in rural Burkina Faso

Müller O, Garenne M, Reitmaier P, Baltussen van Zweeden A, Kouyaté B, Becher H

Int J Epidemiol. 2003 Dec; 32(6): 1098-102

Reprinted with permission from Oxford University Press

PAEDIATRIC EPIDEMIOLOGY

Effect of zinc supplementation on growth in West African children: a randomized double-blind placebo-controlled trial in rural Burkina Faso

O Müller,[1] M Garenne,[2] P Reitmaier,[1] A Baltussen van Zweeden,[3] B Kouyate[3] and H Becher[1]

Accepted	31 March 2003
Objective	To analyse the effects of zinc supplementation on growth parameters in a representative sample of young children in rural Burkina Faso.
Design	Randomized, double-blind, placebo-controlled efficacy trial.
Setting	Eighteen villages in rural northwestern Burkina Faso.
Subjects	In all, 709 children aged 6–31 months were enrolled; 685 completed the trial.
Intervention	Supplementation with zinc (12.5 mg zinc sulphate) or placebo daily for 6 days a week for 6 months.
Outcomes	Weight, length/height, mid-arm circumference, and serum zinc.
Results	In a representative subsample of study children, 72% were zinc-deficient at baseline. After supplementation, serum zinc increased in zinc-supplemented but not in control children of the subsample. No significant differences between groups were observed during follow-up regarding length/height, weight, mid-arm circumference, and z scores for height-for-age, weight-for-age, and weight-for-height.
Conclusions	We conclude that zinc supplementation does not have an effect of public health importance on growth in West African populations of young children with a high prevalence of malnutrition. Multinutrient interventions are likely to be more effective.
Keywords	Zinc, growth, malnutrition, children, Africa, Burkina Faso

Malnutrition and micronutrient deficiencies are highly prevalent in developing countries, and it has been estimated that malnutrition is the underlying cause for up to 50% of all deaths among children in these populations.[1–5] Zinc is important for a number of biological functions, and zinc deficiency has been associated with complications in pregnancy and childbirth, lower birthweight and poor growth in childhood, reduced immuno-competence, and increased infectious disease morbidity.[6–8] As there are no reliable biochemical indices of marginal zinc status, controlled supplementation trials are the best method to study the relation between zinc deficiency and health parameters in human populations.[9] A number of such trials have consistently demonstrated an association between zinc supplementation and major reductions of morbidity due to respiratory infections and diarrhoea in young children of developing countries.[10] More recently, a controlled trial on zinc supplementation during pregnancy has been able to demonstrate a reduced frequency of diarrhoea, dysentery, and impetigo in low birthweight infants born to mothers in the zinc-supplemented group.[11]

The impact of zinc supplementation on growth parameters has also been studied in countries of Asia, Latin America, and Africa. Trials in different populations of young children from

---

[1] Department of Tropical Hygiene and Public Health, Ruprecht-Karls-University Heidelberg, Medical School, Heidelberg, Germany.
[2] Centre Francais sur la Population et le Development, Paris, France.
[3] Centre de Recherche en Santé de Nouna, Nouna, Burkina Faso.
Correspondence: Dr Olaf Müller, Division of Epidemiology, Biostatistics and Disease Control, Department of Tropical Hygiene and Public Health, Ruprecht-Karls-University, Im Neuenheimer Feld 324, 69120 Heidelberg, Germany. E-mail: olaf.mueller@urz.uni-heidelberg.de

these countries have provided conflicting results on the effects of zinc supplementation on growth. While some have found no effect, others provided evidence for zinc supplementation increasing growth velocity.[12–20] In a meta analysis of 25 studies, there were small but highly significant effect sizes for changes in height and weight of +0.22 SD and 0.26 SD respectively with zinc supplementation.[12]

We undertook a randomized placebo-controlled zinc supplementation trial in young children of rural Burkina Faso. Results on morbidity outcome have been published elsewhere.[21] Here we report our findings on anthropometric measurements associated with zinc supplementation during this trial.

Subjects and Methods

Study area
The study area was in the Nouna Health District in northwestern Burkina Faso. The trial took place June–December 1999. The Nouna area is a dry orchard savanna, populated almost exclusively by subsistance farmers of different ethnic groups. The rainy season usually lasts from June until October, and the average annual rainfall is 700 mm. The main staple food in the study area is millet, with young children usually receiving a diet that contains very little protein. Traditional rearing of animals is practised mainly for income generation. During the rainy season, when villager's workload as well as disease incidence are high, food intake is particularly low.[22]

Study design
The study design has been described in detail.[21] In brief, children aged 6–31 months at enrolment were recruited by lottery from 18 villages of the study area of the *Centre de Recherche en Santé de Nouna* (CRSN).[23] Children found to have serious underlying illness were excluded from enrolment. Children were individually allocated supplementation with zinc or placebo in blocks of 30 (15 zinc, 15 placebo) by computer-generated randomly permutated codes (prepared by WHO/Geneva). Study children were supplemented with 12.5 mg (half of a 25-mg tablet) of zinc sulphate or placebo every morning (except Sundays) during a 6-month period. Zinc and placebo tablets were identical in appearance and taste (Biolectra Zinc, Hermes Arzneimittel GMBH, München, Germany). Supplementation was done through village-based fieldworkers supervized through specific fieldsupervisors and a Nouna-based study physician (AB). Compliance with the supplementation was systematically investigated in all study children in October 1999. On a semi-quantitative measurement scale (very good, good, acceptable, difficult, bad) and based on specific standard guidelines, compliance was judged as acceptable or better in 80% of study children by the responsible field staff.

For surveillance of morbidity, mortality, and periods of absence, children were seen daily except Sundays by their respective fieldworker. In addition, three cross-sectional surveys were undertaken at baseline (June), mid study (September), and end of study (December). Children were seen and examined by the same physician (OM) during all survey visits. Anthropometric measurements were made on all children, while serum zinc level was measured in a random subsample of 100 children.

Laboratory procedures
Venous blood taken during the surveys was kept in a cold box until centrifugation, which was done on the same day in Nouna. Serum samples were stored at −20°C until zinc determination took place at the Heidelberg University laboratory by flame atomic absorption spectrometry (Perkin-Elmer 1100 B, Germany).

Anthropometry
Weight and mid-upper-arm circumference (MUAC) were measured during each of the three surveys, while height/length was measured only at baseline (before supplementation) and the end-of-study survey. Weight was measured with one Salter hanging spring scale with 100-g gradations which was calibrated and controlled daily before and after use. Children were allowed to wear a minimum of light clothes. Recumbent length and standing height were measured with a locally produced length board with an upright wooden base and a moveable headpiece and a simple anthropometer respectively. MUAC was taken with a flexible non-stretch measuring tape.[24] Measures included weight to the nearest 0.1 kg, height/length to the nearest 1.0 cm, and MUAC to the nearest 0.5 cm. Anthropometric measurements were usually performed by the same fieldworker following standard techniques.[25] The SD scores for height-for-age (HAZ), weight-for-age (WAZ), and weight-for-height (WHZ) were calculated in comparison to the National Center for Health Statistics (NCHS) standard population, using Epi Info, version 6.0.[26] Age calculations were based on the precise information available through the existing demographic surveillance system in the study area.[24] Stunting, underweight, and wasting were defined as HAZ $\leqslant -2$, WAZ $\leqslant -2$, and WHZ $\leqslant -2$ respectively.[27]

Statistical analysis and data management
Field data forms were checked manually by supervisors for completeness before independent computer entry (Microsoft ACCESS, version 97) at the *Centre de Recherche en Santé de Nouna*. All data were checked for range and consistency, and survey data were double-entered. Any differences were resolved by checking against the original case record forms. The randomization code was broken after the database was closed.

All analyses were done with SAS (version 8.1). Differences among zinc supplementation and placebo group with respect to the anthropometric measures were analysed as follows. For each child we calculated the individual 6-month difference. The effect of zinc supplementation as well as possible confounding factors (age, sex, height and weight at baseline, ethnic group) on these differences were investigated using a linear regression model (SAS PROC REG). Changes in anthropometric measures were also analysed seperately for children who were stunted at baseline (HAZ <-2).

Ethical aspects
Approval was granted by the Ethical Committee of the Heidelberg University Medical School and the Ministry of Health in Burkina Faso. The trial was explained in detail to local authorities, to study village populations and to the respective head of each participating compound. Oral consent was sought from the parents and caretakers of study children before enrolment.

Results

The trial profile is given in Figure 1. Of 713 children eligible for the study (one small village only had 23 children of the required age group), 709 children were enrolled and randomized to supplementation with zinc (n = 356) or placebo (n = 353). Children were not supplemented on 4349 days in total due to absence: average 6.3 days missing for each child (2163 zinc, 2186 placebo). During cross-sectional surveys, 661/685 (96%) of study children were examined at baseline, mid study, and end of study respectively.

Baseline data

In June 1999, the overall age distribution of study children was as follows: 26% were 6–12 months, 27% were 13–18 months, 26% were 19–24 months, and 21% were 25–31 months old. Of zinc supplemented children, 165/332 (50%) and 160/329 (49%) of placebo children were male. Overall, 304/661 (46%), 129/661 (20%), 130/661 (20%), and 77/661 (12%) of study children belonged to the ethnic group of Marka, Mossi, Bwaba, and Peulh respectively. Zinc and placebo groups were similar at baseline regarding all demographic parameters, except that zinc children were slightly older compared with placebo children (18.7 versus 17.6 months).

The prevalence of malnutrition was high at baseline, with 36.3% of children below –2 z score for height for age (stunting) and 24.6% below the –2 z score for weight for height (wasting). The children in our study were not significantly different from the normally poor nutritional status in the Sahel region.[28] Baseline characteristics of study children by treatment group are shown in Table 1.

Follow-up data

Paired serum zinc values for June and September (baseline and mid-study survey) were available for 81 (41 zinc, 40 placebo) of study children. Mean zinc levels at baseline were 11.7 µmol/l with no differences between zinc and placebo group, and 72% of study children were zinc deficient according to the reference laboratory defined threshold value of 13.0 µmol/l. In September (mid-study survey), after 3 months of supplementation, children in the zinc group had significantly higher values compared with placebo children (15.3 versus 12.4 µmol/l, $P = 0.005$) and the proportion of zinc-deficient children has significantly declined in the zinc but not the placebo group (11/41 versus 28/40, $P = 0.0001$).

Changes in length/height, weight, MUAC, and scores for WAZ/HAZ/WHZ after 6 months of intervention are shown in Table 2. Linear growth averaged 5 cm over the 6-month period, which can be considered as normal. However, weight gains were rather low (about 1 kg) so that gains in weight for age, weight for height, and arm circumference tended to be negative. There were however no significant differences between treatment and placebo groups, even after controlling for sex, ethnic group, age, weight, and height at baseline. When considering changes in anthropometric indicators for stunted children only (HAZ <–2), there was again no significant effect of zinc on growth parameters.

Table 1 Baseline characteristics of study children in intervention and control group

	Zinc (n = 332)	Placebo (n = 329)
Age (months)	18.7 ± 7.0	17.6 ± 6.5
Height (cm)	76.0 ± 6.7	75.3 ± 6.5
Weight (kg)	8.8 ± 1.8	8.6 ± 1.9
MUAC[a] (cm)	13.6 ± 1.3	13.6 ± 1.5
HAZ[b]	–1.6 ± 1.3	–1.5 ± 1.6
WAZ[c]	–2.0 ± 1.1	–2.0 ± 1.3
WHZ[d]	–1.2 ± 1.0	–1.3 ± 1.0

Data are mean ±SD.
[a] Mid-upper-arm circumference.
[b] Height-for-age Z score.
[c] Weight-for-age Z score.
[d] Weight-for-height Z score.

A few study children were missing individual measurements for length (n = 37), weight (n = 32), MUAC (n = 31), HAZ (n = 37), WAZ (n = 32), and WHZ (n = 40).

Discussion

It has been estimated that 42% of children less than 5 years old who are living in low-income countries are stunted (HAZ <–2), a situation which has changed little over recent decades.[3] High incidence rates of infectious diseases in combination with poor nutritional quality of traditional diets contributing to insufficient food intake are considered the main causes of malnutrition in such populations.[1,29]

We also found a high prevalence of stunting in this rural West African study area, a situation furthermore complicated by a high prevalence of wasting. The nutritional indicators were particularly bad in children aged 12–24 months (data not shown), which is typical for young children in rural Africa where bulky weaning diets of low energy density prevail.

Given the low intake of animal products in the study area, the existence of a high prevalence of zinc deficiency in young children is very likely. This is supported by the finding of low serum zinc levels in the study population, and by the significant increase of serum zinc levels in children supplemented with zinc compared to control children.

In this study, we have not found any significant effect of zinc supplementation on nutritional indicators at a level verifiable with standard anthropometric equipment in developing

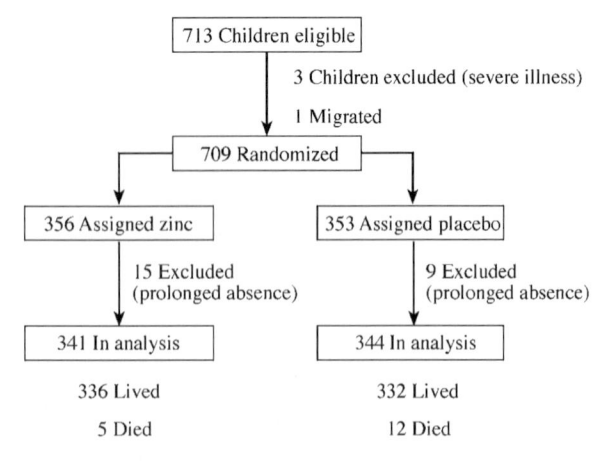

Figure 1 Trial profile

- 713 Children eligible
  - 3 Children excluded (severe illness)
  - 1 Migrated
- 709 Randomized
  - 356 Assigned zinc
    - 15 Excluded (prolonged absence)
    - 341 In analysis
      - 336 Lived
      - 5 Died
  - 353 Assigned placebo
    - 9 Excluded (prolonged absence)
    - 344 In analysis
      - 332 Lived
      - 12 Died

Table 2 Effect of zinc supplementation on growth velocity of study children in intervention and control group

	All children			HAZa ≤−2 baseline		
	Zinc (n = 332)	Placebo (n = 329)	P-value[b]	Zinc (n = 119)	Placebo (n = 112)	P-value[b]
	Difference		(95% CI)	Difference		(95% CI)
Gain in height (cm/6 months)	5.0 ± 2.2 0.13	4.9 ± 2.1	0.45 (−0.21, 0.48)	5.1 ± 2.5 0.22	4.8 ± 2.4	0.52 (−0.44, 0.88)
Gain in weight (kg/6 months)	1.0 ± 0.7 0.08	0.9 ± 0.7	0.16 (−0.03, 0.18)	1.1 ± 0.7 0.16	0.9 ± 0.7	0.11 (−0.034, 0.35)
Change in MUAC[c] (cm/6 months)	−0.3 ± 1.0 0.13	−0.4 ± 1.1	0.13 (−0.04, 0.29)	−0.1 ± 1.0 0.17	−0.3 ± 1.1	0.22 (−0.11, 0.45)
Change in HAZ	0.06 ± 0.8 0.08	−0.02 ± 0.8	0.24 (−0.05, 0.20)	0.3 ± 0.8 0.08	0.3 ± 0.8	0.46 (−0.13–0.29)
Change in WAZ[d]	−0.002 ± 0.6 0.08	−0.08 ± 0.6	0.13 (−0.02, 0.18)	0.2 ± 0.6 0.13	0.07 ± 0.6	0.12 (−0.032, 0.30)
Change in WHZ[e]	−0.09 ± 0.8 0.02	−0.1 ± 0.7	0.72 (−0.10, 0.15)	−0.01 ± 0.9 0.11	−0.1 ± 0.8	0.38 (−0.13, 0.34)

Data are mean ±SD.
[a] Height-for-age Z score.
[b] Effect of zinc on anthropometric variables by t-test.
[c] Mid-upper-arm circumference.
[d] Weight-for-age Z score.
[e] Weight-for-height Z score.

countries. However, these results have to be interpreted with caution, as the study was not primarily designed to measure the nutritional effects of zinc.[21] Moreover, the pattern of observed growth velocity is not usual in this age range, and is due primarily to the heavy presence of malaria during the rainy season.

The differences between zinc and placebo groups were indeed remarkably small, so that if there is any nutritional impact of zinc supplementation it is likely to be of small magnitude. However, it should be noted that differences tended to be in the expected direction, that is slightly higher weight and height gains and smaller losses in MUAC in zinc-supplemented compared with not zinc-supplemented children, especially in the subgroup of stunted children. It remains therefore possible that a larger trial might have detected minor differences between groups in favour of zinc supplementation.

Small but real effects of zinc on nutritional improvement have been considered likely in a recent meta-analysis of published studies.[12] Moreover, there is evidence for such effects primarily being attributed to the effects of zinc on increasing appetite and decreasing infectious disease morbidity.[20] Growth velocity changes, that might be associated with the reduced diarrhoea morbidity observed in our study population, appear to have been small and were not detected by our anthropometric procedures followed here.[21]

There is now increasing evidence for a number of micronutrients being implicated in linear growth, not just zinc.[30] Consequently, it has been shown in a Chinese population that supplementation with zinc plus other micronutrients was superior compared with zinc alone in increasing growth velocity.[16] It has furthermore been shown that zinc was an effective micronutrient in children with relatively better nutritional status, whereas those with poorer nutritional status were deficient in other nutrients that limited the response to zinc supplementation.[15] As the nutritional status of our study children was rather poor, this might further explain our non-significant results. Such an interpretation is furthermore supported by the lack of an effect on growth velocity in children of all three zinc supplementation trials from Africa which were included in the meta-analysis,[12] as well as by newer studies on children with a poor nutritional status from Mexico and Jamaica.[14,31] The obvious policy implications would be to avoid single-nutrient interventions in favour of multinutrient programmes in populations of young children with a high prevalence of malnutrition.

It is noteworthy to comment on our results in the light of the meta-analysis by Brown et al.[12] In our study the estimated effect of zinc supplementation on change in weight is +0.08 kg with 95% CI (−0.03, 0.18) which corresponds to 0.11 SD. Given the study size of our trial, an observed difference of about 0.14 SD of weight gain would appear significant with $P = 0.05$. In the meta-analysis an effect size of 0.26 SD was calculated (95% CI: 0.17, 0.36). Although our results are in line with several of the studies included, overall our study therefore does not support the general conclusion of the meta-analysis. For height we have a similar result. Since our study appears larger than each single study, inclusion would have a considerable impact towards a lower overall effect.

In conclusion, zinc supplementation had no measurable effect on growth velocity in young children in rural Burkina Faso. If a small but real effect of zinc on nutritional development exists, such an effect will not be of major public health importance.

Acknowledgements

The study was funded by the World Health Organisation (Department of Child and Adolescent Health and Development), and by the Deutsche Forschungsgemeinschaft (SFB 544, Control of Tropical Infectious Diseases). We thank Walter Fiehn of the Heidelberg Medical School laboratory for determination of serum zinc values. Gabriele Stieglbauer is gratefully acknowledged for her assistance with data management in Heidelberg. We thank the staff of the Centre de Recherche en Sante de Nouna for their enthusiasm and support. We are particularly grateful to the children and the parents who participated in the study.

References

[1] Pinstrup-Andersen P, Burger S, Habicht JP, Peterson K. Protein-energy malnutrition. In: Jamison DT, Mosley WH, Measham AR, Bobadilla JL (eds). *Disease Control Priorities in Developing Countries.* Oxford: Oxford University Press, 1993, pp. 391–420.

[2] Levin HM, Pollitt E, Galloway R, McGuire J. Micronutrient Deficiency Disorders. In: Jamison DT, Mosley WH, Measham AR, Bobadilla JL (eds). *Disease Control Priorities in Developing Countries.* Oxford: Oxford University Press, 1993, pp. 421–51.

[3] De Onis M, Monteiro C, Akre J, Clugston G. The worldwide magnitude of protein-energy malnutrition: an overview from the WHO Global Database on Child Growth. *Bull World Health Organ* 1993;**71:**703–12.

[4] World Health Organization. Integrated management of the sick child. *Bull World Health Organ* 1995;**73:**735–40.

[5] Rice AL, Sacco L, Hyder A, Black RE. Malnutrition as an underlying cause of childhood deaths associated with infectious diseases in developing countries. *Bull World Health Organ* 2000;**78:**1207–21.

[6] Shankar AH, Prasad AS. Zinc and immune function: the biological basis of altered resistance to infection. *Am J Clin Nutr* 1998;**68(Suppl.):**447S–63S.

[7] Aggett PJ. Severe zinc deficiency. In: Mills CF (ed.). *Zinc in Human Biology.* Berlin and Heidelberg: Springer-Verlag, 1989, pp. 259–79.

[8] Black RE. Therapeutic and preventive effects of zinc on serious childhood infectious diseases in developing countries. *Am J Clin Nutr* 1998;**68(Suppl.):**476–79.

[9] Brown KH. Effect of infections on plasma zinc concentration and implications for zinc status assessment in low-income countries. *Am J Clin Nutr* 1998;**68(Suppl.):**425–29.

[10] Zinc Investigators' Collaborative Group: Bhutta ZA, Black RE, Brown KH *et al.* Prevention of diarrhea and pneumonia by zinc supplementation in children in developing countries: pooled analysis of randomized controlled trials. *J Pediatr* 1999;**135:**689–97.

[11] Osendarp SJM, van Raaij JMA, Darmstadt GL, Baqui AH, Hautvast JGAJ, Fuchs GJ. Zinc supplementation during pregnancy and effects on growth and morbidity in low birthweight infants: a randomised placebo controlled trial. *Lancet* 2001;**357:**1080–85.

[12] Brown KH, Peerson JM, Allen LH. Effect of zinc supplementation on children's growth: a meta-analysis of intervention trials. *Bibl Nutr Dieta* 1998;**54:**76–83.

[13] Friis H, Ndhlovu P, Mduluza T *et al.* The importance of zinc supplementation on growth and body composition: a randomised, controlled trial among rural Zimbabwean schoolchildren. *Eur J Clin Nutr* 1997;**51:**38–45.

[14] Rosado JL, Lopez P, Munoz E, Martinez H, Allen LH. Zinc supplementation reduced morbidity, but neither zinc nor iron supplementation affected growth or body composition of Mexican preschoolers. *Am J Clin Nutr* 1997;**65:**13.

[15] Kikafunda JK, Walker AF, Allen EF, Tumwine JK. Effect of zinc supplementation on growth and body composition of Ugandan preschool children: a randomised, controlled, intervention trial. *Am J Clin Nutr* 1998;**68:**1261–66.

[16] Sandstead HH, Penland JG, Alcock NW *et al.* Effects of repletion with zinc and other micronutrients on neuropsychological performance and growth in Chinese children. *Am J Clin Nutr* 1998;**68(Suppl.):** 470–75.

[17] Lira PIC, Ashworth A, Morris SS. Effect of zinc supplementation on the morbidity, immune function, and growth of low-birth-weight, full-term infants in northeast Brazil. *Am J Clin Nutr* 1998;**68(Suppl.):** 418–24.

[18] Clark PJ, Eastell R, Barker ME. Zinc supplementation and bone growth in pubertal girls. *Lancet* 1999;**354:**485.

[19] Roy SK, Tomkins AM, Haider R, Akramuzzaman SM, Behrens RH, Mahalanabis D. Impact of zinc supplementation on subsequent growth and morbidity in Bangladeshi children with acute diarrhea. *Eur J Clin Nutr* 1999;**53:**529–34.

[20] Umeta M, West CE, Haidar J, Deurenberg P, Hautvast JGAJ. Zinc supplementation and stunted infants in Ethiopia: a randomised controlled trial. *Lancet* 2000;**355:**2021–26.

[21] Müller O, Becher H, Baltussen A *et al.* Effect of zinc supplementation on malaria morbidity among west African children: a randomized double-blind placebo-controlled trial. *BMJ* 2001;**322:**1567–70.

[22] Sauerborn R, Nougtara A, Diesfeld HJ (eds). Les couts economiques de la maladie pour les menages au milieu rural du Burkina Faso. Frankfurt: Peter Lang Verlag, 1996.

[23] Kouyaté B, Traoré C, Kielmann K, Müller O. North and South: bridging the information gap. *Lancet* 2000;**356:**1035.

[24] Benzler J, Sauerborn R. Rapid risk household screening by neonatal arm circumference: results from a cohort study in rural Burkina Faso. *Trop Med Int Health* 1999;**3:**962–74.

[25] United Nations. *National Household Survey Capability Programme. Annex I: How to Weigh and Measure Children.* New York: United Nations, Department of Technical Co-operation for Development and Statistical Office, 1986.

[26] Dibley MJ, Goldsby JB, Staehling NW, Trowbridge FL. Development of normalized curves for the international growth reference: historical and technical considerations. *Am J Clin Nutr* 1987;**46:**736–48.

[27] World Health Organization Working Group. Use and interpretation of anthropometric indicators of nutritional status. *Bull World Health Organ* 1986;**64:**929–41.

[28] McGregor IA. Morbidity and mortality at Keneba, The Gambia, 1950–75. In: Feachem RG, Jamison DT (eds). *Disease and Mortality in Sub-Saharan Africa.* Oxford: Oxford University Press, 1991, pp. 306–24.

[29] Waterlow JC. Causes and mechanisms of linear growth retardation (stunting). *Eur J Clin Nutr* 1994;**48(Suppl.1):**S1–4.

[30] Solomons NW, Ruz M, Gibson RS. Single-nutrient interventions with zinc. *Am J Clin Nutr* 1999;**70:**111–13.

[31] Meeks Gardner JM, Witter MM, Ramdath DD. Zinc supplementation: effects of the growth and morbidity of undernourished Jamaican children. *Eur J Clin Nutr* 1998;**52:**34–39.

2.8 Efficacy of pyrimethamine-sulfadoxine in young children with uncomplicated falciparum malaria in rural Burkina Faso

MÜLLER O, TRAORE C, KOUYATÉ B

Malar J 2004 May 11; 3(1):10

Reprinted with permission from BioMed Central Ltd.

Malaria Journal

Research

Efficacy of pyrimethamine-sulfadoxine in young children with uncomplicated falciparum malaria in rural Burkina Faso

Olaf Müller*[1], Corneille Traore[2] and Bocar Kouyate[2]

Address: [1]Department of Tropical Hygiene and Public Health of the Ruprecht-Karls-University Heidelberg, Heidelberg, Germany and [2]Centre de Recherche en Santé de Nouna, Nouna, Burkina Faso

Email: Olaf Müller* - olaf.mueller@urz.uni-heidelberg.de; Corneille Traore - corneille.traore@yahoo.com; Bocar Kouyate - bocar.crsn@fasonet.bf

* Corresponding author

Published: 11 May 2004

Malaria Journal 2004, **3**:10

Received: 16 January 2004
Accepted: 11 May 2004

This article is available from: http://www.malariajournal.com/content/3/1/10

© 2004 Müller et al; licensee BioMed Central Ltd. This is an Open Access article: verbatim copying and redistribution of this article are permitted in all media for any purpose, provided this notice is preserved along with the article's original URL.

Abstract

The efficacy of pyrimethamine-sulfadoxine in the treatment of uncomplicated falciparum malaria in young children of a malaria holoendemic area in rural Burkina Faso is reported. Of 28 children treated with a standard single dose of pyrimethamine-sulfadoxine and followed-up over 14 days, only one Late Treatment Failure and four Late Parasitological Failures were observed, all with low-grade parasitaemia. In this area of very restricted use of pyrimethamine-sulfadoxine, the drug appears to be still sufficiently effective in the treatment of malaria. These findings provide further evidence for the justification of continued use of pyrimethamine-sulfadoxine as a second-line treatment for malaria in Burkina Faso.

Background

The first cases of *in vitro* and *in vivo* chloroquine resistance in Burkina Faso were seen in 1983 and 1988, respectively, and reported clinical failure rates after use of chloroquine for treatment of uncomplicated malaria in children were already around 5% in the early 1990s [1]. More recently, the clinical failure rate of chloroquine in pre-school children was shown to be around 10% in western Burkina Faso [2,3]. These findings have led to the conclusion that chloroquine still remains sufficiently effective after many years of resistance occurrence in this part of West Africa.

Little information exists on the dynamics of resistance development towards pyrimethamine-sulfadoxine, the usual second-line treatment choice in African countries with moderate chloroquine resistance. In Burkina Faso, only very low parasitological and clinical failure rates during use of have been reported in the past [1,2].

The efficacy of pyrimethamine-sulfadoxine in a rural area of north-western Burkina Faso is reported.

Methods

The study took place in six representative villages of the research area of the *Centre de Recherche en Santé* de Nouna (CRSN) in north-western Burkina Faso [4]. The Nouna area is a dry orchard savanna, populated mainly by subsistence farmers of different ethnic groups. Malaria is holoendemic but highly seasonal in the study area [4].

The study was nested into an ongoing insecticide-treated bed net (ITN) study [5]. All ITN cohort children from the six villages visited during a cross-sectional survey in October 2002 were enrolled if they fulfilled the following inclusion criteria: age >6 months, falciparum malaria (≥37.5°C axillary temperature + ≥2.000 *Plasmodium falciparum* parasites/µl blood in the absence of another obvious fever cause), absence of antimalarial treatment during previous two weeks, informed oral consent. All study children received a fully supervised single-drug treatment with 1/2 tablet Fansidar (12.5 mg pyrimethamine plus 250 mg sulfadoxine), taken from the essential drug stock of Nouna Health District. Children were observed for an hour after treatment. In the event of vomiting, they received another 1/2 tablet Fansidar.

Enrolled children were seen daily by village-based field staff over a 14-day period and, in case of fever (≥37.5°C axillary temperature), blood films were taken. Systematic blood slides were taken from all study children on day 0, 3, 7 and 14. Blood films were examined by two experienced laboratory technicians of the CRSN.

For the evaluation of treatment outcome, a modified definition of the WHO protocol for assessment of therapeutic efficacy of anti-malarial drugs in areas with intense transmission was used [6]. Early Treatment Failure (ETF) was defined as development of severe malaria on days 1–3 or axillary temperature ≥37.5°C on day 3 in the presence of parasitaemia, and Late Treatment Failure (LTF) as development of severe malaria and/or axillary temperature ≥37.5°C on days 4–14 in the presence of parasitaemia without previously meeting the criteria of ETF. Late Parasitological Failure (LPF) was defined as the presence of parasitaemia on day 7 and/or day 14. Approval for the study was granted by the Ethical Committee of the Heidelberg University Medical School and the Ministry of Health in Burkina Faso.

Results
Of 357 cohort children seen during the survey, 40 children (11%) were febrile and of those only 4 children had no detectable malaria parasitaemia. Overall, 28 children met the inclusion criteria and were enrolled into the study. At baseline, the mean age of these study children was 23 months (range 9–32), 17/28 (61%) were male, the mean temperature was 38.1°C (range 37.5–39.9), and the mean weight was 9.5 kg (range 5.5–12.9). The median baseline number of $P.\ falciparum$ trophozoites was 13.100/µl (range 2.000–177.000), and 9/28 (32%) study children had $P.\ falciparum$ gametocytes on day 0.

There was no loss to follow-up. No ETF was observed and only one LTF occurred in a 26 months old and 10.0 kg weighing male child, who had fever (38.7°C) and a low-grade parasitaemia (50/µl) on day 14. In addition, 7/28 (25%) study children still had measurable parasitaemia on day 3 (50–475/µl) without fever, and 4/28 (14%) study children had a LPF with low-grade parasitaemias (75–250/µl), two on day 7 and two on day 14 (all male). On day 7 and/or day 14, $P.\ falciparum$ gametozytes were seen in 19/28 (68%) of study children.

Discussion
The findings from this study confirm the still very low level of resistance to pyrimethamine-sulfadoxine in West Africa [2,7-9]. The likely reason for the continued efficacy of pyrimethamine-sulfadoxine is the low level of drug pressure in these areas, where the large majority of malaria cases is still treated with chloroquine [10]. These findings justify continued use of pyrimethamine-sulfadoxine for malaria second-line treatment in Burkina Faso, as in most of West Africa.

However, the question of which drug or drug combination should be the successor of chloroquine for malaria first-line treatment once this has reached unacceptable high failure rates remains largely unsolved for the poor malaria-endemic countries in sub-Saharan Africa (SSA) [11,12]. Although, with regard to its still high efficacy, pyrimethamine-sulfadoxine would be a promising candidate for replacing chloroquine in West Africa, resistance is predicted to occur rapidly when the drug is used alone [11,13]. Artemisinin combination therapy (ACT) is now recommended by the World Health Organization as a first-line treatment for malaria, but these combinations are comparably very expensive and their use in malaria control programmes will thus not be possible in many countries of SSA without sustainable external support [11,14]. The combination of amodiaquine and pyrimethamine-sulfadoxine has recently been shown to be even more effective than ACT, and this combination has now been chosen as a pragmatic interim solution by some countries of SSA [15,16]. Finally, the implications on the long-term effectiveness of intermittent pyrimethamine-sulfadoxine preventive treatment during pregnancy need to be taken seriously into consideration when using pyrimethamine-sulfadoxine as a first-line malaria therapy regimens in SSA [17].

Authors' contributions
OM was the Principal Investigator of the study. He was responsible for the design of the study, drafted the manuscript and made all necessary corrections. CT was responsible for the fieldwork during data collection and supervised data entry. BK was responsible for the overall organisation in Burkina Faso and contributed to data analysis. All co-authors contributed to the writing of the paper.

Competing interests
None declared.

Acknowledgments
The study was funded by the Deutsche Forschungsgemeinschaft (SFB 544, Control of Tropical Infectious Diseases).

References

1. Guigemdé TR, Aoba A, Ouedraogo JB, Lamizana L: **Ten year surveillance of drug-resistant malaria in Burkina Faso (1982–1991).** *Am J Trop Med Hyg* 1994, **50:**699-704.
2. Tinto H, Zoungrana EB, Coulibaly SO, Ouedraogo JB, Traoré M, Guigemdé TR, Van Marck E, D'Alessandro U: **Chloroquine and sulphadoxine-pyrimethamine efficacy for uncomplicated malaria treatment and haematological recovery in children in Bobo-Dioulasso, Burkina Faso during a 3-year period 1998–2000.** *Trop Med Int Hlth* 2002, **7:**925-30.
3. Muller O, Traoré C, Kouyaté B: **Clinical efficacy of chloroquine in young children with uncomplicated falciparum malaria – a community-based study in rural Burkina Faso.** *Trop Med Int Health* 2003, **8:**202-203.
4. Müller O, Becher H, Baltussen A, Ye Y, Diallo D, Konate M, Gbangou A, Kouyate B, Garenne M: **Effect of zinc supplementation on malaria morbidity among West African children: a randomized double-blind placebo-controlled trial.** *B M J* 2001, **322:**1567-1572.
5. Müller O, Traoré C, Kouyaté B, Becher H: **Effects of insecticide-treated mosquito nets (ITN) on malaria morbidity and all-cause mortality in infants of a malaria holoendemic area in rural Burkina Faso.** *Acta Trop* 2002, **83(supplement):**71-72.
6. WHO: **Assessment of therapeutic efficacy of antimalarial drugs for uncomplicated Falciparum malaria in areas with intense transmission.** *World Health Organization, Geneva, WHO/MAL/96.1077* 1996.
7. Müller O, Boele van Hensbroek M, Jaffar S, Drakeley C, Okorie C, Joof D, Pinder M, Greenwood B: **A randomized trial of chloroquine, amodiaquine, and pyrimethamine-sulfadoxine in Gambian children with uncomplicated malaria.** *Trop Med Int Hlth* 1996, **1:**124-132.
8. Diourté Y, Djimdé A, Doumbo O: **Pyrimethamine-sulfadoxine efficacy and selection for mutations in *Plasmodium falciparum* dihydrofolate and dyhydropterate synthetase in Mali.** *Am J Trop Med Hyg* 1999, **60:**475-78.
9. Von Seidlein L, Ouilligan P, Pinder M, Bojang K, Anyalebechi C, Gosling R, Coleman R, Ude JI, Sadiq A, Duraisingh M, Warhust D, Alloueche A, Targett G, McAdam K, Greenwood B, Walraven G, Olliaro P, Doherty T: **Efficacy of artesunate plus pyrimthamine-sulfadoxine for uncomplicated malaria in Gambian children: a double-blind, randomised, controlled trial.** *Lancet* 2000, **355:**352-57.
10. Müller O, Traoré C, Becher H, Kouyaté B: **Malaria morbidity, treatment seeking behaviour, and mortality in a cohort of young children in rural Burkina Faso.** *Trop Med Int Health* 2003, **8:**290-296.
11. Bloland PB, Ettling M, Meek S: **Combination therapy for malaria in Africa: hype or hope?** *Bull World Health Organ* 2000, **78:**1378-88.
12. Winstanley P: **Modern chemotherapeutic options for malaria.** *Lancet Inf Dis* 2001, **1:**242-50.
13. Greenwood B: **Treating malaria in Africa.** *Br Med J* 2004, **328:**534-35.
14. International Artemisinin Study Group: **Artesunate combinations for treatment of malaria: meta-analysis.** *Lancet* 2004, **363:**9-17.
15. Dorsey G, Njama D, Kamya R, Cattamanchi A, Kyabayinze D, Staedke SG, Gasasira A, Rosenthal PJ: **Sulfadoxine/pyrimethamine alone or with amodiaquine or artesunate for treatment of uncomplicated malaria: a longitudinal randomised trial.** *Lancet* 2002, **360:**2031-38.
16. Abacassamo F, Enosse S, Aponte JJ, Gómez-Olivé FX, Quintó L, Mabunda S, Barreto A, Magnussen P, Ronn AM, Thompson R, Alonso PL: **Efficacy of chloroquine, amodiaquine, sulfadoxine-pyrimethamine and combination therapy with artesunate in Mozambican children with non-complicated malaria.** *Trop Med Int Hlth* 2004, **9:**200-08.
17. Goodman CA, Coleman PG, Mills AJ: **The cost-effectiveness of antenatal malaria prevention in sub-Saharan Africa.** *Am J Trop Med Hyg* 2001, **64(1-2 Suppl):**45-56.

3 Epidemiological Studies

HEIKO BECHER[1], GAEL HAMMER[1], GISELA KYNAST-WOLF[1], BOCAR KOUYATÉ[2] AND FLORENT SOME[2]

[1]*University of Heidelberg, Department of Tropical Hygiene and Public Health, Im Neuenheimer Feld 324, 69120 Heidelberg, Germany*

Tel.: +49 6221 565031

Email: Heiko.becher@urz.uni-heidelberg.de

[2]*Centre de Recherche en Santé de Nouna,, BP 02 Nouna, Burkina Faso*

Tel.: +226-20-537043

Email: bocar.crsn@fasonet.bf

3.1 Introduction

During the last five years, in collaboration between CRSN and Heidelberg University, a number of epidemiological studies have been performed, are ongoing, or are in the planning stage. The epidemiologists have benefited from the Nouna DSS, which provides a rich database and is ideally suited as a sampling frame for various epidemiological studies. The DSS procedures for data entry, data checking and data exchange between the partner institutions are described in chapter 1.2.

There are common sequences of epidemiologic research: Often, in a first descriptive part standard measures such as incidence, prevalence and mortality are presented. This is usually followed by an analytical part in which risk factors for total mortality or specific diseases are identified and quantified. However, before epidemiological research is possible, basic conditions have to be fulfilled like, for example, the accessibility to the field. This has been made possible through the setup of the DSS.

A full sequence of this kind has been gone through since the foundation of CRSN: The DSS data had been collected for several years and were waiting for epidemiological analysis. Since data on morbidity and mortality are sparse in developing countries, DSS data provide a valuable source. The description of mortality of the population in space and time was a relevant topic which has been addressed in the joint epidemiologic investigations. Results from these studies are presented in chapters 3.2, 3.4 and 3.5. In a further analytical step, risk factors of childhood mortality were identified and quantified in a paper given in chapter 3.7, and a detailed analysis of malaria morbidity and mortality in a cohort of young children was described in another paper, given in chapter 3.6.

The analysis of the longitudinal DSS data showed a high infant and childhood mortality, comparable to other West African countries.

In the following section, some of the ongoing studies and recent results are outlined.

Ongoing epidemiological studies

Risk factors for childhood mortality in Burkina Faso: a comparison of data from a national survey and information from the Nouna DSS

This investigation is part of the second round of the collaborative research grant SFB 544 described above. In this study, we evaluated the accuracy of data obtained from a Demographic and Health Survey (DHS) with regard to risk factors for childhood mortality, using information gained from the Nouna Demographic Surveillance System (DSS) run by the CRSN. Using birth histories available from the DHS survey Burkina Faso 1998-99, a household survey which was planned to be representative for the whole country, we performed a survival analysis of childhood births in a similar fashion as had already been done for DSS data alone. All live births of the period 1994-98 (n=5953) were taken into account and a distinction was made between urban and rural areas. Similar information (on 12905 children) is available from the Nouna DSS, which now includes a total population of about 60 000 inhabitants. We used all-cause childhood mortality as outcome variable (877 and 932 deaths from DHS and DSS).

A simultaneous estimation of hazard rate ratios by a Cox regression model yields similar estimates for the DHS and DSS data, in line with previous findings. Moreover, we estimate that the mothers of 1.5% of children of the DSS were deceased, thus underreporting of child deaths in DHS surveys is not very high.

These findings demonstrate that, despite some limitations, DHS surveys are broadly comparable to the presumably more precise DSS data, and are therefore a valuable tool for assessing the importance of risk factors for childhood mortality in sub-Saharan Africa. This will help us to investigate new methods of estimating childhood mortality for a whole country, based on DSS data and knowledge about the distribution of the main risk factors.

Seasonal patterns of mortality in the Nouna DSS

Few data exist on the seasonal pattern of mortality in sub-Saharan Africa. Yet age-specific mortality data and these data are both needed to inform health policy and target specific interventions.
We analyzed the mortality data from the Nouna DSS. During the nine-year observation period from 1993 to 2001, a total number of 4098 deaths were recorded in 39 villages with a population of around 32000. We investigated seasonal patterns of mortality by (i) date of death and (ii) date of birth for five different age groups: infants (<1 year), children (1-4), young people (5-14), adults (15-59), and older people >60 years. Calculating age-specific death rates by month of death is straightforward. We assessed the relative effect of each month of death using the floating relative risk method. Additionally, we modeled the seasonal effect with Poisson regression using a sine function with a 12-month period. To investigate the effect of date of birth, we calculated age specific death rates for cohorts born in different months. We applied a method which allows the calculation of a mean in circular distributions to detect date of birth as a mortality indicator.

The crude mortality is 14.5/1000 (95% CI 14.1-15.0). Overall mortality is consistently higher during the dry season (November until May) compared to the rainy season (June until October) (see figure 1). Mortality peaks in the early dry season for all age groups except in infants, where the highest mortality rates are observed around the end of the rainy season. Children aged 1-4 years have an intermediate pattern with highest mortality rates around the end of the rainy season but additionally also during the early dry season. For infants, we found a strong association between being born during the period September to February and mortality.

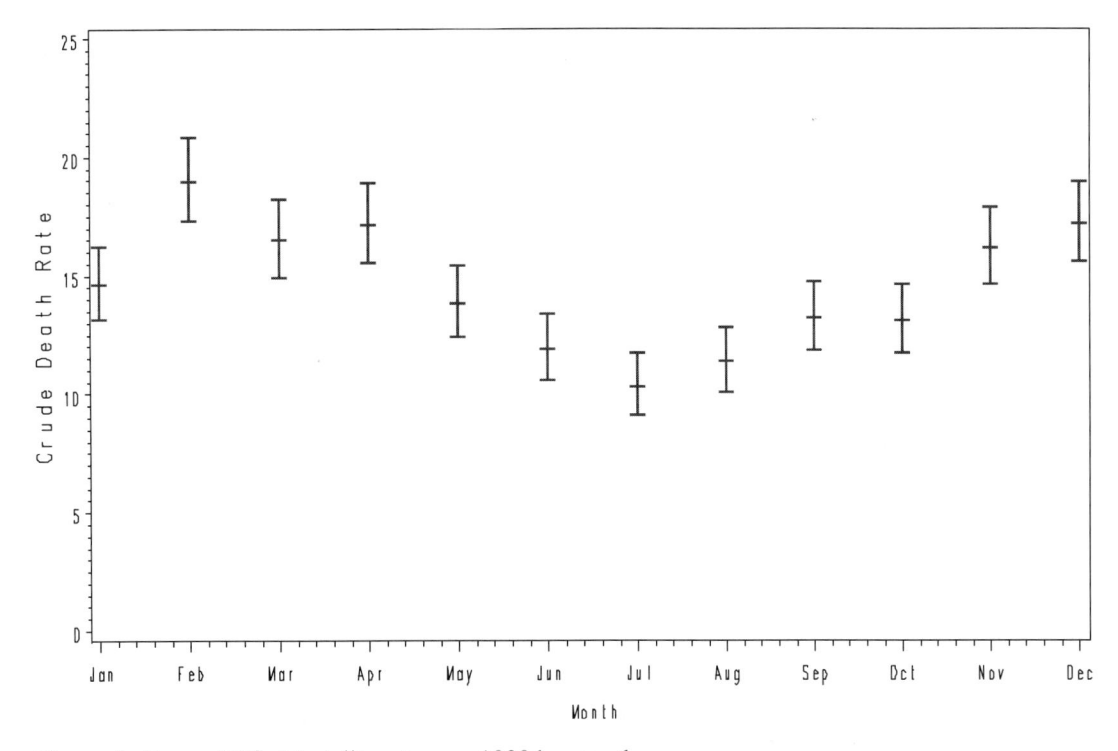

Figure 1: Nouna DSS, Mortality rates per 1000 by month

Infectious diseases and particularly malaria can explain this excess mortality in young children around the end of the rainy season. In contrast, the excess mortality in the other age groups during the early dry season remains largely unexplained. Specific infectious diseases, such as meningitis and pneumonia, are likely to be its main causes. The association between being born around the end of the rainy season and mortality in infant is likely due to malaria deaths in areas of high transmission intensity occurring in the second half of infancy.

Bayesian and GIS mapping of childhood mortality

Various geographic information systems (GIS) are now widely used to map the distribution of diseases and mortality. However, the mapping of raw mortality rates has been found to be inappropriate since it does not account for the spatial heterogeneity of the population at risk. Therefore, Bayesian techniques have been suggested as a solution to the problem.

The original death rates are presented in a map in figure 2.

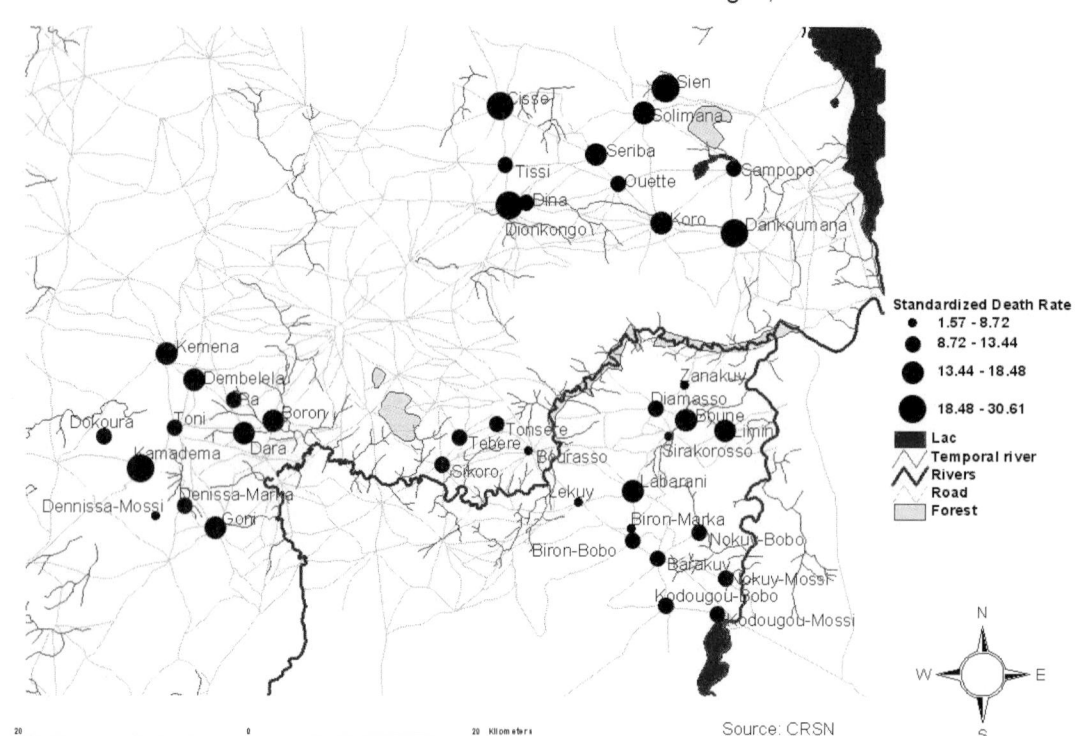

Distribution of Standardized Death Rate in Nouna DSS villages, from 1993 to 1998

Figure 2: Distribution of standardized death rates in the Nouna DSS villages, averaged over the period 1993 to 1998.

We calculated annual mortality rates for each of the 39 villages of the study area using midyear populations of children under five. We then used two mapping techniques. Firstly, we used the GIS software ArcView to map the crude mortality rates. Secondly, we smoothed the data by the method of empirical Bayes estimation. We then made use of the geostatistical prediction method of Kriging to spatially interpolate the data for successive years.

No spatial pattern is identifiable from the circles representing mortality rates drawn on the map using ArcView. The circles are scattered over the study area and comparing annual distributions between them is difficult. The maps produced by the Bayesian technique also do not show a clear spatial trend pattern. However, they indicate the tendency of villages in the north-eastern region to produce higher incidence or risk values, confirming the results of an earlier study reporting a significant cluster of high childhood mortality in that same area.

When drawing maps, estimates of disease incidence/mortality should account for the difference in population density to reflect the distribution of risk. Raw mortality rates should be first multiplied by a factor, in our case 1000, before they are plotted by any GIS approach. The Bayesian smoothing technique addresses the issue of heterogeneity in the population at risk and it we therefore recommend it for explorative mapping of disease/mortality. In this study, we have seen that the Bayesian method is helpful for visual identification of clustering in the northeastern part of the study region.

Mortality of twins and antenatal care

Only few data on child mortality among twins in sub-Saharan Africa exist. We intend to assess the twinning in rural Burkina Faso with respect to prevalence and mortality. Beyond being an important risk factor for maternal and child mortality, multiple pregnancy has also gained attention as a tracer condition for assessing the quality of antenatal screening and referral.

Thus, the comparison of population-based twinning rates and hospital-based twinning rates reflects the effect of antenatal detection and referral and allows assessing the coverage of obstetric care in this high risk group.

We analyzed population-based data (deliveries, life births, deaths) from the Nouna DSS. All births in the period from 1.1.1993 to 31.12.1998 were included and followed up until the 30.04.2002. 9457 deliveries with 9610 life births were recorded in the surveillance area (population 30988 in 1998) in this study period.

In addition, we derived health service data from a document review in health facilities in Nouna District for the years 1994 to 2001. The District Hospital provides obstetric care for the entire district with its 252,000 population (1998).

We estimated age and sex specific mortality risks, both by standard methods and adjusted mortality risks.

Mortality of twins is high with one out of three dying before reaching the age of five years. This is 2.5 times the mortality risk of singletons. Among twins, mortality is particularly high in the neonatal period (RR 5.16; CI: 3.6 – 7.5) and in twins born to mothers above the age of 35 (RR 5.12; CI: 3.5 – 7.6). The overall population-based twinning rate is 1.6 % (CI: 1.4 - 1.9), compared to a hospital-based twinning rate of 2.8% (CI: 2.2-3.1). Still, most twins (90.5%) were delivered outside a hospital setting. The high neonatal mortality in twins points to the need for special care in pregnancy, childbirth and post partum. Maternity services fail to cover adequately the vast majority of multiple pregnancies.

From epidemiologic research to action: An example

In the final section of this chapter we briefly describe the sequence of action that led from a descriptive epidemiological study to a project in a particular village in the DSS study area.

The analysis of the DSS data showed that infant and childhood mortality in the Nouna region is high, comparable to most countries in Sub-Saharan Africa. However, a closer scrutiny of the data showed that there is a considerable variation in the mortality rates between the 39 villages within the DSS. Using advanced techniques to analyse spatial and time-spatial patterns, we found that the north-east part of the study region had a significantly increased mortality compared to the rest (see chapter 3.2). One particular village, Cissé, had an extremely high death rate for all years within the observation period 1993-1998, with a peak yearly childhood mortality rate of 138.5 per 1000.

To investigate the reasons for this alarming finding, we did the following: We visited the village for a direct inspection of the local living conditions, and we performed a case-control study in which families from Cissé and another village with comparably low childhood mortality were included. Families with a recent death of a child formed the cases, and families with a surviving child of comparable age formed the controls. Case and control families were interviewed on several factors (lifestyle, nutrition etc.) suspected to be related with childhood mortality. From another clinical study (chapter 2.2) which also included children from Cissé, it was found that the children from that village had a significantly lower weight than children from other villages.

While the case-control study – which was not very large – gave some indication on risk factors, the prevalence of these was not that different in both villages as to explain the observed difference in mortality. The visit of the village, however, showed that the water supply in Cissé was worse than in other villages.

A little later a charity organisation was founded in Heidelberg called "Friends of Nouna". The city of Heidelberg as well as several companies were successfully approached to collect funds for projects which may be useful to improve living conditions in the Nouna DSS area. In a local meeting with representatives of the village Cissé and the Friends of Nouna, projects were discussed and it was decided to build a new well in Cissé and to improve the hygienic conditions of the existing wells. In the beginning of 2004, the digging of the well reached ground water in a depth of 38 meters, and the finalisation of the construction was in Summer 2004. In a small ceremony, the well will finally be "opened" in parallel to the symposium to celebrate the 5th anniversary of the CRSN.

3.2 Clustering of childhood mortality in rural Burkina Faso

SANKOH OA, YE Y, SAUERBORN R, MÜLLER O, BECHER H

Int J Epidemiol. 2001 Jun; 30(3):485-92

Reprinted with permission from Oxford University Press

Clustering of childhood mortality in rural Burkina Faso

Osman A Sankoh,[a] Yazoumé Yé,[b] Rainer Sauerborn,[a] Olaf Müller[a] and Heiko Becher[a]

Background	Childhood mortality is a major public health problem in sub-Saharan Africa. For the implementation of efficient public health systems, knowledge of the spatial distribution of mortality is required.
Methods	Data from a demographic surveillance research project were analysed which comprised information obtained for about 30 000 individuals from 39 villages in northwest Burkina Faso (West Africa) in the period 1993–1998. Total childhood mortality rates were calculated and the geographical distribution of total childhood mortality was investigated. In addition, data from a cohort of 686 children sampled from 16/39 of the villages followed up during a randomized controlled trial in 1999 were also used to validate the results from the surveillance data. A spatial scan statistic was used to test for clusters of total childhood mortality in both space and time.
Results	Several statistically significant clusters of higher childhood mortality rates comprising different sets of villages were identified; one specific village was consistently identified in both study populations indicating non-random distribution of childhood mortality. Potential risk factors which were available in the database (ethnicity, religion, distance to nearest health centre) did not explain the spatial pattern.
Conclusion	The findings indicate non-random clustering of total childhood mortality in the study area. The study may be regarded as a first step in prioritizing areas for follow-up public health efforts.
Keywords	Childhood mortality, clustering, demographic surveillance, spatio-temporal analysis
Accepted	15 February 2001

In the developing world, morbidity and mortality continue to show a pattern characterized by high childhood mortality, mainly due to infectious diseases. The World Health Organization[1] states that 'despite the extraordinary advances of the 20th century, a significant component of the burden of illness globally still remains attributable to infectious diseases …' It therefore states the need to develop more effective health systems as one of the challenges to be addressed in order to improve the world's health. 'The goal must be to create health systems that can: improve health status; reduce health inequalities; enhance responsiveness to legitimate expectations; increase efficiency; protect individuals, families and communities from financial loss; and enhance fairness in the financing and delivery of health care'.

Until now, there is no routine registration of births and deaths in most of the developing world. Information on basic demographic measures often stems from demographic surveillance systems (DSS). Usually, these systems are based on initial census of a population of limited size, often in the order of some ten thousands of individuals, followed by an active follow-up in which births, deaths, in- and out-migration are recorded. Active follow-up consists of information from specific community informants or regular house-to-house visits to the respective population at which events in the period since the preceding visit are obtained.

The development and evaluation of effective programmes to reduce the burden of disease requires a detailed knowledge of disease or mortality distribution and causal pathways. This knowledge could be derived from analytical epidemiological

---

[a] Department of Tropical Hygiene and Public Health, University of Heidelberg Medical School, Heidelberg, Germany.

[b] Centre de Recherche en Santé de Nouna (CRSN), BP 02, Nouna, Burkina Faso.

Correspondence: Prof. Heiko Becher, Department of Tropical Hygiene and Public Health, University of Heidelberg Medical School, Im Neuenheimer Feld 324, D-69120 Heidelberg, Germany. E-mail: heiko.becher@urz.uni-heidelberg.de

studies that use as a platform large-scale health surveys and the above described demographic surveillance systems (DSS) in which causal relationships between risk factors and diseases or mortality are investigated. Benzler and Sauerborn[2] recommend that in cases where general population-wide intervention programmes are too expensive to implement, it is necessary to limit such programmes to high risk units where certain adverse health effects are more likely to occur. Therefore, investigating whether the distribution of adverse health outcomes in a population are either random or not should be an important primary objective before starting a programme for primary and secondary prevention of infectious diseases. It is necessary to determine whether there are clusters where adverse health outcomes seem to aggregate. If this is the case, there is need to identify the causes of such clustering, to enable local health personnel to identify them by means of simplified scores, and to develop specific health care strategies targeted at these clusters.

Statistical methodology to identify disease clusters is under constant development. A general review of clustering methods is provided by Hertz-Piciotto[3] and examples of specific applications are given by Hjalmars et al.,[4] Britton,[5] Kulldorff et al.[6] and Kulldorff.[7] In this paper we employ the Kulldorff spatial scan statistic[8] for the identification of and testing for clusters of childhood mortality.

The paper is organized as follows: First, we describe the main characteristics of the DSS population on which most of the analyses are based. We then describe the study population from a controlled trial[9] which turned out to be useful for supporting the findings and give an outline of the statistical methods used. Following the results we discuss our findings in the light of immediate and future impact on public health and their possible limitations.

Study populations

Geographical description

The study area is within the rural province of Kossi in northwest Burkina Faso with the town of Nouna as its administrative headquarters (Figure 1). Burkina Faso is a landlocked country in West Africa with an estimated gross domestic product (GDP) per capita purchasing power parity of $1000 (CIA[10]), and an estimated cumulative mortality rate up to age 5 years of 182 for males and 172 for females (World Health Report[11]). The population is about 11 million (1997), with 56% children under 15 years, and an annual population growth rate of 2.6%. The country is predominantly rural; about 80% of the population live in rural areas. The rural provinces have an inadequate health delivery system compared to the urban areas.

With an area of 7464.44 km^2, Kossi province has a population of 240 000 and a population density of 32 inhabitants per square kilometre. Of the population, 50.16% are female and 49.84% male. In all, 18.7% of the population are projected to be children aged 0–5 years in 2000.

The DSS population

The DSS in rural Burkina Faso comprises the entire population of 39 villages with approximately 30 000 people and approximately 4800 households within the province of Kossi. The villages are in the catchment area of three dispensaries with attached maternity clinics staffed by a nurse and a midwife. In 1992, the first census was carried out. A control census was held in 1993, and a further complete census was held in 1998. Since 1992 Vital Events Registrations (VEE) have been carried out through the visits of trained interviewers to each village. These interviewers ask three key informants if any deaths, births or in- and out-migration have occurred in the preceding month since the previous visit.[12] In the VEE, births, deaths and migrations were recorded with the cause of death determined by verbal autopsy according to the method of Anker et al.[13] The database for this paper included a follow-up of the population until 31 December 1998.

Randomized controlled trial cohort

In June 1999, a cohort of 686 children aged 6–31 months in a subsample of the DSS study villages was enrolled for a randomized placebo-controlled trial on zinc supplementation in which a possible effect on frequency of malaria episodes was investigated.[9] Children for the study were recruited from 16 out of 39 study villages (blocks of 30 and 60 children randomly sampled from small and big villages respectively), and prospectively followed up for a period of 6 months through daily household visits. Information on deaths was recorded during this trial. The data of this study are used here for the purpose of validating the results from the DSS database.

Statistical methods

Mortality ratios for the DSS data

We calculated the childhood death rates (DR) by village i, $i = 1,...,39$ for years j, $j = 1993,...,1998$ using $DR_{ij} = \frac{d_{ij}}{n_{ij}}$ where n_{ij} denotes the midyear population of children aged 0–4 years in village i at year j, and d_{ij} the corresponding observed number of deaths. In order to identify villages in which the death rate was significantly above average, an exact 95% CI for each rate was based on the Poisson distribution of the observed number of deaths.[14] A rate was considered significantly above average if the overall rate of the respective year was below the lower value of the confidence interval of the village rate, a procedure commonly used in descriptive epidemiology.[15] An overall temporal trend in rates was analysed by applying a Poisson regression model of the form $d_{ij} = \log(n_{ij}) + \mu + \beta \cdot j$ where $i = 1,...,39$, $j = 1993, 1994,...,1998$ and tested for $H_0 : \beta = 0$[16] using the software package EGRET.[17]

Method to investigate disease clustering

As briefly outlined in the introduction, several methods for disease cluster analysis have been suggested. We chose the Kulldorff spatial scan statistic[8] in which the spatial distribution of the population is taken into consideration as follows.

A circular window is imposed on a map by the spatial scan statistic and it allows the centre of the circle to move across the study region. For any given position of the centre, the radius of the circle changes continuously so that it can take any value between zero and some upper limit. The circle is therefore able to include different sets of neighbouring villages. A village is captured if it lies in the circle.

The method creates a set containing an infinite number of distinct circles. Each of these circles could contain a different set of neighbouring villages and each of the circles is a potential cluster of childhood mortality in the Kossi study area. For each circle, the spatial scan statistic calculates the likelihood of observing the observed number of cases inside and outside the circle. The circle with the maximum likelihood is defined as the most likely cluster, implying that it is least likely to have occurred by chance. For each circle, the method tests the null hypothesis against the alternative hypothesis that there is at least one circle for which the underlying risk of mortality is higher inside the circle as compared to outside. Generally, the method tests the null hypothesis that the risk of children dying is the same in all villages in the study area.

Let N be the total number of deaths in the study area, n the observed number of deaths within the circle, and λ the expected number of deaths in the circle under the null hypothesis. Let the number of deaths in each village follow a Poisson distribution. Hence the likelihood ratio for a specific circle is therefore proportional to

$$\frac{L_A(D)}{L_0} \propto \left(\frac{n}{\lambda}\right)^n \left(\frac{N-n}{N-\lambda}\right)^{N-n} I(n > \lambda), \quad (1)$$

where $L_A(D)$ is the likelihood under the alternative hypothesis that there is a cluster of elevated annual mortality rates in age group 0–4 in a specific circle D, L_0 is the likelihood under the null hypothesis, and I is an indicator function that is equal to 1 when the circle has more deaths than expected under the null hypothesis, and 0 otherwise. Maximizing (1) over all circles results in the one that constitutes the most likely mortality cluster. The test statistic is

$$\max_D \frac{L_A(D)}{L_0} \quad (2)$$

Kulldorff[8] has derived the likelihood ratio test and provided the properties of the test statistic. We have used SaTScan 2.1[18] to perform the calculations. The P-value of the statistic is obtained through Monte Carlo hypothesis testing, where the null hypothesis of no clusters is rejected at an α level of 0.05 exactly if the simulated P-value is ≤ 0.05 for the most likely cluster. The program gives the most likely cluster with the corresponding P-value. If other clusters not overlapping with the most likely cluster are identified, these are also given by the program with their corresponding P-values. We applied this method both to the DSS population (each year separately) and to the zinc study population.

Kulldorff et al.[4] have extended the spatial scan statistic into a space-time scan statistic. In this case, the window imposed on the study area by the statistic is cylindrical with a circular geographical base and with height corresponding to time. The centre of the base is one of several possible centroids located throughout the study area and the height reflects any possible time interval. The cylindrical window is then moved in space and time. This was applied to the DSS data for the time window 1993–1998.

Results

The focus of this section is on the results from the DSS data. As noted earlier, the results from the randomized control cohort study are used here to validate the results from the DSS database.

The DSS population

Table 1 provides summary data for all 39 villages in the study area. The average yearly death rate (per 1000) for children under 5 for the 6-year period was 35. This corresponds to a cumulative rate up to age 5 years of $1-\exp(-5 \times 0.035) = 0.16$ which is close to the estimated country-wide rate reported by the WHO. There is a decline towards the end of the observation period. We investigated whether there is a trend in the rates. Using the full observation period, no significant trend was observed. However, considering the possibility of some under-reporting of deaths in the first year (1993) of observation which may have resulted in the course of establishing the field procedures, we omitted the first year from the analysis and found a highly significant decreasing trend in mortality ($P < 0.001$).

Table 2 shows crude death rates (per 1000) per year for each of the 39 villages in Kossi province (ordered according to the population size in the villages).

We calculated the death rates (per 1000) per year for each of the 39 villages in Kossi province and the confidence intervals for the rates. We then checked whether or not these contained the overall average. In the second column of Table 2 are mean midyear populations of children under 5 years old. Although there was some variation in the number of children within a village over the years, the population between the villages differed up to a factor of about 15. The variation in rates in almost all the villages can mainly be attributed to chance. An exception is the village of Cissé which has rates significantly above average in the last three years of the observation period (1996–1998). The fact that these rates for Cissé appeared consistent for consecutive years gives a first hint that chance alone cannot explain these patterns. The following analysis further strengthens this point.

Space and space-time scan statistic results of the DSS population

Table 3 presents the results of the purely spatial analysis scanning for high rates using the Poisson model for 1993 to1998. No statistically significant cluster was identified for 1993. A statistically significant cluster ($P = 0.0051$) comprised of

Table 1 Total childhood mortality in the study area. (Summary data for all 39 villages.) Demographic surveillance systems study population

	1993	1994	1995	1996	1997	1998	Total (1993–1998)
Total no. of deaths	151	195	172	204	147	162	1031
Midyear population children <5	4720	4786	4899	4840	4895	5323	29 463
Death rate (per 1000)	35.0	44.7	38.6	46.2	32.8	33.5	35.0
95% CI[a]	29.91–40.11	38.94–50.38	33.37–43.87	40.38–51.94	27.96–37.66	28.78–38.16	32.89–37.09

[a] Based on normal approximation.

Table 2 Total childhood mortality in 39 villages in the Kossi province. Demographic surveillance systems study population

Name of village	Total no. of deaths	Mean population size[a]	Death Rate (per 1000)					
			1993	1994	1995	1996	1997	1998
Goni	86	405	52.6	36.8	43.3	43.8	12.2	24.2
Koro	73	319	36.7	41.3	41.0	56.8	19.5	26.0
Kemena	72	310	40.8	19.4	28.2	48.8	60.6	33.3
Toni	34	255	10.5	15.0	19.5	41.0	34.2	16.5
Kamadema	64	244	50.3	79.4	55.6	71.7	64.3	60.6
Bourasso	40	237	33.5	30.2	40.4	23.5	17.0	26.4
Solimana	47	230	37.2	63.1	39.5	31.0	13.5	60.4
Kodougou-B	32	194	5.0	20.4	19.3	58.2	17.4	40.6
Nokuy-Bobo	35	189	11.2	31.4	25.1	55.0	34.1	29.1
Ouette	31	166	6.6	85.5	55.9	5.8	23.7	15.5
Sobon	42	161	41.4	73.8	40.0	25.2	59.8	43.0
Seriba	42	150	68.8	50.0	45.8	50.7	20.0	43.5
Pa	40	141	22.2	44.8	58.4	53.7	35.7	6.6
Sikoro	18	137	14.6	15.2	6.6	78.7	8.1	13.4
Cissé	76	135	80.7	51.9	69.9	**138.5**	**131.8**	**80.5**
Tissi	16	133	15.9	37.0	23.6	37.0	0.0	22.6
Lekuy	13	126	15.4	31.8	23.1	32.5	17.0	7.9
Sampopo	18	109	29.1	56.6	19.4	9.3	26.1	25.0
Dionkongo	33	107	46.3	75.5	77.8	46.7	26.8	42.4
Labarani	25	104	86.2	**120.0**	27.3	19.4	29.4	26.3
Dankoumana	28	90	13.7	68.5	68.2	93.0	40.8	37.4
Boune	27	86	76.1	75.0	66.7	34.5	74.1	11.4
Tebere	14	84	0.0	40.5	12.4	22.7	32.3	52.1
Biron-Marka	6	83	11.6	11.8	11.5	12.2	0.0	12.4
Dennissa-M	3	83	0.0	25.6	0.0	12.2	0.0	0.0
Barakuy	6	81	0.0	0.0	11.4	11.4	26.0	24.1
Boron	14	73	50.0	30.3	54.8	0.0	25.3	23.8
Dembelela	12	67	29.4	29.0	27.8	31.8	33.9	28.2
Dokoura	12	59	55.6	50.0	0.0	31.8	50.9	17.9
Tonsere	12	56	40.0	40.0	18.2	17.9	67.8	31.8
Diamasso	6	52	20.4	0.0	18.9	62.5	0.0	17.9
Limini	7	51	21.3	20.4	40.0	37.0	0.0	18.5
Denissa-Marka	6	40	45.5	0.0	54.1	0.0	0.0	0.0
Sirakorosso	2	33	0.0	27.8	0.0	27.8	0.0	0.0
Zanakuy	1	31	0.0	0.0	0.0	0.0	33.3	0.0
Dina	5	26	41.7	41.7	41.7	0.0	37.0	32.3
Lei	4	25	0.0	40.0	95.2	0.0	0.0	31.3
Sien	5	24	0.0	55.6	43.5	90.9	0.0	29.4
Biron-Bobo	3	17	0.0	0.0	100.0	0.0	0.0	0.0
OVERALL		4911	35.0	44.67	38.6	46.2	32.8	33.5

Bold numbers indicate mortality rates significantly ($P \leq 0.05$) above average in the respective year.

[a] Arithmetic mean of midyear populations.

Villages in bold print were selected for the Zinc Study.

the census areas of 15 villages including Cissé and Labarani was identified for 1994. In all 106 cases of childhood mortality were observed (78.2 expected) and the cluster had a relative risk of 1.4. No statistically significant cluster was identified for 1995. For 1996 the identified statistically significant cluster ($P < 0.001$) comprises the village of Cissé; 18 childhood mortality cases were observed (5.5 expected) with a high relative risk of 3.3. Cissé was also identified as a statistically significant cluster ($P < 0.001$) for 1997 (17 childhood mortality cases observed, 3.9 expected, overall relative risk 4.4). A significant second cluster ($P < 0.001$) was identified for 1997. This cluster comprises seven villages (61 cases observed, 37.4 expected, relative risk 1.6). For 1998, the statistically significant cluster ($P < 0.001$) identified comprises the census areas of five villages including Cissé and Solimana (37 cases observed, 18 expected, relative risk of 2.0).

The scan statistic was thereafter applied to perform a spatio-temporal analysis. The results are presented in Table 4. It is seen

Table 3 Total childhood mortality in Kossi province for 1993–1998 using purely spatial analysis scanning for high rates; Demographic surveillance system study population

Year	Type	Location	Cases	Expected	Relative risk	P-value
1993	Most likely	Lei, Sien, Solimana Seriba, **Cissé**	29	17.6	1.7	0.26
1994	Most likely	Dankouma, Sampopo, Koro, Ouette, Zanakuy, Sien, Boune, Limini, Sirakorosso, Dina, Dionkongo, Tissi, Lei, **Cissé**, Labarani	106	78.2	1.4	**0.01**
1995	Most likely	Sampopo, Dankouma, Koro, Sien, Ouette, Lei, Seriba, Dina, Solimana, Dionkongo, Tissi, **Cissé**, Diamasso, Boune, Limini	79	62.0	1.3	0.31
1996	Most likely	**Cissé**	18	5.5	3.3	**<0.001**
1997	Most likely	**Cissé**	17	3.9	4.4	**<0.001**
	Secondary	Toni, Dembelela, Kamadema, Pa, Sobon, Dokoura, Kemena	61	37.4	1.6	**<0.001**
1998	Most likely	Lei, Sien, Solimana, Seriba, **Cissé**	37	18.4	2.0	**<0.001**

Table 4 Total childhood mortality in Kossi province for 1993–1998 using space-time analysis scanning for high rates; Demographic surveillance system study population

Type	Location	Time frame	Cases	Expected	Relative risk	P-value
Most likely	Cissé	1996–1998	47	14.4	3.3	<0.001
Secondary	Kamadema	1994–1996	48	24.2	2.0	0.02

that the village of Cissé was identified as a statistically significant cluster ($P < 0.001$) for the period covering 1996–1998 (47 cases observed, 14.4 expected, overall relative risk for this period 3.3). The identified statistically significant secondary clusters were the village of Kamadema ($P = 0.02$) for the 1994–1996 period (48 cases, 25.2 expected, relative risk 2.0).

Since the village of Cissé was consistently identified as belonging to clusters of significantly higher childhood mortality, we decided to omit this village and apply the statistic again. Only the following two statistically significant clusters were identified. For 1994, a significant cluster ($P = 0.01$) included the villages of Dankoumana, Sampopo, Koro, Ouette, Zanakuy, Sien, Seriba, Solimana, Diamasso, Boune, Limini, Sirakorosso, Dina, Dionkongo, Tissi, Lei and Labarani (97 cases, 71.2 expected, overall relative risk 1.3). This is the northwestern region of the study area to which Cissé also belongs. For 1997, a significant cluster ($P < 0.001$) included the villages of Kenema, Dembelela, Toni, Pa, Sobon, Dakoura and Kamadema (61 cases, 34.0 expected, overall relative risk 1.8). This cluster has also been identified as a secondary cluster in the first analysis. For all other years, no significant clusters were found. In Figure 1 the clusters are displayed.

The results after omitting Cissé show that the significant cluster in 1994 remains unaffected (the same villages except Cissé form a cluster, $P = 0.01$). For 1995 and 1996 no significant cluster was identified. For 1997 the previously identified secondary cluster was identified. For 1998 the previously identified cluster except Cissé (Solimana, Sien, Seriba) was again identified, however not significant ($P = 0.1$). These results show that while Cissé seems to be the village with the strongest increase in mortality, the whole subregion appears to be conspicuous.

The scan statistic was also applied to scan for clusters of significantly lower mortality. No such cluster was identified. This may provide a good evidence of no systematic under-reporting in certain villages versus others.

The DSS database provides information on some other variables possibly linked to childhood mortality. In particular, we investigated the variables 'distance to next health centre', 'religion' and 'ethnicity'. The increased risk for children in Cissé appeared to be independent of these factors: The nearest health centre to Cissé is 18 km away, only slightly above average for all villages (range: 0–34 km, mean 11.3 km). The predominant ethnic group in Cissé is the Peulh in contrast to the surrounding villages. However, the Peulh have an overall childhood mortality which is below average. The most frequent religion in Cissé is Islam (94.3% in Cissé, 60.5% in the total study region). However, the overall mortality in Muslims is below average. Thus, all these factors do not explain the increased risk.

The randomized controlled trial cohort

Table 5 shows the data from the Zinc study. We observed 17 deaths in the observation period, which corresponds to a mortality rate of 57 per 1000 person-years (95% CI: 32.7–89.3). We did not distinguish between treatment and placebo groups because (1) zinc supplement was not shown to have an effect on malaria mortality or morbidity and (2) the randomization unit was the child and not the village. This is higher than the rate for the age group 0–4 in the total DSS population, which may partly be explained by the lower age of this cohort. In all, 13 out of the 17 deaths are concentrated in the two villages in the study area (Cissé [7 deaths] and Solimana [6 deaths]).

Space scan statistic results of the randomized controlled trial cohort
Using data from the Zinc study shown in Table 5, a purely spatial analysis scanning for high rates was carried out. The statistically significant most likely cluster ($P < 0.001$) of childhood mortality identified comprises the villages of Cissé, Tissi, Dionkongo, Sériba and Solimana (14 cases recorded, 5.7 expected). The cluster has a high relative risk of 2.4. All the five

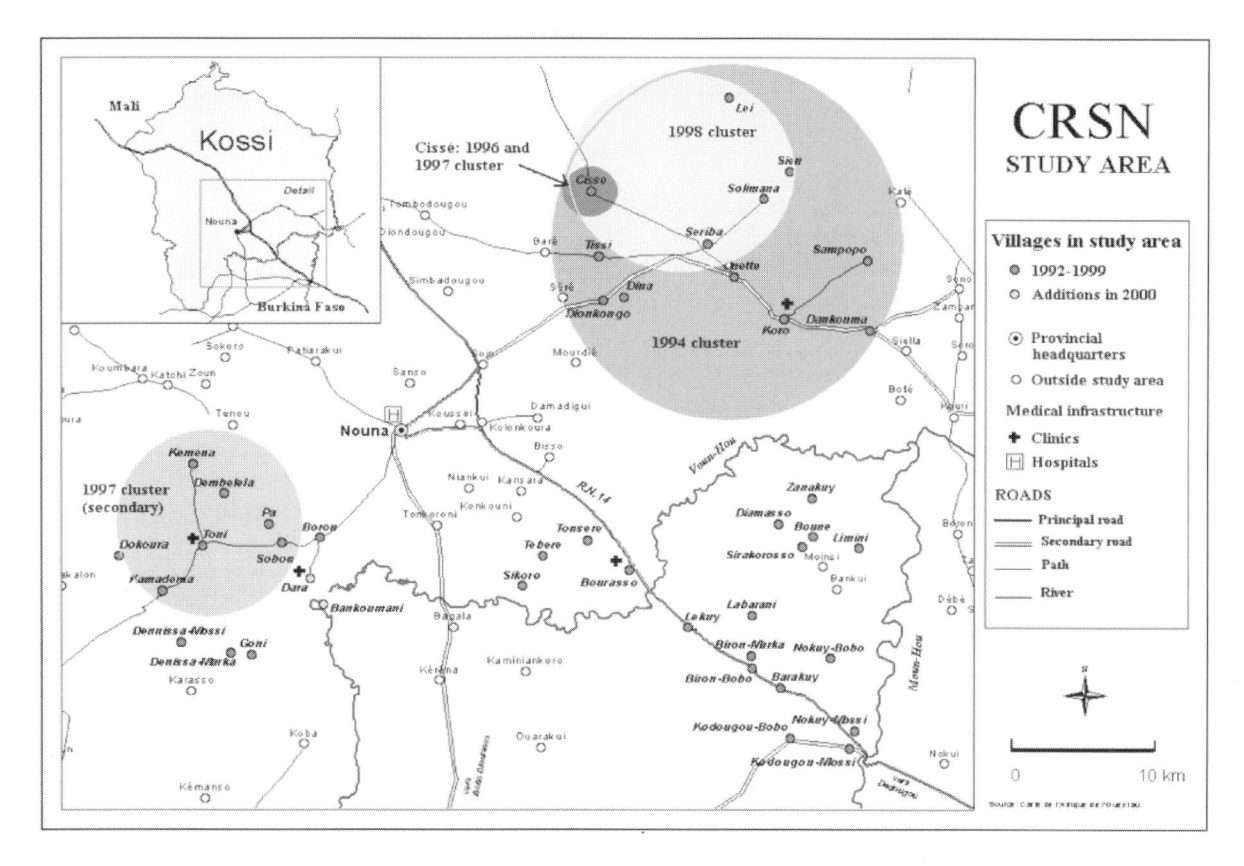

Figure 1 Map of study area showing location of significant clusters of higher total childhood mortality rates in 1994, 1996, 1997 and 1998

Table 5 Study population and number of deaths by village. Randomized controlled trial cohort

Name of village	No. died during study period	Total no. of children in the study
Biron Marka	0	26
Bourasso	0	59
Cissé	7	60
Dankoumana	0	29
Dionkongo	1	30
Kodougou Bobo	0	57
Koro	0	55
Labarani	0	30
Nokuy Bobo	2	53
Ouette	0	30
Sampopo	0	30
Seriba	0	60
Sikoro	0	57
Solimana	6	52
Tebere	1	29
Tissi	0	29
OVERALL	17	686

villages are located in the northeastern part of the study area and are close to each other (Figure 1).

Discussion

Data from this DSS have been collected since 1993, and many efforts have been made to provide as complete and accurate a database as possible. For example, in order to minimize errors in data collection, interviewers use pre-printed database registration forms. Three field supervisors examine the questionnaires in the field to check if the data collected by the interviewer makes sense. Among several steps, the supervisors take a sample of the completed questionnaires and return to the households to verify the information they contain.

However, irrespective of the above efforts, the conditions for data collection in rural parts of developing countries have their limitations. It is not possible to achieve a record of all deaths. The question is whether underreporting of cases or other incomplete recording of events (birth, in- and out-migration) could have had an impact on our results. If, for example, in several villages a constant underreporting of cases had occurred, this would have an immediate effect on our results. Although we cannot rule out the possibility that some infant deaths remained unreported, we do not have evidence of differential underreporting of cases between the villages. The non-existence of clusters with significantly lower total childhood mortality in the study area indicates that there was no systematic underreporting in some villages.

The following characteristics hold in the whole study region and not specifically in some parts of it: (1) the death rates obtained from the DSS are well within the order of magnitude expected, when compared with other DSS results (e.g. Bergane et al.[19]). (2) The interviewers who visited the villages and collected the information were well trained according to standardized procedures. (3) The information used in this paper was total mortality only, rather than cause-specific mortality. The latter was much more difficult to obtain from the data set with sufficient reliability, as the causes of death were basically obtained by verbal autopsy from the mother, and it is often difficult to decide on a particular cause of death from that information. In several cases, the cause of death is unknown. However, the majority of cases included in this analysis were from infectious diseases (malaria, diarrhoea), often in combination with malnutrition. As an immediate consequence from our findings, a qualitative study is underway with the aim to scrutinize possible causal factors with in-depth interviews.

Using the method for analysing temporal trend described above, we found a significant decrease in childhood mortality over the observation period when omitting the birth year (1992) from the analysis. However, this was a data-driven procedure as the rate for 1993 was found to be considerably lower than in the years after. Therefore, the significant finding of a decreased trend must be considered as a trend rather than a definite finding, and more years of observation are needed before one can conclude that the childhood mortality in the DSS catchment area is decreasing significantly.

In the study by Benzler and Sauerborn[2] which used the main components of the DSS in Nouna, several attributes of newborns and households were used as potential predictors of childhood death in a cohort of 1367 newborn children in the study area from 1992 to 1994. The authors found an average mortality rate of 6.8% per year. However, specific patterns of death rates by village have not been reported in their analysis.

In our study we analysed the DSS data as to a possible spatial-temporal pattern of mortality. The result of a very pronounced cluster of higher rates with the centre of the cluster being the village of Cissé is rather alarming. This finding is supported by the results from the randomized controlled trial described above as in this trial excess mortality was again observed in the village of Cissé. Thus, we strongly believe that our finding on clustering of total childhood mortality in the Nouna region is indeed real and not due to systematic bias. We looked at the distribution of exact date of death, in particular in the village of Cissé, to look for seasonal peaks in mortality. We found a surprisingly uniform distribution over the years which does not support the hypothesis that an infectious disease outbreak has occurred causing the excess mortality.

A possible drawback of the analysis using the Kulldorff method is that clusters are defined as circles. This feature has some implications which must be considered in the interpretation of the results: (1) if a village with low mortality is surrounded by villages with high mortality, it is always included in the cluster although some characteristics of this village may be different than the others; and (2) if a clustering of cases is, say, along a river, a circle is not the appropriate form to detect it. The first feature can be observed in the analysis of the controlled trial cohort, where the two villages with high numbers of deaths are surrounded by others in which no deaths or only one death was recorded. By construction of the test statistic, all these were also included in the cluster identified.

This study may be regarded as a first step in prioritizing areas for analytical studies. In general, malnutrition, malaria, diarrhoea, measles, and acute respiratory infections remain the major causes of childhood disease and death in most of rural Africa.[20] Childhood mortality is also on the increase in many parts of Africa, partly due to the consequences of the AIDS epidemic and partly due to increasing resistance of malaria parasites to the main first-line therapy drug chloroquine.[21] Although little is known about the prevalence of HIV in the Nouna study area, there is little evidence today to suggest that HIV/AIDS contributes much to childhood mortality in rural Kossi province.

Studies in other parts of Africa have documented significant space-time clustering of malaria. For instance, Snow et al.[22] report a space-time clustering of severe childhood malaria on the Coast of Kenya with seasonal peaks in incidence of severe malaria comprising discrete mini-epidemics. Similar studies on the microepidemiology of malaria are now underway in the Nouna study area, and the results are likely to help us better understand the observed clustering of mortality in the area. There is some evidence that the cultural pattern of hygiene and health-seeking behaviour contributing to the observed differences in health outcomes (Müller, unpublished results) in the Nouna study area.

Acknowledgements

This work was supported by the Deutsche Forschungsgemeinschaft, SFB 544 'Control of tropical infectious diseases'. The authors would like to thank Dr Martin Kulldorff (National Cancer Institute, Bethesda, MD, USA) for his advice and for providing the SaTScan software, Ralf Würthwein at the University of Heidelberg, and anonymous referees for their helpful comments. We also thank Ms Gabriele Stieglbauer at the University of Heidelberg for her assistance in preparing the data set for the analysis. Last but not least the authors would like to thank the people from the Nouna study area, both the villagers and the field staff, for their indefatigable contribution to our data collection.

KEY MESSAGES
- A demographic surveillance system in a rural area in Burkina Faso provides data for childhood mortality analysis (1993–1998).
- The spatial scan statistic was used to identify spatial and space-time clustering of childhood mortality.
- Regions of different sizes, however, always including one particular village with significantly increased mortality, were identified.
- Data from a controlled trial which included this particular village showed a similar result.
- Available demographic and other variables (e.g. ethnicity, religion) did not explain the finding.

References

[1] World Health Organization. *The World Health Report 1999—Making a Difference.* Geneva, 1999.

[2] Benzler J, Sauerborn R. Rapid risk household screening by neonatal arm circumference. Results from a cohort study in Burkina Faso. *Trop Med Int Health* 1998;**3**:962–74.

[3] Hertz-Piciotto I. Environmental epidemiology. In: Rothman KJ, Greenland S (eds). *Modern Epidemiology, 2nd Edn.* Lippincott-Raven, 1998, pp.555–84.

[4] Hjalmars U, Kulldorff M, Gustafsson G, Nagarwalla N. Childhood leukemia in Sweden: Using GIS and a spatial scan statistic for cluster detection. *Stat Med* 1996;**15**:707–15.

[5] Britton T. Tests to detect clustering of infected individuals within families. *Biometrics* 1997;**53**:98–109.

[6] Kulldorff M, Athas WF, Feuer EJ, Miller BA, Key CR. Evaluating luster alarms: a space-time scan statistic and brain cancer in Los Alamos, New Mexico. *Am J Public Health* 1998;**88**:1377–80.

[7] Kulldorff M. Statistical evaluation of disease cluster alarms. In: Lawson AB *et al.* (eds). *Disease Mapping and Risk Assessment for Public Health.* John Wiley & Sons Ltd, 1999.

[8] Kulldorff M. A spatial scan statistic. *Communications in Statistics—Theory and Methods* 1997;**26**:1481–96.

[9] Müller O, Becher H, Baltussen A *et al.* Effect of zinc supplementation on malaria morbidity in Westafrican children: A randomized double-blind placebo-controlled trial. *BMJ* (In Press), 2001.

[10] Central Intelligence Agency (CIA). *The World Factbook 2000.* http://www.odci.gov/cia/publications/factbook/index.html

[11] World Health Organization. *Statistics World Health Report 2000.* http://www.who.int/whr/2000/en/statistics.htm

[12] Sauerborn R, Berman P, Nougtara A. Age bias, but not gender bias, in the intra-household resource allocation for health care in rural Burkina Faso. *Health Transit Rev* 1996;**6**:131–45.

[13] Anker M, Black RE, Coldham C *et al.* Verbal *Autopsy Method for Investigating Causes of Death in Infants and Children.* Geneva: World Health Organization, 1999.

[14] Estève J, Benhamou E, Raymond L. *Statistical Methods in Cancer Research, Vol. IV, Descriptive Epidemiology.* International Agency for Research on Cancer (IARC), Lyon, France, 1994.

[15] Pickle LW, Mason TJ, Howard N, Hoover RR, Fraumeni JF. *Atlas of US Cancer Mortality among Whites: 1950–1980.* DHHS Publication No (NIH) 87–2900, 1987.

[16] dos Santos Silva, I. *Cancer Epidemiology: Principles and Methods.* International Agency for Research on Cancer (IARC), Lyon, 1999.

[17] *EGRET Reference Manual, Rev. 4.* Cytel Software Corporation, 1997.

[18] Kulldorff M, Rand K, Gherman G, Williams G, DeFrancesco D. *SatSCan—Software for the Spatial and Space-time Scan Statistics, Version 2.1.* Bethesda, Madison: National Cancer Institute, 1998b.

[19] Bergane Y, Wall S, Kebede D *et al.* Establishing an epidemiological field laboratory in rural areas—potentials for public health research and interventions. *Ethiop J Health Dev* 1999;**13**:1–47.

[20] Jaffar S, Leach A, Greenwood AM *et al.* Changes in the pattern of infant and childhood mortality in Upper River Division, The Gambia, from 1989 to 1993. *Trop Med Int Health* 1997;**2**:28–37.

[21] Müller O, Garenne M. Childhood mortality in sub-Saharan Africa. *Lancet* 1999;**353**:673.

[22] Snow RW, Armstrong-Schellenberg JRM, Peshu N *et al.* Periodicity and space-time clustering of severe childhood malaria on the coast of Kenya. *Trans R Soc Trop Med Hyg* 1993;**87**:386–90.

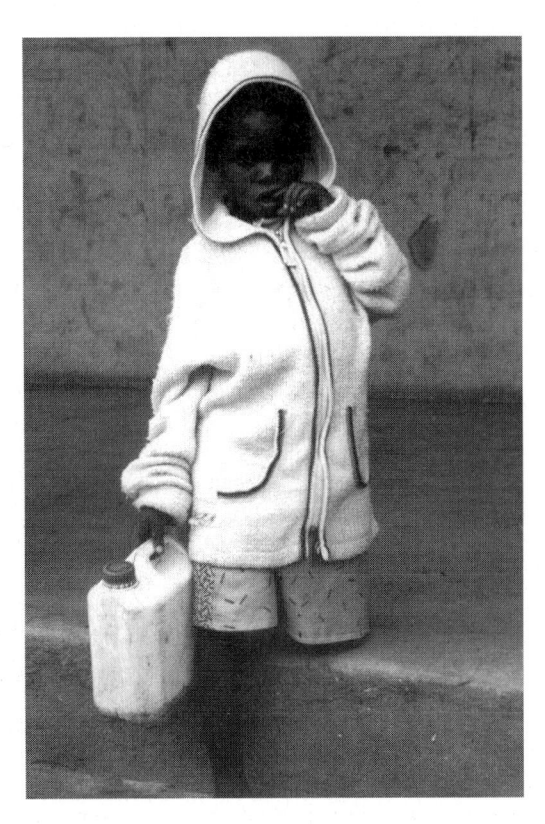

Photography: Debbie Lawlor

3.3 Community factors associated with malaria prevention by mosquito nets: an exploratory study in rural Burkina Faso

OKRAH J, TRAORE C, PALE A, SOMMERFELD J, MÜLLER O

Trop Med Int Health. 2002 Mar; 7(3): 240-8

Reprinted with permission from Blackwell Publishers Ltd.

Community factors associated with malaria prevention by mosquito nets: an exploratory study in rural Burkina Faso

Jane Okrah[1], Corneille Traoré[2], Augustin Palé[2], Johannes Sommerfeld[3] and Olaf Müller[3]

1 Ministry of Health, Public Health Division, Accra, Ghana
2 Centre de Recherche en Santé de Nouna, Nouna, Burkina Faso
3 Department of Tropical Hygiene and Public Health, Ruprecht-Karls-University, Heidelberg, Germany

Summary Malaria-related knowledge, attitudes and practices (KAP) were examined in a rural and partly urban multiethnic population of Kossi province in north-western Burkina Faso prior to the establishment of a local insecticide-treated bednet (ITN) programme. Various individual and group interviews were conducted, and a structured questionnaire was administered to a random sample of 210 heads of households in selected villages and the provincial capital of Nouna. *Soumaya*, the local illness concept closest to the biomedical term malaria, covers a broad range of recognized signs and symptoms. Aetiologically, *soumaya* is associated with mosquito bites but also with a number of other perceived causes. The disease entity is perceived as a major burden to the community and is usually treated by both traditional and western methods. Malaria preventive practices are restricted to limited chloroquine prophylaxis in pregnant women. Protective measures against mosquitoes are, however, widespread through the use of mosquito nets, mosquito coils, insecticide sprays and traditional repellents. Mosquito nets are mainly used during the rainy season and most of the existing nets are used by adults, particularly heads of households. Mosquito nets treated with insecticide (ITN) are known to the population through various information channels. People are willing to treat existing nets and to buy ITNs, but only if such services would be offered at reduced prices and in closer proximity to the households. These findings have practical implications for the design of ITN programmes in rural areas of sub-Saharan Africa (SSA).

keywords Africa, malaria control, mosquito nets, insecticide, community, Burkina Faso

correspondence Olaf Müller, Department of Tropical Hygiene and Public Health, Ruprecht-Karls-University, Im Neuenheimer Feld 324, 69120 Heidelberg, Germany. E-mail: Olaf.Mueller@urz.uni-heidelberg.de

Introduction

Of the estimated annual 300–500 million clinical malaria cases and 1.5–2.7 million deaths that are directly attributable to malaria, the great majority occur in young children of remote rural areas of sub-Saharan Africa (SSA) (WHO 1997; Snow *et al.* 1999). As malaria control mainly relies on early diagnosis and prompt treatment with effective and affordable first-line antimalarial drugs, the rapidly increasing level of resistance to chloroquine in SSA is likely to contribute substantially to observed reversals in child mortality rates (Müller & Garenne 1999; Trape 2001).

For more than two decades now, insecticide-impregnated bednets and curtains (ITN) have raised renewed interest as a tool in malaria control. In Africa, five major trials in areas of different malaria transmission intensities have documented a reduction in all-cause mortality of young children associated with ITN protection (Alonso *et al.* 1991; D'Alessandro *et al.* 1995; Nevill *et al.* 1996; Binka *et al.* 1997; Habluetzel *et al.* 1997). A meta-analysis of all randomized controlled trials showed an overall protective efficacy against all-cause mortality and malaria disease episodes of 18 and 45%, respectively (Lengeler 1998).

ITNs have since become an integral part of the global malaria control strategy and the global 'Roll Back Malaria' partnership (World Bank 1993; Nabarro & Tayler 1998). Until today, the distribution of ITN through the governmental health system and the sale through the private sector by a social marketing approach are the two major strategies for implementing community-based ITN interventions in SSA (Lines 1996).

To date, however, experience with local factors influencing the effectiveness and sustainability of ITN programmes remains limited. In the Gambian National Impregnated Bednet Programme (NIBP), the introduction of fee-for-service was accompanied by a sharp drop in impregnation coverage from 85% during the first year to 14% in the second year (D'Alessandro et al. 1995). An evaluation of the activities of the NIBP during its third year showed that offering insecticide through private channels leads to increased impregnation coverage, and that providing insecticide through maternal and child health services is effective in targeting young children (Müller et al. 1997). More recently, in Tanzania, a major ITN social marketing pilot project achieved high coverage of the intervention, which was associated with a substantial reduction in malaria morbidity in young children (Armstrong-Schellenberg et al. 1999; Abdulla et al. 2001).

Prior to the intervention, a number of ITN programmes conducted community-based research to elucidate community knowledge, attitudes, and practices (Procacci et al. 1991; Aikins et al. 1993, 1994; Ettling et al. 1994; Gyapong et al. 1996; Van Bortel et al. 1996; Vundule & Mharakurwa 1996). Much of this research was based exclusively on survey research. Only in the late 1990s, triangulated public health research using both qualitative and quantitative approaches to data collection was promoted (Agyepong et al. 1995; Gyapong et al. 1996; Agyepong & Manderson 1999; Rashed et al. 1999) and anthropologically informed studies were undertaken (Agyepong 1992; Winch et al. 1994; Makemba et al. 1996; Winch et al. 1996; Binka & Adongo 1997; Winch et al. 1997). Profound, long-term ethnographic research related to malaria and its prevention is still an exception and much needed (Hausmann Muela et al. 1998).

This body of research suggests that mosquito nuisance, perceived malaria risk, household income and other household variables such as ethnicity, age and gender are the most important determinants of mosquito net ownership and use (Aikins et al. 1993, 1994; Winch et al. 1994; Gyapong et al. 1996; Zimicki 1996). As mosquito nuisance is one of the major determinants for use of mosquito nets, compliance is usually much lower during the dry season than the rainy seasons (Winch et al. 1994; Zimicki 1996; Binka & Adongo 1997).

As an exploratory study prior to a district-based ITN programme in northwestern Burkina Faso, we conducted descriptive research on community factors associated with malaria prevention including mosquito net use. We also examined issues of acceptability of ITNs by the local population.

Methods

Study area

Our study was conducted in the research zone of the *Centre de Recherche en Santé de Nouna* (CRSN), Burkina Faso (Kouyaté et al. 2000). Nouna, the capital of Kossi province, is situated about 280 km northwest of Ouagadougou. The CRSN study area comprises Nouna town (20 000 population) and a rural area of 41 villages (35 000 population). Most of the population belongs to the Marka, Mossi, Bwaba, Peulh and Samo ethnic groups. The main socio-economic activity is subsistance farming. Malaria is holoendemic but markedly seasonal, with most transmission and disease occurring at the end of the rainy season, which usually lasts from June to October (Müller et al. 2001).

The study focused on 10 of the 41 rural CRSN study villages and all sectors of Nouna town. The villages were purposely selected to represent the rural study population in its socio-cultural, demographic and geographical diversity.

Study design

The study was exploratory and descriptive in nature, using both qualitative and quantitative approaches to data collection. The research team comprised of the investigators and four trained interviewers who were familiar with the local setting and the local languages. All questionnaires were translated into Dioula, the lingua franca of the study area, and were pre-tested before being administered. The survey instrument was informed by findings of the qualitative research.

Qualitative research

Focus group discussions (FGD), individual interviews and key informant interviews were conducted in four of the 10 study villages and in Nouna town. Ten FGDs (five with men and five with women) were held with groups of 10 participants each. We selected participants with at least one child below 5 years in their household, because we felt that they would have more specific experience with malaria and would be able to contribute more to the discussions. The discussions dealt with community knowledge of malaria-related concepts, and attitudes and practices regarding malaria prevention and treatment. We deliberately focused on naturalistic illness concepts close to the biomedical concept of malaria, relevant and amenable to the mosquito net programme as a public health intervention, at the expense of a more elaborate ethnographic investigation of local illness terminologies and taxonomies, supernatural aetiologies and their ethnographic context (Hausmann Muela et al. 1998). The local illness terminology reported by FGD participants was supplemented by information from semistructured interviews with 40 persons of mixed ethnicities in Nouna town. We also conducted nine key informant interviews with medical personnel, local tailors and traders of mosquito nets, users of mosquito nets, traditional healers and ambulant drug peddlers. The interviews assessed the respondents' beliefs concerning malaria aetiology, nosology and prevention, and their practices on current malaria prevention and treatment measures including pattern of mosquito net ownership and use.

Raw field notes and tape recordings were first transcribed and translated. The data were processed and analysed with ATLAS.ti, a software package for qualitative data analysis, using a pre-established code list (ATLAS.ti 1997).

Quantitative research

Concepts and categories emerging from qualitative research informed the construction of the survey instrument, notably the definition of variables. Respondents were sampled through a modified Expanded Programme for Immunization (EPI) cluster sampling methodology. This was carried out by first dividing the CRSN study area into two geographical clusters, urban and rural. The urban cluster comprised Nouna town while the rural cluster comprised a random sample of six of the 10 purposely selected villages for this study. In the second stage, the urban cluster was subdivided into seven subclusters (all seven Nouna sectors), and the rural cluster into six subclusters (all six study villages). Overall, 210 households were selected proportional to the size of the geographical cluster, and the participating households were finally chosen at random in each cluster. A structured questionnaire was administered to the heads of the selected households. The questions focused on socio-demographic characteristics, ownership and use of mosquito nets, factors determining the possession and use of mosquito nets, knowledge and acceptability of insecticide-impregnated mosquito nets and the knowledge and practice of other malaria prevention and treatment methods.

The data were analysed with the Statistical Package for Social Sciences (SPSS) for Windows 95. Simple proportions were used to describe the parameters investigated.

Approval was granted by the Ethical Committee of the Heidelberg University Medical School and the Ministry of Health in Burkina Faso.

Results

Description of the study population

Most of the study population was within the age range 20–40 years and the great majority was illiterate. All respondents in the qualitative research with the exception of two FGD participants and four key informants were farmers, with different ethnic background. While roughly half of the participants on the qualitative interviews and discussions were females, the great majority (87%) of the heads of households interviewed during the survey were males. Of those, 80/210 (38%) were from Nouna town and 130/210 (62%) were from the six villages. The distribution of ethnicity was as follows: Bwaba 71/210 (34%), Marka 55/210 (26%), Mossi 46/210 (22%), Samo 26/210 (12%), Peulh 9/210 (4%) and others 3/210 (1%). Most respondents were married (190/210 90%) and most were in a monogamous union (137/190 72%).

Knowledge and awareness of malaria

There is no one-to-one equivalent for the biomedical concept of malaria in any of the local languages. The Djoula term *soumaya*, a broad syndromic entity, is closest, and generally used in public health discourse to communicate with the population on malaria-related matters. *Soumaya* literally means 'a state of being cold'. Although most people acknowledge that mosquitoes can transmit *soumaya*, other aetiological factors such as humidity, exposure to rain and cold are widely being held as causative factors.

Soumaya is unanimously considered a serious illness, as expressed by the following citation from one of our FGDs: 'When we hear of *soumaya*, it is a serious illness Because it is the mother of all illnesses. All illnesses which have not yet developed, begin to appear when you have *soumaya*. Headache, backache, constipation, all come from *soumaya*.'

Soumaya is perceived to manifest through different signs and symptoms, the more general ones being headaches, constipation, muscle weakness, eye pains, stomach pains, fever, tiredness, cold, itching of hands, neck and back pain. According to our respondents, these symptoms indicate a simple type of malaria common to adults as well as children. The more serious reported manifestations of *soumaya* are jaundice, dizziness and joint pains. The latter symptoms were associated with the Djoula term *djokadjo*, which means 'yellow eyes'. All the ethnic groups further knew of *djokadjo* as an illness common in adults and children.

Virulent fevers with convulsions during childhood are often interpreted as resulting from an ibou bird (translated as *kono* in local language and *engoulevent* in French language) flying during full moon over the village taking away the soul of the child. A variety of preventive efforts are undertaken to avoid this, for example, women clap their hands when they see an ibou flying over a village at night. Pregnant women are forbidden to sleep outside during full moon.

The serious types of malaria were perceived as very problematic and characterized by severe suffering of victims. Participants of our FGDs considered the disease very disturbing, especially in households with children. Some of their typical statements are captured in the following citations: 'When we hear of *soumaya*, and we have children, our heart is not at peace. *Soumaya* in any way is a true problem among us here If your child is sick and lying down how do you get money to care for him. You either think of the work on the farm or the child and you must leave one to do the other *Soumaya* is a big thing because a lot of our children are losing their lives from it '

Some of the reported impact is economic and social distress and hardship, including the inability to work. During our FGDs, it was emphasized that *soumaya* is an illness burden particularly during the high time of agricultural activities when households have depleted most of their food stocks and have neither time nor money for transport and treatment.

Most FGD participants stated that mosquitoes cause *soumaya*. This was partly explained by mosquitoes transmitting the disease from a sick person to a healthy one, and partly through dirty water deposits responsible. Typical statements were as follows: 'There are also a lot of mosquitoes here, if they bite you, after biting a sick person, you know that the sickness has come. The wicked *soumaya* does not leave any part. It is the mosquito, which brings all that ' 'The mosquitoes which live in water, when they bite you, they leave the water under your skin. That can also give you *soumaya*'.

The interview participants reported a number of other causes for *soumaya*, ranging from specific food to hygiene and poverty (Table 1).

Malaria treatment and prevention

Malaria treatment was often reported to be a combination of both modern and traditional methods. Depending on the type of malaria and its severity, people usually started with some traditional therapy, followed by modern treatment in case of failure. For serious disease, the nearest health centre was the most frequently cited option.

Malaria was reportedly cured with 'anti malaria drugs' such as chloroquine, paracetamol and aspirin, which were bought from merchants or governmental health services.

Table 1 Perceptions of the causes and the mechanisms of *soumaya*

Perceived causes of *soumaya*	Perceived causal mechanisms involved	Number of times mentioned during FGDs (n 10)	
		Frequency	%
Mosquitoes	Sucking blood	10	100
	Deposition of dirty water under the skin of victims	6	60
Poverty and lack of means	Inability to provide good care, to prevent disease or to purchase treatment	10	100
Poor personal and environmental hygiene	Favours indirectly the growth of various parasites	6	60
Fruits (i.e. mangoes), shea nut, leaves of fresh beans, sugary foods, condiments (i.e. Maggi)	Eating food items considered cold in terms of property	6	60
Kono (bird)	Flies over the house at night	5	50
Fatigue	Weakening of the body	4	40
Dirty food	Eating	3	30
Dust	Entering one's chest	2	20
Cold, particularly cold rains	Cold temperatures, rain water falling on 'chilling' persons	2	20
Inheritance + environmental factors	Sick mother gives birth to sick child	1	10

Although there was evidence for incorrect dosages in several instances, perceived effectiveness was emphasized by many respondents: 'We often treat malaria by taking antimalaria drugs. That is to say, you can even have the germ in the organism, but if you take antimalaria products, they completely neutralize the germ.'

Most respondents reported the regular use of traditional treatments like flowers of eucalyptus plants, acacia, citronella, papaya, guava and leaves and roots of the neem tree. The herbs were used in various combinations, the common one being eucalyptus plants with acacia and neem leaves. They are reportedly boiled, and the concoctions drunk, bathed in or perfused, depending on the perceived severity of the illness. However, unlike biomedical drugs, the effectiveness of the herbal treatments was considered uncertain, as expressed by some respondents: 'When one has *soumaya*, we uproot the leaves and bathe it is a question of chance. For some people it works, others use the traditional plants in vain and go to the hospital.'

Specific malaria prevention measures reported during the FGD were the use of chloroquine for pregnant women, the use of mosquito nets, the evacuation of dirty stagnant water, and the use of a specific plant (Djoula: Fariwêgnè yiri) as an insect repellent in rooms. The most frequently mentioned specific practice against mosquitoes reported from participants in the survey was the use of mosquito coils (142/210 68%). Mosquito coils and insecticide sprays were sold, under various brand names, in the local markets. Most of the measures against mosquitoes targeted at the perceived mosquito nuisance rather than for malaria prevention.

A statement from a key informant, a health officer, is summarized below: 'As for the preventive measures in general, it is individual protection. At the moment, where we can say something better is only with pregnant women. All the rest, we cannot say that any measure is in place '

Mosquito net prevalence, characteristics and use

Forty-nine percent (103/210) of respondents in the survey reported at least one mosquito net in their household (21% owned one, 13% two, and 15% more than two mosquito nets). More urban households compared with rural households owned mosquito nets (55% *vs.* 34%).

About two-thirds of the nets were rectangular, white and synthetic, of various origins and sold in the local markets. The materials are usually imported from Europe or Asia, and the mosquito nets produced by local tailors. Some were locally made mosquito nets and curtains, made from thick cotton. These were particularly preferred by older individuals, as a means to provide warmth during the colder periods of the year. Most mosquito nets were used for more than 3 years (60/103 58%). Most of households had devices on their walls (77/103 75%) and/or ceiling beams (63/103 62%) for fixing nets. Seventy-three percent (75/103) of respondents used their mosquito nets only during the raining season, only 12/103 (12%) used their nets throughout the year.

Adult men were the group who reportedly used mosquito nets most often (35/103 34%), followed by mothers with young children (20/103 19%) and elderly persons (17/103 17%) (Table 2).

Table 2 Mosquito net use in households by age and sex

Persons using nets	Frequency	%
Children under 15 years alone	4	4
Young children and their mothers	20	19
Adult men alone	35	34
Adult women alone	5	5
Elderly persons	17	16
Couples	12	12
Other	10	10
Total	n 103	100

Cost of mosquito nets and factors associated with net ownership

Most mosquito nets were purchased at local markets and the shops of Nouna, while a few were purchased in the major towns of Bobo Dioulasso and Ouagadougou. The price for a mosquito net ranged from 9 to 22 US$ (mean 9.2 US$), depending on material and size. High costs of these mosquito nets were the most frequently stated reason for not owning nets.

Ninety-five percent (98/103) of households owning mosquito nets used them as a measure against the nuisance of mosquitoes. Only a minority stated other reasons, such as privacy, protection against cold, flies and falling debris (8/103 8%).

Acceptability of insecticide-impregnated mosquito nets

Among the respondents owning mosquito nets, 42/103 (41%) had ever heard about the method of treating nets with insecticide. Of these, 13/42 (31%) obtained the information from health personnel, 11/42 (26%) from friends and neighbours, and 18/42 (42%) from the media (radio, television, newspapers). All these respondents were interested in the future use of treated nets, mostly because they felt it would provide them with better protection against mosquitoes (90/103 87%). Only a minority

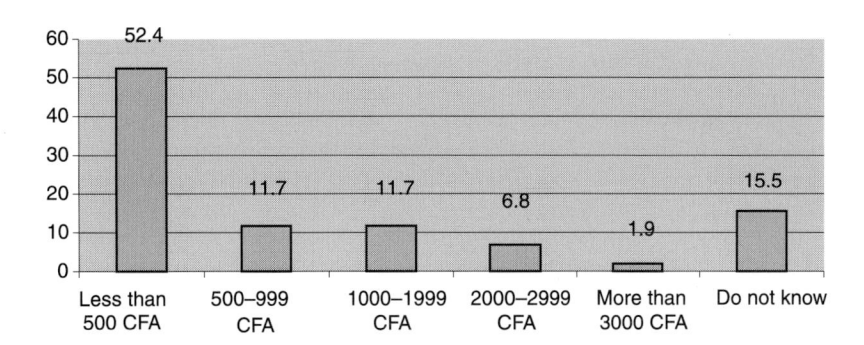

Figure 1 Amount of money mosquito net owners are willing to pay for net treatment with insecticide 1 US$ 650 CFA.

stated that treated nets would provide them with better protection against illnesses (3/103 3%). When asked about how much money they would be willing to spend on net treatment, the majority did not want to spend more than 0.5–1 US$ on treatment (Fig. 1).

Most rural and urban respondents stated that they would prefer to have mosquito net treatment services close to their home (78/103 76%); a few wanted to have such services to be established centrally at Nouna hospital and the surrounding health centres (22/103 21%).

Asked about the type of assistance needed to enable them to acquire new mosquito nets and/or to get existing ones treated with insecticide, 38/103 (37%) of respondents wanted them for free, 46/103 (45%) indicated their preference for reduced prices, and 10/103 (10%) preferred the nets to be provided on credit.

Discussion

Soumaya, the local equivalent to malaria, is considered a widespread and important health problem in northwestern Burkina Faso. As particularly young children of this area are experiencing a number of *soumaya* episodes during each rainy season, a significant additional burden is put on families at the time when agricultural work is most demanding and resources are most limited (Sauerborn et al. 1996; Müller et al. 2001). *Soumaya* manifests through various signs and symptoms. Although the majority of our study population knew that mosquitoes cause malaria, other natural and supernatural causes for malaria were frequently stated during interviews. These local perceptions of malaria are strikingly similar to findings from other malaria-endemic areas of SSA (Makemba et al. 1996; Ahorlu et al. 1997; Minja et al. 2001; Tarimo et al. 2000).

As in most of SSA and depending on accessibility, costs and on whether the entity is perceived as a 'normal' or an 'out of order' illness, malaria symptoms in our study area were usually first treated with traditional herbal remedies and/or available western drugs (Deming et al. 1989; Guiguemde et al. 1994; Ruebush et al. 1995; Djimde et al. 1998; Nsimba et al. 1999; Hausmann Muela et al. 2000; Thera et al. 2000). Only in case of non-response or clinical deterioration, and depending on distance to the next health care facility, as well as on funds and time available for transport and treatment, patients visited formal health services. Although it is reassuring that western drugs are considered more effective as compared with traditional treatment, the fact that most villages in our study area are several kilometres away from the next health centre results in the great majority of illness episodes not being seen by trained health staff. There are major problems associated with this type of treatment-seeking behaviour. First, few cases are treated with an effective antimalarial drug in a timely manner (chloroquine is the officially recommended first line treatment in Burkina Faso). Second, biomedical drugs are frequently dosed incorrectly. For example, chloroquine is often given as a single dose, but sometimes daily for weeks. Third, dangerous drugs are frequently administered, for example aspirin and tetracycline are often given to children in case of fever. As a result, it is rather common that patients present with already advanced disease at health centres or hospital (unpublished observations).

However, it has repeatedly been demonstrated that the effectiveness of malaria control in SSA can be increased substantially through involving communities and particularly through training of the mothers of young children on correct antimalarial drug use (Menon et al. 1988; Pagnoni et al. 1997; Kidane & Morrow 2000). In our study area, a project focusing on training of village-based women groups in malaria treatment has recently shown to be feasible (Gerhardus et al. 2000).

Malaria prevention in our holoendemic study area is restricted to prescription of chloroquine prophylaxis to pregnant women during antenatal care visits. In reality, antenatal care coverage is strongly associated with living in Nouna town or in one of the few villages with a health centre (unpublished observations). Prevention of mosquito bites through use of specific repellent plants, burning of mosquito coils and use of mosquito bednets is common. However, as also reported from many other places in SSA, these measures are primarily targeted against the nuisance of mosquitos and not against malaria (Aikins *et al.* 1994; Van Bortel *et al.* 1996; Zimicki 1996).

There are great variations in the proportions of households using mosquito nets in malaria-endemic communities of SSA (Zimicki 1996). While some countries such as The Gambia have a strong tradition of using mosquito nets for several purposes, mosquito net use is not very common in Ghana and Malawi (Binka *et al.* 1994; D'Alessandro *et al.* 1994; Ziba *et al.* 1994). Thus, the households of CRSN study area demonstrate intermediate rates of mosquito net ownership in the SSA context. Our findings confirm the higher mosquito net ownership rates in urban compared with rural areas observed in other SSA countries (Zimicki 1996).

In our study area the majority of existing mosquito nets were used by adult male heads of households instead of those at greatest risk for severe malaria, namely young children and pregnant women. A predominance of mosquito net use by male adults has also been observed in other SSA countries like Ghana and Tanzania, while in The Gambia young children and pregnant women were more frequently protected with mosquito nets than older children and non-pregnant adults (Aikins *et al.* 1994; D'Alessandro *et al.* 1994; Zimicki 1996). We also found that only a minority of households which own mosquito nets in our study area use them throughout the year. This supports similar findings regarding the influence of seasonal variations on mosquito net use from other SSA countries (Winch *et al.* 1994; Zimicki 1996; Binka & Adongo 1997). These findings have to be taken into consideration during the design of information/education/communication (IEC) messages within the framework of ITN programmes.

Mosquito nets are rather expensive in Burkina Faso, and this was the most important reason for households not owning mosquito nets. Many respondents had already heard about the benefits of treating mosquito nets with insecticides, the majority through the media, and all were interested in impregnation. When asked about their willingness to pay for treatment of existing mosquito nets, the majority were prepared to pay up to around 1 US$ for this service and most would like to find the service close to their homes. There was also a strong argument for subsidy of mosquito net purchase and treatment. These findings demonstrate the barrier of existing high prices on mosquito net coverage in poor rural communities of SSA and have to be taken into consideration during implementation of ITN programmes.

Acknowledgements

We thank the staff of the Centre de Recherche en Santé de Nouna and the population of the Nouna study area for their support. The study was funded by the Deutsche Forschungsgemeinschaft (SFB 544, Control of Tropical Infectious Diseases). Jane Okrah was supported by a grant from the German Academic Exchange Service (Deutscher Akademischer Austauschdienst, DAAD, Germany.

References

Abdulla S, Armstrong Schellenberg J, Nathan R *et al.* (2001) Impact on malaria morbidity of a programme supplying insecticide treated nets in children aged under 2 years in Tanzania: community cross sectional study. *British Medical Journal* 322, 270–273.

Agyepong IA (1992) Malaria: ethnomedical perceptions and practice in an Adangbe farming community and implications for control. *Social Science and Medicine* 35, 131–137.

Agyepong IA, Aryee B, Dzikunu H & Manderson L (1995) *The Malaria Manual. Guidelines for the Rapid Assessment of Social, Economic and Cultural Aspects of Malaria.* UNDP/World Bank/WHO Special Programme for Research and Training in Tropical Diseases, (TDR), Geneva.

Agyepong IA & Manderson L (1999) Mosquito avoidance and bed net use in the Greater Accra region, Ghana. *Journal of Biosocial Science* 31, 79–92.

Ahorlu CK, Dunyo SK, Afari EA, Koram KA & Nkrumah FK (1997) Malaria-related beliefs and behaviour in southern Ghana: implications for treatment, prevention and control. *Tropical Medicine and International Health* 2, 488–498.

Aikins MK, Pickering H, Alonso PL *et al.* (1993) A malaria control trial using insecticide-treated bednets and targeted chemoprophylaxis in a rural area of the Gambia, West Africa. Perceptions of the causes of malaria and of its treatment and prevention in the study area. *Transactions of the Royal Society of Tropical Medicine* 87 (Suppl. 2), 25–30.

Aikins MK, Pickering H & Greenwood BM (1994) Attitudes to malaria, traditional practices and bednets (mosquito nets) as vector control measures: a comparative study in five West African countries. *Journal of Tropical Medicine and Hygiene* 97, 81–86.

Alonso PL, Lindsay SW, Armstrong JRM *et al.* (1991) The effect of insecticide-treated bednets on mortality in Gambian children. *Lancet* 337, 1499–1502.

Armstrong-Schellenberg J, Abdulla S, Minja H *et al.* (1999) KINET: a social marketing programme of treated nets and net treatment for malaria control in Tanzania, with evaluation of child health and long-term survival. *Transactions of the Royal Society of Tropical Medicine* 93, 225–231.

ATLAS.ti (1997) *Visual Qualitative Data Analysis, Management and Model Building in Education, Research and Business*, Version 4.1. for Windows 95, Scientific Software Development, Berlin (www.atlasti.de).

Binka FM & Adongo P (1997) Acceptability and use of insecticide impregnated bednets in northern Ghana. *Tropical Medicine and International Health* **2**, 499–507.

Binka FN, Kubaje A, Adjuik M *et al.* (1997) Impact of permethrin-impregnated bednets on child mortality in Kassena Nankana district, Ghana: a randomized controlled trial. *Tropical Medicine and International Health* **1**, 147–154.

Binka FN, Morris S, Ross DA, Arthur P & Aryeetey ME (1994) Patterns of malaria morbidity and mortality in children in northern Ghana. *Transactions of the Royal Society of Tropical Medicine and Hygiene* **88**, 381–385.

D'Alessandro U, Aikins MK, Langerock P, Bennett S & Greenwood BM (1994) Nationwide survey of bednet use in rural Gambia. *Bulletin of the World Health Organization* **72**, 391–394.

D'Alessandro U, Olaleye B, McGuire W *et al.* (1995) Mortality and morbidity from malaria in Gambian children after introduction of an impregnated bednet programme. *Lancet* **345**, 479–483.

Deming MS, Gayibor A, Murphy K, Jones TS & Karsa T (1989) Home treatment of febrile children with antimalarial drugs in Togo. *Bulletin of the World Health Organization* **67**, 695–700.

Djimde A, Plowe CV, Diop S *et al.* (1998) Use of antimalarial drugs in Mali: policy versus reality. *American Journal of Tropical Medicine and Hygiene* **59**, 376–379.

Ettling M, Steketee RW, Macheso A, Schultz LJ, Nyasulu Y & Chitsulo L (1994) Malaria knowledge, attitudes and practices in Malawi: survey population characteristics. *Tropical Medicine and Parasitology* **45**, 57–60.

Gerhardus A, Kielmann K & Sanou A (2000) The use of research for decision-making in the health sector: the case of 'Shared Care' in Burkina Faso. In: *Lessons in Research to Action and Policy*. COHRED, Document, The Council on Health Research for Development, Geneva, Switzerland, pp. 19–27.

Guiguemde TR, Dao F, Curtis V *et al.* (1994) Household expenditure on malaria prevention and treatment for families in the town of Bobo-Dioulasso, Burkina Faso. *Transactions of the Royal Society of Tropical Medicine and Hygiene* **88**, 285–287.

Gyapong M, Gyapong JO, Amankwa JA *et al.* (1996) Introducing insecticide impregnated bednets in area of low bednet usage: an exploratory study in northwest Ghana. *Tropical Medicine and International Health* **1**, 328–333.

Habluetzel A, Diallo DA, Esposito F *et al.* (1997) Do insecticide-treated curtains reduce all-cause child mortality in Burkina Faso? *Tropical Medicine and International Health* **2**, 855–862.

Hausmann Muela S, Muela Ribera J & Tanner M (1998) Fake malaria and hidden parasites – the ambiguity of malaria. *Anthropology and Medicine* **5**, 43–61.

Hausmann Muela S, Mushi AK & Muela Ribera J (2000) The paradox of the cost and affordability of traditional and government health services in Tanzania. *Health Policy and Planning* **15**, 296–302.

Kidane G & Morrow RH (2000) Teaching mothers to provide home treatment of malaria in Tigray, Ethiopia: a randomised trial. *Lancet* **356**, 550–555.

Kouyaté B, Traore C, Kielmann K & Mueller O (2000) North and South: bridging the Information gap. *Lancet* **356**, 1034–1035.

Lengeler C (1998) Insecticide treated bednets and curtains for malaria control (Cochrane Review). In: *The Cochrane Library*, Issue, 3. Update Software, Oxford.

Lines J (1996) Mosquito nets and insecticides for net treatment: a discussion of existing and potential distribution systems in Africa. *Tropical Medicine and International Health* **1**, 616–632.

Makemba AM, Winch PJ, Makame VM *et al.* (1996) Treatment practices for *degedege*, a locally recognized febrile illness, and implications for strategies to decrease mortality from severe malaria in Bagamoyo District, Tanzania. *Tropical Medicine and International Health* **1**, 305–313.

Menon A, Joof D, Rowan KM & Greenwood BM (1988) Maternal administration of chloroquine: an unexplored aspect of malaria control. *Journal of Tropical Medicine and Hygiene* **91**, 49–54.

Minja H, Schellenberg JA, Mukasa O *et al.* (2001) Introducing insecticide-treated nets in the Kilombero Valley, Tanzania: the relevance of local knowledge and practice for an Information, Education and Communication (IEC) campaign. *Tropical Medicine and International Health* **6**, 614–623.

Müller O, Becher H, Baltussen A *et al.* (2001) Effect of zinc supplementation on malaria morbidity among Westafrican children: a randomized double-blind placebo-controlled trial. *British Medical Journal* **322**, 1–6.

Müller O, Cham K, Jaffar S & Greenwood BM (1997) The Gambian National Impregnated Bednet Programme: evaluation of the 1994 cost-recovery trial. *Social Science and Medicine* **44**, 1903–1909.

Müller O & Garenne M (1999) Childhood mortality in sub-Saharan Africa. *Lancet* **353**, 673.

Nabarro DN & Tayler EM (1998) The 'Roll Back Malaria' Campaign. *Science* **280**, 2067–2068.

Nevill CG, Some E, Mungala V *et al.* (1996) Insecticide-treated bednets reduce mortality and severe morbidity from malaria among children on the Kenyan coast. *Tropical Medicine and International Health* **1**, 139–146.

Nsimba SED, Warsame M, Tomson G, Massale AY & Mbatiya ZA (1999) A household survey of source, availability, and use of antimalarials in a rural area of Tanzania. *Drug Information Journal* **33**, 1025–1032.

Pagnoni F, Convelbo N, Tiendrebeogo J, Cousens S & Esposito F (1997) A community-based programme to provide prompt and adequate treatment of presumptive malaria in children. *Transactions of the Royal Society of Tropical Medicine and Hygiene* **91**, 512–517.

Procacci PG, Lamizana L, Pietra V, Di Russo C & Rotigliano G (1991) Utilisation de rideaux imprégnés de permethrine par les habitants d'une communauté rurale du Burkina Faso. *Parassitologia* **33**, 93–98.

Rashed S, Johnson H, Dongier P *et al.* (1999) Determinants of the permethrin impregnated bednets (PIB) in the Republic of Benin: the role of women in the acquisition and utilisation of PIBs. *Social Science and Medicine* **49**, 993–1005.

Ruebush TK, Kern MK, Campbell CC & Oloo AJ (1995) Self-treatment of malaria in a rural area of western Kenya. *Bulletin of the World Health Organization* **73**, 229–236.

Sauerborn R, Nougtara A, Hien M & Diesfeld HJ (1996) Seasonal variations of the household costs of illness in Burkina Faso. *Social Science and Medicine* **43**, 281–290.

Snow RW, Craig M, Deichmann U & Marsh K (1999) Estimating mortality and disability due to malaria among non-pregnant population. *Bulletin of the World Health Organization* **77**, 624–640.

Tarimo DS, Lwihula GK, Minjas JN & Bygbjerg IC (2000) Mothers' perceptions and knowledge on childhood malaria in the holoendemic Kibaha district, Tanzania: implications for malaria control and the IMCI strategy. *Tropical Medicine and International Health* **5**, 179–184.

Thera MA, D'Alessandro U, Thiero M *et al.* (2000) Child malaria treatment practices among mothers in the district of Yanfolila, Sikasso region, Mali. *Tropical Medicine and International Health* **5**, 876–881.

Trape JF (2001) The public health impact of chloroquine resistance in Africa. *American Journal of Tropical Medicine and Hygiene* **64** (Suppl.), 12–17.

Van Bortel W, Barutwanayo M, Delacollette C & Coosemans M (1996) Motivation à l'acquisition et à l'utilisation des moustiquaires imprégnées dans une zone à paludisme stable au Burundi. *Tropical Medicine and International Health* **1**, 71–80.

Vundule C & Mharakurwa S (1996) Knowledge, practices, and perceptions about malaria in rural communities of Zimbabwe: relevance to malaria control. *Bulletin of the World Health Organization* **74**, 55–60.

Winch PJ, Makemba AM, Kamazima SR *et al.* (1994) Seasonal variation in the perceived risk of malaria: implications for the promotion of insecticide-impregnated bed nets. *Social Science and Medicine* **39**, 63–75.

Winch PJ, Makemba AM, Kamazima SR *et al.* (1996) Local terminology for febrile illnesses in Bagamoyo district, Tanzania and its impact on the design of a community-based malaria control programme. *Social Science and Medicine* **42**, 1057–1067.

Winch PJ, Makemba AM, Kamazima SR *et al.* (1997) Social and cultural factors affecting rates of regular retreatment of mosquito nets with insecticide in Bagamoyo District, Tanzania. *Tropical Medicine and International Health* **2**, 760–770.

World Bank (1993) *World Development Report: Investing in Health.* Oxford University Press, New York.

World Health Organization (1997) World malaria situation in 1994. *Weekly Epidemiological Record* **72**, 269–276.

Ziba C, Slutsker L, Chitsulo L *et al.* (1994) Use of malaria prevention measures in Malawian households. *Tropical Medicine and Parasitology* **45**, 70–73.

Zimicki S (1996) Promotion in Sub-Saharan Africa. In: *Net Gain. A New Method for Preventing Malaria Deaths* (eds C Lengeler, J Cattani & D de Savigny) World Health Organization, Geneva, pp. 111–148.

3.4 Mortality patterns, 1993-98, in a rural area of Burkina Faso, West Africa, based on the Nouna demographic surveillance system

Kynast-wolf G, Sankoh oA, Gbangou A, Kouyate B, Becher H

Trop Med Int Health. 2002 Apr; 7(4): 349-56

Reprinted with permission from Blackwell Publishers Ltd.

Mortality patterns, 1993–98, in a rural area of Burkina Faso, West Africa, based on the Nouna demographic surveillance system

G. Kynast-Wolf[1], O. A. Sankoh[1], A. Gbangou[2], B. Kouyaté[2] and H. Becher[1]

1 Department of Tropical Hygiene and Public Health, University of Heidelberg Medical School, Heidelberg, Germany
2 Centre de Recherche en Santé de Nouna, Nouna, Burkina Faso, West Africa

Summary The Nouna demographic surveillance system database was analysed for the period 1993–98. Basic demographic parameters, age-specific and age-standardized mortality rates were calculated and a seasonal variation in mortality was analysed. Poisson regression was used to model the calculated mortality rates and to investigate the seasonal mortality pattern. Both the population distribution by age and the mortality rates reflect a typical pattern of population structures and total mortality in rural Africa as a whole: high childhood mortality and a young population (about 60% are up to age 25; about 10% above age 64). We identified a significant seasonal pattern with highest mortality rates in February. Demographic surveillance systems in Africa provide a viable method for the collection of reliable data on vital events in rural Africa and should therefore be established and supported.

keywords demographic surveillance, Poisson regression, sub-Saharan Africa, total mortality

correspondence Prof. H. Becher, Department of Tropical Hygiene and Public Health, University of Heidelberg Medical School, Im Neuenheimer Feld 324, 69120 Heidelberg, Germany.
E-mail: heiko.becher@urz.uni-heidelberg.de

Introduction

In 1978, African delegates joined the representatives of other nations in endorsing the Alma Ata Declaration, which committed all governments to the common goal of achieving 'Health for all' by the year 2000. A major task of epidemiologists is to assess to what extent this ambitious target has been realized.

Good descriptive epidemiological data are required, and the difficult task of collecting and presenting them was started in a rather heterogeneous way in Africa. A comprehensive volume on mortality and morbidity data in sub-Saharan Africa (Feachem & Jamison 1991) highlighted achievements in the 1980s and shortcomings in terms of lack of data for a large number of countries. During the 1990s, the white spots on mortality maps gradually became smaller, but most estimates of overall mortality are subject to error and bias – especially for sub-Saharan Africa – as reliable mortality statistics covering the total population hardly exist (Cooper et al. 1998). Consequently, many countries in Africa are now taking steps towards providing a reliable information base to support health development. An increasing number of field sites operating demographic surveillance systems (DSS) is being established in rural areas to continuously monitor geographically defined populations. To coordinate the activities of the sites, an International Network of Field Sites with Continuous Demographic Evaluation of Populations and THeir Health in Developing Countries (INDEPTH; see http://www.indepth-network.org for the vision and goals of the network as well as its current activities) was established in Dar es Salaam, Tanzania, in 1998. Many DSS sites in Africa collaborate with international research institutions. For example, the Nouna DSS in Burkina Faso, on which this study is based, collaborates with the Department of Tropical Hygiene and Public Health at the University of Heidelberg in Germany.

Sankoh et al. (2001) analyse a subset of the Nouna DSS data by concentrating on the clustering of children under five in the study area. They use a space and space–time scan statistic proposed by Kulldorff (1997) to identify clusters and test for their statistical significance. The paper reports several statistically significant clusters of higher childhood mortality rates comprising different sets of villages; one specific village was consistently identified in the study population, indicating non-random distribution of childhood mortality. The authors conclude that their 'study may be regarded as a first step in prioritizing areas for follow-up public health efforts'.

In another study, Würthwein *et al.* (2001) discuss the measurement of the local burden of disease (BOD) with respect to years of life lost (YLL) using the same DSS population. The DSS data exhibit the same qualitative BOD pattern as the Global Burden of Disease Study (GBDS) although with different ranking of the diseases. Würthwein *et al.* recommend that 'local health policy should be based on local BOD measurement, rather than on extrapolations that might not represent the true BOD structure by cause'.

Unlike the aforementioned studies, this paper attempts a descriptive statistical analysis of data from the Nouna DSS in order to get a general picture of total mortality in the study area for the observation period, 1993–98. Various statistical methods used to analyse total mortality (i.e. mortality without reference to specific cause) are presented. We briefly describe the study population, discuss the statistical method used, present basic demographic parameters including age-specific and age-standardized mortality rates and discuss the results of an analysis of seasonal variation in mortality in the study area for the observation period.

Materials and methods

Study area and population

A comprehensive description of the study area and study population can be found elsewhere (Baltussen *et al.* 2000; Sankoh *et al.* 2001; Würthwein *et al.* 2001). Briefly, Nouna Health Research Center (Centre de Recherche en Santé de Nouna, CRSN) is located in the Nouna Health District in the northwest of Burkina Faso. With an area of 7464 km^2, Nouna Health District, which is identical to the administrative province of Kossi, has a population of 240 000 inhabitants and a population density of 32 inhabitants/km^2. It covers 16 basic health facilities referred to as *Centre de Santé et de Promotion Sociale* (CSPS), one district hospital, and one medical centre. The main ethnic groups in are Dafing, Bwaba, Mossi, Peulh and Samo. The Dioula language serves as *lingua franca*.

The predominantly rural study area includes the semi-urban town of Nouna. It is dry orchard savanna, populated almost exclusively by subsistence farmers and cattle keepers. The region has a sub-Sahelian climate with a mean annual rainfall of 796 mm (range 483–1083 over the past five decades). Although formal schools have existed in the area since 1935, most children do not attend them; many attend informal koranic schools. More than 70% of the population are illiterate.

The DSS of the CRSN has conducted regular population censuses since 1992. In 1992, the study population consisted of 26 626 individuals. By 1998, this number had risen to 31 782. During the study period of this paper (1993–98), the DSS covered 39 villages, the catchment area of three CSPS. In 2000, a new census enhanced the DSS, which now includes the semiurban town of Nouna and two additional villages, representing the catchment area of the district hospital in Nouna and four CSPS after a redistribution of responsibilities. The total population of the DSS is now about 55 000, and it further comprises a vital events registration (VER) system recording births, deaths, and in- and out-migration and routine verbal autopsy (VA) interviews to be able to analyse mortality data by cause of death (Chandramohan *et al.* 1998; Anker *et al.* 1999; Würthwein *et al.* 2001).

To ensure data reliability, quality control procedures were implemented at various stages of the survey during the field phase in Nouna. Generally, in all surveys of the CRSN, a random sample of 5–10% of the households was re-interviewed by a supervisor. During data entry, a system of systematical, mutual control was implemented and data entry routines contained a set of logical checks and consistency checks for many basic variables, e.g. sex, age and the period of residence in the study area. Multiple entries into the study area and individuals with missing values in the key variables were deleted from the database, or replaced by plausible values if possible.

Statistical methods

In this section, we introduce relevant parameters used for the description of epidemiological and demographic surveillance data. Further details are given in dos Santos Silva (1999).

Mortality rates

Crude death rates, age-specific death rates and age-standardized death rates for appropriate time intervals were calculated based on person-years (PYs) (dos Santos Silva 1999). A PY is the exact time an individual in the study area was under risk. These were exactly calculated for individuals staying in the study area for each year of the observation period using an SAS macro. Crude death rates were standardized by using the Segi world population (Segi 1960; Estève *et al.* 1994). Ninety-five per cent confidence intervals for crude and age-standardized death rates were calculated using the normal approximation.

Poisson-regression model for mortality rates

Poisson regression was used to model the mortality rates (Breslow & Day 1987). We considered the following variables in the analysis: mortality rate as the dependent variable and the sex, age, calendar year and month as explanatory variables. The Poisson model was applied for the entire observation period, 1993–98, as follows.

To assess the effect of age, mortality rates were modelled as a continuous function of age. The method of fractional polynomials (Royston & Altman 1994) was used to identify the model which best describes the data. Other covariables taken are calendar year (as a categorical variable) and sex. The variable calendar year was considered to investigate a time trend.

To investigate whether mortality depends on the season of the year, monthly mortality rates were used. PYs and deaths over the total observation period were calculated for each month. A total of 702 observations were excluded from the analysis because of missing information. The resulting data were used to calculate the monthly age-specific death rates by sex. The null hypothesis was that the value of the mortality rates was independent of the month of the year. This was tested by first estimating the effect of the month as a categorical variable, and a simple function applied to get a continuous description of the effect. We used a sine function of the form

$$g(month) = \sin[(month + k) \times \pi/6], \quad (1)$$

where k can take the value 1, ..., 6 (assuming a period of 12 months). For this analysis, we assumed a constant mortality rate over the observation period. A similar model but with calendar year as additional covariable was also fitted. The Poisson regression analysis was carried out using the SAS-procedure PROC GENMOD with a log-link function (SAS Institute 1997).

Results

Basic demographic parameters

Table 1 shows the population distribution by age and sex at two specific time points, 31 December 1993 and 31 December 1998. The age distribution for both males and females is similar. More than 60% of the population is below 25 years of age. From 1992 to 1998, the population of both sexes rose steadily from 26 626 to 31 782 persons. This is an increase of 19.4%, with a mean yearly population growth rate of 3.0%.

For the entire observation period, 1993–98, the Nouna DSS data set comprised a total of 41 915 individuals

Table 1 Population distribution for the Nouna DSS at the end of 1993 and 1998

	31 December 1993				31 December 1998			
	Males		Females		Males		Females	
Age group	n	%	n	%	n	%	n	%
<1	549	3.9	489	3.6	661	4.1	675	4.3
1–4	2094	15.0	2024	14.8	2360	14.7	2236	14.3
5–9	2366	16.9	2276	16.6	2578	16.0	2385	15.2
10–14	1868	13.4	1632	11.9	2309	14.3	2108	13.4
15–19	1517	10.9	1419	10.4	1666	10.4	1457	9.3
20–24	1035	7.4	983	7.2	1278	7.9	1256	8.0
25–29	838	6.0	880	6.4	978	6.1	970	6.2
30–34	784	5.6	769	5.6	783	4.9	872	5.6
35–39	567	4.1	617	4.5	780	4.8	766	4.9
40–44	470	3.4	523	3.8	542	3.4	605	3.9
45–49	433	3.1	478	3.5	476	3.0	528	3.4
50–54	354	2.5	434	3.2	432	2.7	459	2.9
55–59	284	2.0	310	2.3	353	2.2	425	2.7
60–64	295	2.1	322	2.4	273	1.7	272	1.7
65–69	219	1.6	216	1.6	258	1.6	285	1.8
70–74	146	1.0	168	1.2	175	1.1	171	1.1
75–79	82	0.6	86	0.6	104	0.6	116	0.7
80–84	54	0.4	60	0.4	51	0.3	55	0.4
85+	21	0.2	15	0.1	39	0.2	45	0.3
Total	13 976	100	13 701	100	16 096	100	15 686	100

(20 432 males, 21 483 females, i.e. a male/female ratio of 0.95). A total of 135 individuals with missing sex or age were excluded from the data set. A total of 4886 individuals immigrated into the study area and 5640 individuals emigrated. The PYs of emigrating people were calculated up to the date of emigration. In the end the 41 915 individuals included in the analysis contributed collectively to 174 445 PYs (88 464 for males and 85 981 for females). The overall mean follow-up time is 4.1 with median 5.0 (range 0–6) years. On average 1355 births were registered per year. The distribution of PYs in the age groups is as follows: 18.3% fall in the age group 0–4 years, 40.0% in the age group 5–19, 37.7% in the age group 20–64 and 4.0% in the age group 65+.

Figure 1 shows the age pyramid of the population of Nouna DSS for 1993–98 based on the average PYs of each age group by sex over the years 1993–98. The pyramid looks typical for sub-Saharan Africa: many young and few old people.

Overall mortality

A total of 1274 male and 1217 female deaths were recorded during the observation period 1993–98. Taking into account the 174 903 PYs (including the few persons with unknown ages), a crude death rate of 14.4/1000 for males and 14.1/1000 for females was calculated. The under-five mortality rate (U5MR) is 33.6/1000 for the same period. Male and female crude death rates are similar over the observation period.

The annual PYs, deaths and crude death rates (Kynast-Wolf et al. 2001) show that the highest crude death rates were observed in 1994 and 1995, with a peak in 1994 for females (16.6/1000) and in 1995 for males (15.6/1000). They were standardized using the Segi world population to get the age-standardized death rates shown in the tables. In most cases, crude death rates are slightly lower than age-specific death rates.

Figure 2a,b illustrates age-specific death rates of males and females for two calendar periods (1993–95, 1996–98). Death rates among infants and children under 5 are high: about 40% (for males often well over 40% but slightly under 40% for the last two years 1997 and 1998) of all deaths per year. Infant death rates are higher in males than in females. About 20% of the deaths occur at ages above 65. For these age groups, however, the mortality rates differ substantially by year, possibly because of the small numbers of individuals in these age groups that invariably yield large random variations between years.

Table 2 shows the crude and age-standardized death rates by sex for both calendar periods. The age-standardized

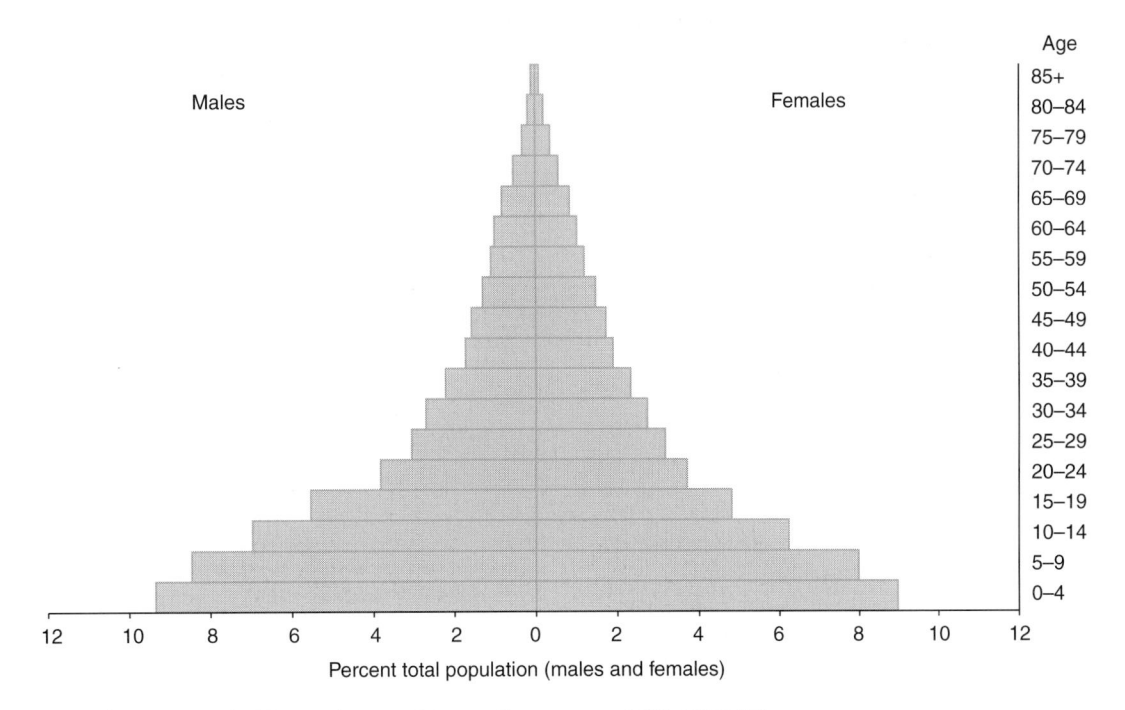

Figure 1 Population pyramid of Nouna demographic surveillance system (DSS) (1993–98).

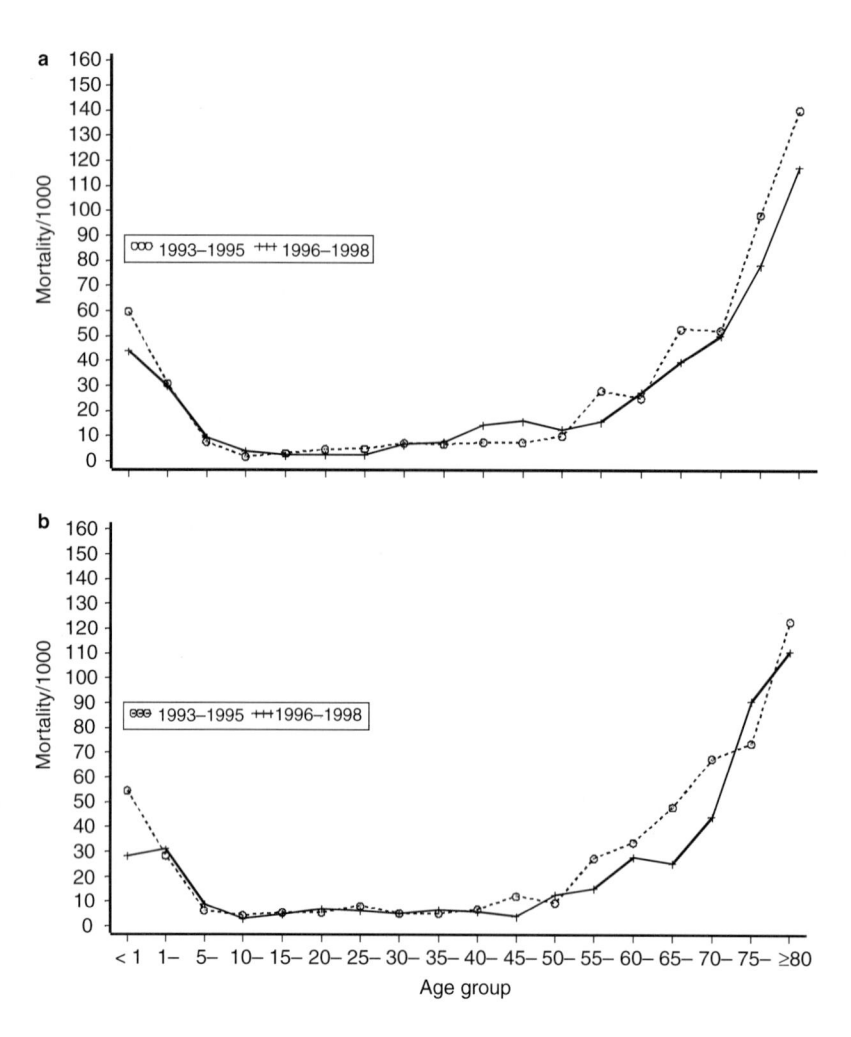

Figure 2 Annual mortality by age for 1993–98: (a) males, Nouna DSS; (b) females, Nouna DSS.

death rate for females dropped from 16.7/1000, 95% CI (15.3, 18.2), in the first period (1993–95) to 13.6/1000, 95% CI (12.4, 14.8), in the second period (1996–98). Mortality for both male and female infants fell considerably (males: 59.8/1000 to 44.0/1000; females: 54.6/1000 to 28.4/1000). Childhood mortality (age 1–4) remained relatively unchanged in both periods. The rates for the succeeding seven age groups maintained a similar slowly decreasing pattern with increasing age for both males and females. We found a decreasing trend in mortality for the two periods 1993–95 and 1996–98 ($P = 0.04$).

The results of the Poisson regression show that the risk of mortality is not significantly associated with sex ($P = 0.46$). Hence, we omitted these variables from the model. Testing second-degree fractional polynomials, we found one which yielded the best fit for the data. The estimated regression coefficients led to the following function of the rate by age:

$$\text{Rate}(\text{age}) = \exp(-2.6565 + 0.0010 \times \text{age}^2 - 0.6459 \times \sqrt{\text{age}}). \tag{2}$$

The result is displayed in Figure 3. The fit is very good and shows the usual bathtub shape of rates.

Seasonal variation in mortality

With the assumption that the two main seasons in Burkina Faso (rainy season June–October and dry season November–May) may have some effect on mortality, we investigated possible seasonal variability in the rates. We calculated the age-standardized death rates and crude death rates for each month by sex for the entire observation period (Kynast-Wolf et al. 2001); the latter are plotted in Figure 4 with 95% confidence intervals.

The data and their illustration in Figure 4 show a distinct pattern. For males and females, the mortality rates

Table 2 Person-years, crude and age-standardized death rates by calendar period

	Males		Females	
	1993–95	1996–98	1993–95	1996–98
Person-years	42 547	46 076	41 567	44 713
Crude death rate (SE)	14.7 (0.59)	14.1 (0.55)	15.0 (0.60)	13.3 (0.55)
95% CI	13.5–15.9	13.0–15.2	13.8–16.2	12.2–14.4
Age standardized* death rate (SE)	15.8 (0.72)	15.2 (0.68)	16.7 (0.74)	13.6 (0.62)
95% CI	14.4–17.2	13.9–16.5	15.3–18.2	12.4–14.8

*Standardization according to the Segi world population.

were high in the months of November until May and relatively low in the months of June until October. There was a peak in the month of September. We assumed that this pattern could have been affected by the data of the first age group (<1 year), but when we excluded infants from the data and repeated the analysis, this did not affect the seasonal pattern. We also investigated age groups (1–4, 5–19, 20–64, 65+) separately (data not shown), and a similar seasonal trend was observed in all although because of smaller numbers the effects were not as clear as for the total group.

The identified seasonal pattern was then modelled using Poisson regression. The function describing the rate ratio (RR) depending on months was estimated as:

$$\log RR(\text{month}) = 0.31 \times \sin[(\text{month} + k) \times \pi/6]. \quad (3)$$

The best fit of the model was got when the constant k was taken as 1. The results indicate a highly significant ($P < 0.001$) monthly effect on mortality in the study area with the highest mortality observed in February and the lowest in July and August. Figure 5 illustrates the RRs for each month using the sine function (1).

Discussion

Descriptive epidemiological studies play an important role in medical research: information on mortality patterns is needed for the evaluation of health politics, identification of health hazards, planning of public health activities, and for many other issues. Such studies are very valuable especially where few epidemiological and demographic data exist. This study contributes to knowledge on general mortality in Burkina Faso and confirms the relevance of DSS as a viable means for collecting valid data on Africa's rural populations. As many such systems are established, new sets of valid data on Africa's populations will replace the 'guesstimates' which have so far been characteristic of international publications on Africa's rural populations.

The population is ascertained by field workers who visit households and collect the data. Newborns who die within the first days of life may not always be recorded (Kouyaté, personal communication), and infant mortality may therefore be slightly underestimated. Another study is underway to estimate the magnitude of this possible bias.

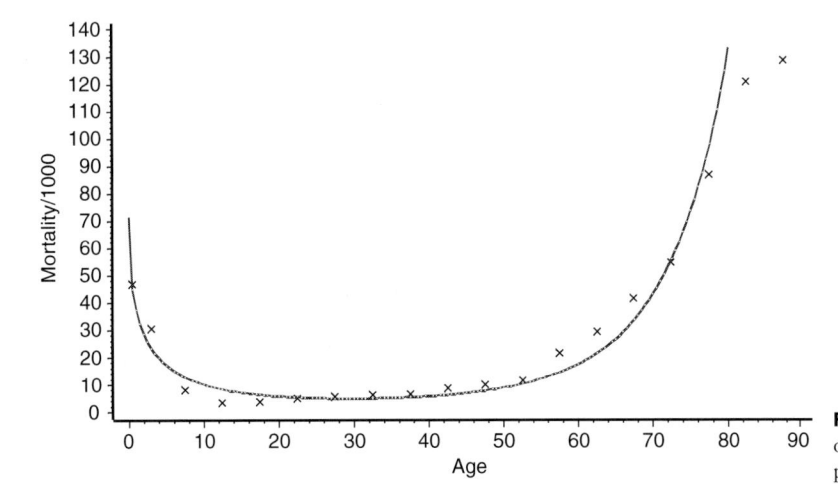

Figure 3 Mortality rates by age, continuous and categorical, males and females, DSS population, Nouna DSS, 1993–98.

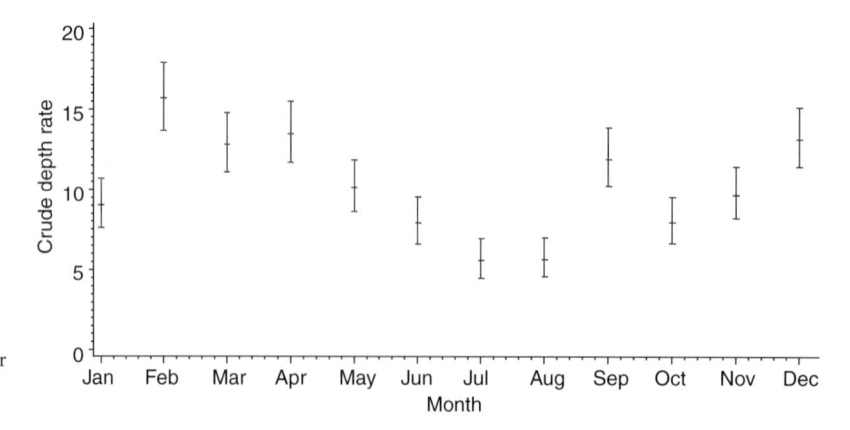

Figure 4 Crude death rates by months for the years 1993–98 (males and females combined).

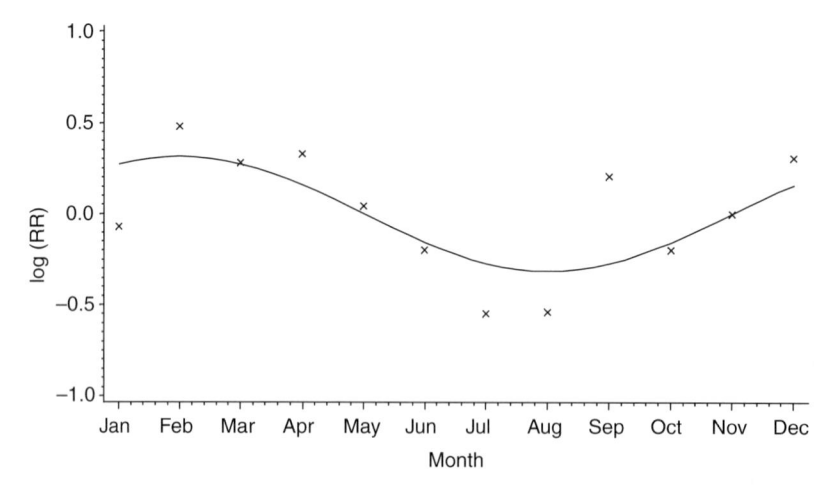

Figure 5 Seasonal-dependent rate ratios using a Poisson model adjusted for sex and age.

We used the Segi world population to standardize calculated crude death rates because most published rates are based on it and thus the results of this paper can be compared directly with previously published work. For developing countries in particular and in the absence of a standard population for Africa, the Segi population is a good choice because its artificial distribution is similar to that found in developing countries. As a result, calculated crude and standardized rates are rather similar. The WHO has recently introduced a new standard to replace it to take into account the increasing life expectancy in the last decades in most countries. However, the age structure of this new population differs from those in the countries in sub-Saharan Africa.

Poisson regression modelling was a useful means to describe mortality rates from DSS. It provides a convenient and intuitively appealing method to graphically illustrate mortality patterns. Appropriate software for its implementation is readily available.

High childhood mortality continues to be a disturbing feature of public health in many developing countries. However, in Nouna infant mortality decreased over the observation period, which was confirmed by Sankoh *et al.* (2001). This promising sign needs to be verified in the next few years. Mortality rates for the age groups 5–14 and 15–64 did not change; those for people above 64 showed a decline, but the numbers are too small to allow firm conclusions. Remarkably, males and females in Nouna showed a very similar mortality pattern across all age groups.

As reported in the results, a highly significant seasonal effect on mortality was identified. Our observation of high mortality rates in the dry season contrasts with a previous study in The Gambia (Jaffar *et al.* 1997) which reports high mortality rates in the rainy season. The reasons for this difference are still unclear. A cause-specific analysis in further investigations may bring some light to this finding. This paper has considered all-cause mortality. To determine the cause of mortality, VA are used in the Nouna DSS. This method is useful for a number of diseases, even infectious ones (Garenne et al. 2000). Cause-specific mortality will be reported in forthcoming publications.

Acknowledgements

Many thanks to Prof. Dr Rainer Sauerborn, Head of the Department of Tropical Hygiene and Public Health at the University of Heidelberg who promoted this research in many ways, and to the field staff in Nouna/Burkina Faso. The authors would like to thank Jörg Langohr and Prof. Dr Maria Blettner (University of Bielefeld, Germany) for providing the SAS-macro used to calculate the person-years. We would also like to thank Ms Gabriele Stieglbauer in our unit for her assistance in preparing the data set. This work was supported by the collaborative research grant SFB 544 'Kontrolle tropischer Infektionskrankheiten' of the German Research Foundation (DFG).

References

Anker M, Black RE, Coldham C et al. (1999) *A Standard Verbal Autopsy Method for Investigating Causes of Death in Infants and Children*. World Health Organization, Geneva.

Baltussen RMPM, Sanon M, Sommerfeld J & Würthwein R (2000) *Eliciting Disability Weights Using a Culturally-Adapted Visual Analogue Scale (VAS) in Rural Burkina Faso*. Discussion Paper 03/2000, SFB 544. University of Heidelberg, Heidelberg, Germany.

Breslow NE & Day NE (1987) *Statistical Methods in Cancer Research. Vol. II. The Design and Analysis of Cohort Studies*. International Agency for Research on Cancer, Lyon, France.

Chandramohan D, Maude GH, Rodrigues LC & Hayes RJ (1998) Verbal autopsies for adult deaths: their development and validation in a multicentre study. *Tropical Medicine and International Health* **3**, 436–446.

Cooper RS, Osotimehin B, Kaufman JS & Forrester T (1998) Disease burden in sub-Saharan Africa: what should we conclude in the absence of data? *Lancet* **351**, 208–210.

dos Santos Silva I (1999) *Cancer Epidemiology: Principles and Methods*. International Agency for Research on Cancer (IARC), Lyon, France.

Estève J, Benhamou E & Raymond L (1994) *Statistical Methods in Cancer Research, Vol. IV, Descriptive Epidemiology*. International Agency for Research on Cancer (IARC), Lyon, France.

Feachem RG & Jamison DT (1991) *Disease and Mortality in Sub-Saharan Africa*. Oxford University Press, New York.

Garenne M, Kahn K, Tollmann St & Gear J (2000) Causes of death in a rural area of South Africa: an international perspective. *Journal of Tropical Pediatrics* **46**, 183–190.

Jaffar S, Leach A, Greenwood AM et al. (1997) Changes in the pattern of infant and childhood mortality in upper river division, The Gambia, from 1989 to 1993. *Tropical Medicine and International Health* **2**, 28–37.

Kulldorff M (1997) A spatial scan statistic. *Communications in Statistics – Theory and Methods* **26**, 1481–1496.

Kynast-Wolf G, Sankoh OA, Stieglbauer G et al. (2001) *Mortality in a Rural Region in Sub-Saharan Africa – Results from a Demographic Surveillance System in Nouna, Burkina Faso*. Discussion Paper 01/2001, SFB 544, University of Heidelberg, Heidelberg, Germany (http://www.hyg.uni-heidelberg.de/sfb544/DP_01_2001.pdf).

Royston P & Altman DG (1994) Regression using fractional polynomials of continuous covariables: parsimonious parametric modelling. *Applied Statistics* **43**, 429–467.

Sankoh OA, Ye Y, Sauerborn R, Müller O & Becher H (2001) Clustering of childhood mortality in rural Burkina Faso. *International Journal of Epidemiology* **30**, 485–492.

SAS Institute (1997) *SAS/STAT Software Changes and Enhancements*. SAS Institute Inc., Cary, NC (SAS/STAT is a submodule of the Statistical Analysis System software package: http://www.sas.com).

Segi M (1960) *Cancer Mortality for Selected Sites in 24 Countries (1950–57)*. Tohoku University School of Public Health, Sendai, Japan.

Würthwein R, Gbangou A, Sauerborn R & Schmidt CM (2001) Measuring the local burden of disease: a study of years of life lost in rural Burkina Faso. *International Journal of Epidemiology* **30**, 501–508.

3.5 Patterns of adult and old-age mortality in rural Burkina Faso

SANKOH OA, KYNAST-WOLF G, KOUYATE B, BECHER H

Journal of Public Health Medicine 2003 Dec; 25(4): 372-6

Reprinted with permission from Oxford University Press.

Patterns of adult and old-age mortality in rural Burkina Faso

Osman A. Sankoh, Gisela Kynast-Wolf, Bocar Kouyaté and Heiko Becher

Summary

Based on a demographic surveillance population from 39 villages in rural Burkina Faso, we describe mortality patterns in adults (15–59 years) and older people (≥60 years), and discuss seasonal trends in mortality. During the study period 1993–1998, 589 deaths in adults and 593 deaths in older people were recorded from an average adult and older people population of 13 550. The crude all-cause mortality rate per 1000 for adults was 7.3 (95 per cent confidence interval (CI) 6.7–7.8) and for older people 55.8 (95 per cent CI 51.3–60.3). The probability of dying before age 60 after reaching age 15 was 34 per cent for males and 32 per cent for females. Malaria and diarrhoea, recorded through verbal autopsy, accounted for 21 per cent of total deaths in adults and 22 per cent in older people. A seasonal trend in mortality for older people with a peak in February was identified. The study shows that malaria is an important cause of death in adulthood.

Keywords: adult mortality, old age mortality, demographic surveillance system, verbal autopsy

Introduction

Unlike childhood mortality, adult (15–59 years) and old-age (≥60 years) mortality has not been a major research focus in sub-Saharan Africa (SSA). Hence, there is little knowledge of the mortality patterns in these groups even though they suffer from a much broader range of communicable and non-communicable diseases (NCDs). For instance, Kaufmann et al.[1] have noted the scarcity of information on cause of death among adults in SSA.

One of the few projects focusing on adults is the Adult Morbidity and Mortality Project (AMMP) in Tanzania, established in 1992 by the Tanzanian Ministry of Health in collaboration with the UK University of Newcastle upon Tyne, to investigate the role of NCDs in the overall disease burden in Tanzania.[2,3] The project estimated for its population in 1997 that 'the proportion of all deaths occurring to those between 15 and 60 years of age may equal or exceed that of deaths to children under 5'.[2]

Based on the Nouna Demographic Surveillance System (DSS) operated since 1992 by the Nouna Health Research Centre in Burkina Faso,[4] we have analysed the mortality patterns of adults and older people in the region. We present the results of a descriptive analysis of all-cause and, to a limited extent, cause-specific mortality patterns in adults and older people for the Nouna health district covered by the Nouna DSS for the period 1993–1998. Only deaths caused by malaria and diarrhoea have been specified.

Materials and methods

Study area

Figure 1 shows the study area in NW Burkina Faso, West Africa, with an estimated population of about 11 million, of whom 80 per cent live in rural areas. Kossi has an area of 7464.44 km^2 and a population of about 240 000.

The study area comprises 39 villages around Nouna town, the headquarters of the Nouna Health District. The distance from village to the few local health centres ranges from 0 to 34 km. The village population ranges from 121 to 2346 persons.

The Demographic Surveillance System (DSS)

The database for this study is based on the DSS of the Nouna Health Research Centre, which has been described before.[4] The variables registered during vital events registration include births, deaths, pregnancies, and migration in and out of the household, as well as information on all the dates related to these events. The DSS database also contains data on household economics and maternal health. The causes of death are determined by the verbal autopsy (VA) method.[5] However, this procedure is currently being implemented in the Nouna DSS, so the percentage of deaths with associated cause is still low. Hence we concentrate on total mortality for most analyses.

---

[1]Department of Tropical Hygiene and Public Health, University of Heidelberg–Medical School, Im Neuenheimer Feld 324, D-69120 Heidelberg, Germany.
[2]INDEPTH Network, P.O. Box KD 213 Kanda, Accra, Ghana.
[3]Nouna Health Research Centre, BP 2, Nouna, Burkina Faso.

Osman A. Sankoh,[1,2] Manager, Communications and External Relations, INDEPTH Network; formerly, Scientist, University of Heidelberg – medical school.
Gisela Kynast-Wolf,[1] Statistician
Bocar Kouyaté,[3] Director
Heiko Becher,[1] Professor of Epidemiology and Biostatistics
Address correspondence to Heiko Becher.
E-mail:heiko.becher@urz.uni-heidelberg.de

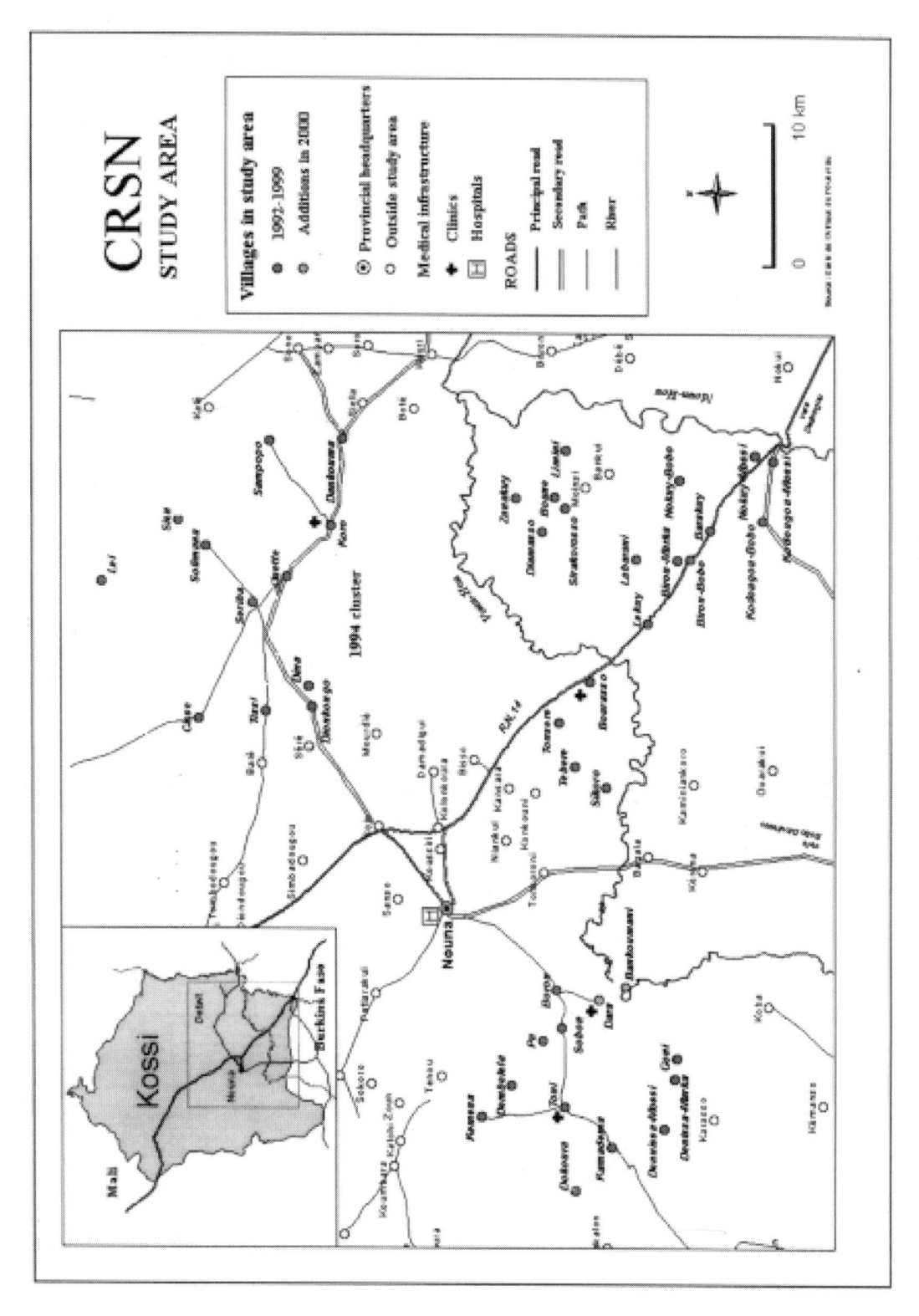

Fig. 1 Map of study area (source: Ref. 9).

Statistical and demographic methods

The methods used are similar to those applied elsewhere to describe infant and childhood mortality[4] in the same area. Briefly, crude death rates and 95 per cent confidence intervals (CIs) were calculated based on the normal approximation, or for smaller sample sizes ($n < 20$) using exact Poisson CIs.[6] Poisson regression modelling[7] was used to investigate patterns of mortality rates (age-specific death rates, ASDR) by season. Life tables were constructed according to Preston et al.[8]

Results

Basic demographic parameters

The total population size (all ages) in 1993–1998 (on 31 December) for both sexes rose steadily by 14.5 per cent from 27 473 persons in 1993 to 31 476 persons in 1998, with a mean yearly population growth rate of 2.8 per cent. The two adult age groups (15–59 and ≥60 years) made up a little more than 50 per cent of the total population. The old-age group (≥60 years) made up about 6 per cent of all adults. The population size of the adult age group (15–59 years) was 12 599 persons in 1993 and rose by 15 per cent to 14 484 in 1998, with a mean annual growth rate of 2.8 per cent. For the old-age group (≥60 years) the population size also rose steadily by 7.3 per cent from 1670 persons in 1993 to 1792 persons in 1998. The mean annual growth rate was 1.4 per cent compared with 27 per cent for the entire country.

All-cause adult and old-age mortality

The Table gives the annual distribution of deaths, midyear populations and mortality rates by sex with their 95 per cent CIs. The all-cause adult death rate of 7.3 per 1000 for the total observation period is much lower than that of 35.0 per 1000 children under five in the same study region and period as reported by Sankoh et al.[9] There were slightly more female adult deaths than male ones, 307 versus 282; this was the case also for the old-age mortality by sex by year (304 versus 289). There is high all-cause old-age mortality of (55.8 per 1000) collectively for 1993–1998. The data show that older women generally have a higher mortality than men.

Cause-specific adult and old-age mortality

As malaria and fever are not easily distinguishable causes through verbal autopsy, they are combined in this analysis. The rest of the causes are put under 'other causes', because for a large percentage of deaths no cause is available. Our results show that both malaria and diarrhoea account for about 39 per cent for female and 33 per cent for male of all deaths of known causes occurring in both adults and old-aged people in the study area.

Seasonal variation in mortality

Figure 2 illustrates the seasonable variation (by month) in the mortality rates with 95 per cent CIs for adults and older people. For the two age groups a trend toward lower rates in the months

Table 1 All-cause adult (15–59 years) and all-cause old-age (≥60 years) mortality by sex in 1993–1998 in the study area

	1993		1994		1995		1996		1997		1998		Total (1993–1998)	
	F	M	F	M	F	M	F	M	F	M	F	M	F	M
Adults (15–59 years)														
Total no. deaths	38	43	60	37	64	57	50	43	43	51	52	51	307	282
Midyear pop.	6370	6233	6587	6506	6726	6797	6810	6836	6939	6972	7258	7263	6781.7	6767.8
Mean age	36.3	35.5	35.6	34.7	34.8	33.6	34.2	33.1	33.5	32.4	32.6	31.5	34.5	33.5
Crude yearly death rate (per 1000)	5.97	6.9	9.11	5.69	9.52	8.39	7.34	6.29	6.20	7.31	7.16	7.02	7.54	6.94
95% CI	4.07–7.87	4.84–8.96	6.81–11.41	3.86–7.52	7.18–11.85	6.21–10.57	5.30–9.38	4.41–8.17	4.35–8.05	5.30–9.32	5.21–9.11	5.09–8.95	6.70–8.38	6.13–7.75
Old age (≥60 years)														
Total no. deaths	50	45	53	46	55	54	41	28	52	38	53	78	304	289
Midyear pop.	865	827	863	843	900	863	924	879	919	896	937	913	901.3	870.2
Mean age	73.2	73.3	73.0	72.8	72.3	72.0	71.6	71.6	71.0	71.0	70.3	70.2	71.9	71.8
Crude yearly death rate (per 1000)	57.8	54.41	61.41	54.57	61.11	62.57	44.37	31.85	56.58	42.41	56.56	85.43	56.21	55.35
95% CI	41.78–73.82	38.51–70.31	44.88–77.94	38.8–70.34	44.96–77.26	45.88–79.26	30.79–57.95	20.05–43.65	41.20–71.96	28.93–55.89	41.33–71.79	66.47–104.39	49.89–62.53	48.97–61.73

F, female; M, male.

May–October (rainy season), and higher rates in November–April was observed.

The mortality rates achieved a peak in February and August. The results indicate a highly significant ($p < 0.001$) seasonal effect on mortality in the study area in the two age groups. The highest mortality rates were observed in the months of February and April and the lowest in the months of July and August. We looked at rate ratios for each month compared with November, used as reference month. Both age groups show a remarkably similar mortality pattern by month.

Life tables

We calculated the probability of dying before age 60 after reaching age 15 to be 34 per cent for males and 32 per cent for females.

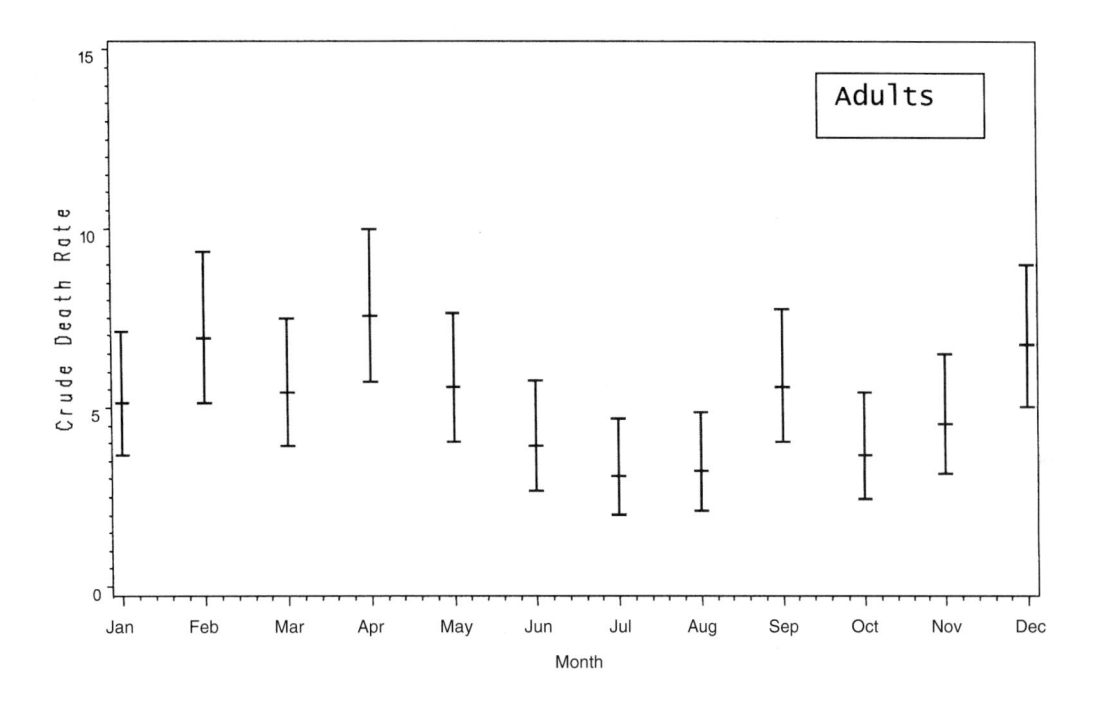

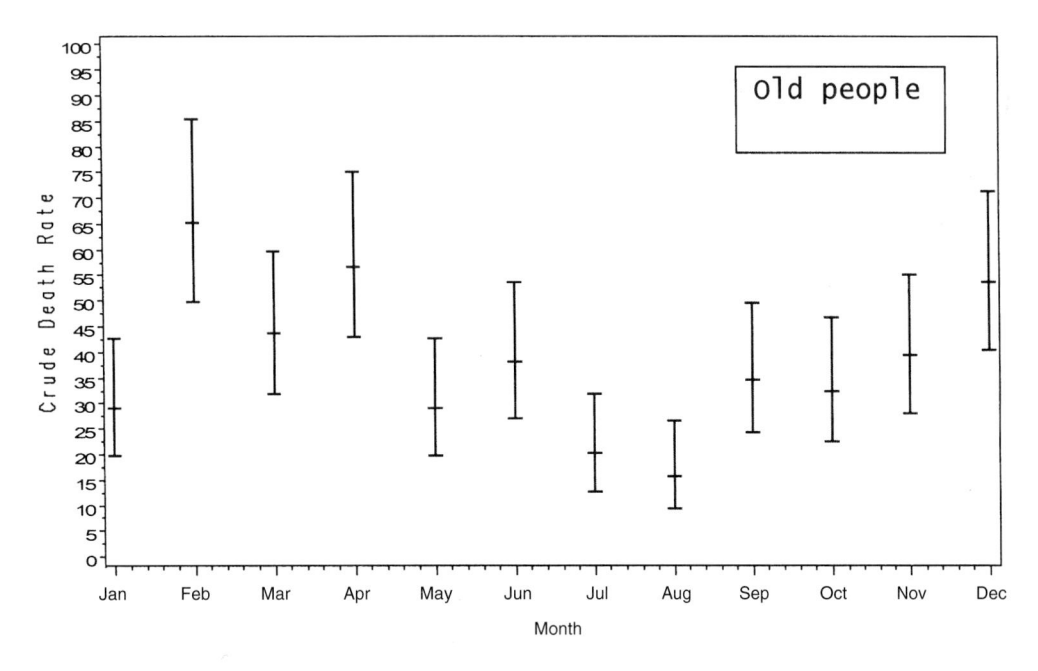

Fig. 2 Death rates by month and 95 per cent CIs for adults (15–60 years) and old people (≥60 years).

The probability of dying in the 5 year age intervals remained less than 10 per cent for both sexes until 50–54 years. It increased steadily to 45 per cent for women and 51 per cent for men in the interval 80–84 years. The life expectancy for females at birth is 51 years, and slightly lower for males. However, given age 15, the expected age at death is 65 years. This clearly shows the large impact of childhood mortality on life expectancy in this population.

Discussion

The adult and old-age mortality patterns identified are largely consistent with the general pattern identifiable in most of SSA. For instance, Kitange et al.[3] reported a crude all-cause adult mortality range of 6.1 per 1000 a year for women in Hai and 15.9 per 1000 a year for men in Morogoro rural area in Tanzania, East Africa. We report an average of 6.9 per 1000 for men and 7.5 per 1000 for women.

A seasonal trend in mortality for older people was identified in the Nouna data: higher rates from November to April with a peak in February and lower rates from May to October. This is strikingly similar to the seasonal trend in mortality in children in the same study region for this DSS population. Kynast-Wolf et al.[4] reported higher total mortality from November to May with a peak in February and lower rates from June to October.

The VA method still remains the most viable option to determine cause of death in rural Africa. In this study, it led to results that reflect the reality of the problem. For instance, about 20 per cent of the adult and old-age deaths in both males and females reported from our analysis are attributable to malaria and diarrhoea. This agrees with Setel et al.,[10] who reported malaria and diarrhoea as among the major causes of adult deaths in three DSS sites in Tanzania.

Finally, although there is some degree of uncertainty resulting from the probability of underreporting of adult deaths, it is reasonable to conclude that adult mortality in the Nouna DSS has remained low over the years. If the impact of the HIV/AIDS epidemic could be contained in the study area, coupled with the implementation of effective interventions to address the devastating impact of malaria, we do not foresee an increase in adult mortality in the Nouna area in the near future.

Acknowledgements

We would like to thank Pierre Ngom (African Population and Health Research Centre, Nairobi, Kenya) and Sam Clark (Agincourt, South Africa) for their helpful comments on life table analysis. We also thank Gabriele Stieglbauer (medical documentalist) for assisting with the database. This work was supported by research grant SFB 544 (Control of tropical infectious diseases) from the German Research Foundation (DFG).

References

1 Kaufmann JS, Asuzu MC, Rotimi CN, et al. The absence of adult mortality data for sub-Saharan Africa: a practical solution. *Bull WHO* 1997; **75**: 389–395.

2 Adult Morbidity and Mortality Project. *Policy implications of adult morbidity and mortality* 1997. Dar es salaam: AMMP.

3 Kitange, HM, Machibya, H, Black J, et al. Outlook for survivors of childhood in sub-Saharan Africa: adult mortality in Tanzania. *Br Med J* 1996; **312**: 216–220.

4 Kynast-Wolf G, Sankoh OA, Kouyaté B, Becher H. Mortality patterns 1993–1998 in a rural area of Burkina Faso, West Africa, based on the Nouna Demographic Surveillance System. *Trop Med Int Hlth* 2002; **7**: 349–356.

5 Anker M, Black RE, Coldham C, et al. *Verbal autopsy method for investigating causes of death in infants and children*. Geneva: World Health Organization, 1999.

6 dos Santos Silva, I. *Cancer epidemiology: principles and methods*. Lyon: International Agency for Research on Cancer, 1999.

7 Breslow NE, Day NE. *Statistical methods in cancer research. Vol. II. The design and analysis of cohort studies*. Lyon: International Agency for Research on Cancer, 1987.

8 Preston SH, Heuveline P, Guillot M, Guillan M. *Demography: measuring and modeling population processes*. Oxford: Blackwell, 2001.

9 Sankoh, OA, Ye, Y, Sauerborn, R, Müller, O, Becher, H. Clustering of childhood mortality in rural Burkina Faso. *Int J Epidemiol* 2001; **30**: 485–492.

10 Setel, PW, Unwin, N, Alberti KGMM, Hemed, Y, for the AMMP Team. Cause-specific adult mortality: evidence from community-based surveillance – selected sites, Tanzania, 1992–1998. *Morbid Mortal Wkly Rep* 2000; **49**: 416–419.

Accepted on 10 June 2003

3.6 Malaria morbidity, treatment-seeking behaviour, and mortality in a cohort of young children in rural Burkina Faso

MÜLLER O, TRAORE C, BECHER H, KOUYATE B

Trop Med Int Health. 2003 Apr; 8(4): 290-6

Reprinted with permission from Blackwell Publishers Ltd.

Malaria morbidity, treatment-seeking behaviour, and mortality in a cohort of young children in rural Burkina Faso

Olaf Müller[1], Corneille Traoré[2], Heiko Becher[1] and Bocar Kouyaté[2]

1 Department of Tropical Hygiene and Public Health of the Ruprecht-Karls-University, Heidelberg, Germany
2 Centre de Recherche en Santé de Nouna, Nouna, Burkina Faso

Summary

OBJECTIVE To describe the pattern of fever-associated morbidity, treatment-seeking behaviour for fever episodes, and cause-specific mortality in young children of a malaria-holoendemic area in rural Burkina Faso.

METHODS In a longitudinal community-based intervention study, 709 representative children aged 6–31 months were followed daily over 6 months (including the main malaria transmission period) through village-based field staff.

RESULTS Of 1848 disease episodes, 1640 (89%) were fever episodes, and of those, 894 (55%) were attributed to malaria (fever + ≥5000 parasites/μl). Eighty-five percent of fever episodes were treated, mainly with chloroquine and paracetamol, 69% of treatments took place in households, 16% in local health centres, 13% in villages, and 1% in hospitals. Treatment-seeking in a health centre or hospital was associated with accessibility and disease severity. Cerebral malaria and malnutrition-associated diarrhoea were the most frequently diagnosed causes of death. While most children with a post-mortem diagnosis of diarrhoea had not received any treatment, children who died of malaria had often received insufficient treatment. In particular, there was a lack of an appropriate second-line treatment at formal health services after chloroquine treatment had failed to resolve symptoms.

CONCLUSIONS These findings call for more effective prevention and treatment of malaria, malnutrition and diarrhoea in rural African communities, as well as for better supervision of existing malaria treatment guidelines in formal health services.

keywords malaria, cerebral malaria, chloroquine, treatment-seeking behaviour, mortality, diarrhoea, malnutrition, Africa, Burkina Faso

Introduction

Malaria remains the most important parasitic disease and is globally responsible for 300–500 million fever episodes and 1.5–2.7 million deaths per year (WHO 1997). The greatest burden of malaria is in sub-Saharan African (SSA) where it has been estimated that 40% of fever episodes are caused by malaria (Brinkmann & Brinkmann 1991). Most malaria deaths occur in young children of rural SSA areas with little access to health services (Greenwood et al. 1987a; WHO 1997; Snow et al. 1999). This situation is now aggravated through the increasing development of resistance by *Plasmodium falciparum* to existing and affordable first-line drugs such as chloroquine and sulphadoxine–pyrimethamine in most countries of SSA (Trape 2001).

The success of malaria treatment strategies is closely linked to the behaviour of patients and caretakers of young children. Treatment-seeking behaviour usually depends on the local epidemiology of malaria, access to health care providers, costs of services, attitudes towards providers, perceived severity of disease, age, sex, educational level, socio-economic status, and cultural beliefs about the cause and cure of illness (Deming et al. 1989; Greenwood 1989; Reuben 1993; McCombie 1994; Tanner & Vlassoff 1998; Molyneux et al. 1999; Baume et al. 2000). Although it has been suggested that fever is more likely than other symptoms to prompt caregivers to seek treatment in formal health services, self-medication through pharmacies and drug sellers is consistently the most common response when people first experience symptoms that could be malaria (Dabis et al. 1989; McCombie 1994). Underdosing of antimalarials received through public or private sector providers is virtually universal, and costs, side-effects and resistance development of drugs used are of increasing concern (McCombie 1994; Ruebush et al. 1995; Tanner & Vlassoff 1998; Baume et al. 2000; Nshakira et al. 2002). But there is little information on the impact of treatment-seeking behaviour on the outcome of malaria illness. We describe here the pattern of febrile morbidity, treatment-seeking behaviour and cause-specific mortality in a cohort of young children in a rural area of Burkina Faso with high *P. falciparum* transmission intensity.

Methods

Study area

The study was conducted in 18 villages of the research zone of the *Centre de Recherche en Santé de Nouna* (CRSN) in Nouna Health District in north-western Burkina Faso (Kouyaté *et al.* 2000). Nouna is a dry orchard savanna area, populated almost exclusively by subsistence farmers of different ethnic groups. There is a short rainy season which usually lasts from June until October. Malaria is holoendemic and childhood mortality is high, with marked differences between villages (Müller *et al.* 2001; Sankoh *et al.* 2001). Malnutrition in young children is also frequent, with the highest prevalence during the rainy season (Müller *et al.* 2001). Formal health services in the CRSN research zone are restricted to four village-based health centres and the district hospital in Nouna town. The current policy of the Burkina Faso Ministry of Health is for all fever cases with no other obvious cause to be treated presumptively as malaria, with chloroquine as the first-line drug and sulphadoxine–pyrimethamine, second-line.

Study participants

Data for this study were taken from the data bank of a randomized controlled trial (RCT) on the effects of zinc supplementation on malaria morbidity conducted in the CRSN research zone in 1999 (Müller *et al.* 2001). During this trial, a representative sample of 709 children (356 intervention and 353 placebo group) aged 6–31 months (mean 18 months) at enrolment in June 1999 were recruited from 18 villages of two health-centre defined subareas (Koro and Bourasso) and followed over a 6-month period.

Field methods for data collection are described elsewhere (Müller *et al.* 2001). Briefly, study children were visited daily over the main malaria transmission period (June to December) by village-based field staff for temperature measurement and malaria slide preparation from fingerprick blood in case of fever. As the field staff was not medically trained, they did not treat sick children but regularly advised the child's caretaker to seek diagnosis and treatment at the next governmental health centre (where the availability of trained staff and sufficient drug supply is guaranteed). All relevant signs and symptoms of children were recorded in a standard questionnaire during daily visits. Moreover, a comprehensive questionnaire was filled in for each disease episode which included information on specific signs and symptoms as well as place, time and type of treatment received. A disease episode was subjectively defined as any significant impairment of the health of a study child, a fever episode was defined as a disease episode with ≥37.5 °C axillary temperature, and a malaria episode was defined as a fever episode accompanied by a *P. falciparum* parasite density of ≥5000/μl and no other obvious cause for the illness.

All mothers or guardians of study children who had died during the 6-month observation period were interviewed in depth by the study physician shortly after the event. The final post-mortem diagnosis was based on the results of this interview together with the detailed clinical and parasitological information available through the daily visits to all study children. Simple proportions were used to describe the parameters investigated.

Ethical aspects

Approval for the RCT was granted by the Ethical Committee of the Heidelberg University Medical School, the Ethical Committee of the World Health Organization in Geneva and the Ministry of Health in Burkina Faso. Before the study was implemented, the protocol was explained in detail to the communities of the study area, and oral informed consent sought from the community leaders, the heads of households, and the parents of study children. Study children were examined by a physician during three cross-sectional surveys, and sick children were treated in the village or were referred to Nouna Hospital free of charge. In addition, parents were regularly educated regarding prevention and treatment of malnutrition.

Results

Morbidity

Detailed information on morbidity was available from 1848 disease episodes recorded over the 6-month observation period in 666 of the 709 children (median three episodes, range 0–9). Of these, 1640 of 1848 (89%) were fever episodes (median duration 4 days, range 1–96), and 894 of 1640 (55%) of fever episodes were attributable to falciparum malaria. Febrile episodes were frequently accompanied by diarrhoea, vomiting and cough, with vomiting being more frequent in febrile than non-febrile episodes (14% *vs.* 6%) and diarrhoea/dysentery being more frequent in non-febrile than febrile episodes (53% *vs.* 23%). Convulsions and coma were always associated with fever. Accidents (12 of 16 were burns) were rare. The distribution of self-reported morbidity by fever status is shown in Table 1.

Table 1 Distribution of self-reported morbidity by fever status in 1848 disease episodes in a cohort of 709 young children in rural Burkina Faso

	Febrile episodes N = 1640 (%)	Non-febrile episodes N = 208 (%)
Diarrhoea	353 (22)	93 (45)
Dysentery	18 (1)	18 (9)
Vomiting	233 (14)	13 (6)
Cough	232 (14)	38 (18)
Dyspnoea	24 (1)	4 (2)
Rhinitis and/or otitis	73 (4)	15 (7)
Pyodermia	45 (3)	15 (7)
Convulsions	13 (1)	0 (0)
Coma	6 (0.4)	0 (0)
Accidents	0	16 (8)

Table 2 Treatment during fever episodes in a cohort of 709 young children in rural Burkina Faso

Treatment category	No. of episodes	Proportion %
Chloroquine (CQ)	558	40
CQ + antipyretics	266	19
CQ + traditional remedies	67	5
CQ + antipyretics + traditional remedies	28	2
CQ + tetracycline	45	3
CQ + other drugs	53	4
Antipyretics	48	3
Traditional remedies	87	6
Quinine	22	2
Antibiotics	12	1
Others	200	14
Total	1386	100

Treatment-seeking behaviour

Of 1640 recognized fever episodes, 1386 (85%) were treated. Overall, 2228 treatments were provided during these fever episodes: 1541 of 2228 (69%) with drugs or traditional remedies available in the household, 360 of 2228 (16%) in a local health centre, 290 of 2228 (13%) in the village (shops, village health workers, traditional healers), and 20 of 2228 (1%) in a hospital. Treatment-seeking at formal health services (health centre/hospital) was largely influenced by location of the household. The highest frequencies of health centre/hospital visits per child during the 6-month study period were in the two villages with an existing health centre (1.7 in Bourasso and 0.8 in Koro) and in a village close to a hospital of the neighbouring district (1.7 in Nokui-Bobo). The mean number of health centre/hospital visits per child during the 6-month study period was 0.5, ranging from 0.03 to 0.07 in the villages of Sampopo and Cisse, respectively, to 1.7 in Bourasso and in Nokui-Bobo. While there were no differences in the overall number of mean treatments per child between the two study subareas of Bourasso and Koro, the mean number of health centre/hospital visits in Bourasso subarea was higher than in Koro subarea (0.8 vs. 0.3). There was no association between the length of fever episodes and visiting a health centre or hospital, but children with ≥38.5 °C temperature were more likely to visit a health centre or hospital than children with <38.5 °C (19% vs. 12%). Of the few fever episodes with reported convulsions, four of 13 (31%) were treated at a health centre or hospital.

Of 2228 treatments provided during 1386 fever episodes, 1180 (53%) were chloroquine, 426 (19%) were antipyretics (mainly paracetamol), 283 (13%) were traditional remedies, 56 (3%) were oral rehydration solution, 45 (2%) were tetracycline, 43 (2%) were quinine, 30 (1%) were ampicillin/amoxicillin, 29 (1%) were cotrimoxazole, and four (0.2%) were pyrimethamine–sulphadoxine. Overall, 73% of fever episodes were treated with chloroquine alone or in combination with other drugs, mainly antipyretics (Table 2). While chloroquine and antipyretics were usually available at the household/village level, quinine treatment was observed in similar proportions at household/village and health centre/hospital level, and most antibiotic treatment (except tetracycline) and the few treatments with pyrimethamine–sulphadoxine were mainly reported from the health centre/hospital level (Table 3).

Table 3 Proportions of fever treatment provided at household/village level compared with health centre/hospital level by treatment category in a cohort of 709 young children in rural Burkina Faso

Treatment category	Household/village (%)	Health centre/hospital (%)
Chloroquine	1049/1180 (89)	131/1180 (11)
Antipyretics	369/426 (87)	57/426 (13)
Traditional remedies	283/283 (100)	0/283 (0)
Oral rehydration solution	26/56 (46)	30/56 (54)
Tetracycline	45/45 (100)	0/45 (0)
Quinine	22/43 (51)	21/43 (49)
Ampicillin/amoxicillin	3/30 (10)	27/30 (90)
Cotrimoxazole	5/29 (17)	24/29 (83)
Pyrimethamine–sulphadoxine	0/4 (0)	4/4 (100)

Mortality

Of 709 cohort children, 17 children (2.4%) died over the 6-month observation period (median age 20 months, range

11–32). The most frequent post-mortem diagnosis was malaria with 7/17 (41%) and diarrhoea with six of 17 (35%) cases, while malnutrition (mainly marasmus) was documented in six of 17 (35%) children (four of six diarrhoea cases) (Table 4). Of cases with a malaria diagnosis, six of seven showed typical signs of cerebral malaria (fever, convulsions, coma), and three of seven showed signs of respiratory distress. Thirteen of 17 (76%) deaths occurred in just two of 18 villages (Cisse and Solimana) (Table 4).

The median duration of the final disease episode was 5 days (range 1–31), and 10 of 17 (59%) children had not received any specific treatment during those episodes (three of seven malaria cases, five of six diarrhoea cases). Treatments during final disease were chloroquine complemented by traditional remedies (four of seven), paracetamol (three of seven), tetracycline (one of seven), and cotrimoxazole (one of seven). Two children with malaria had also visited a health centre during their final disease episode, and one child had been brought to a hospital. None of the children seen at a health centre had received appropriate second line treatment for malaria (Table 4).

Discussion

This paper describes the pattern of morbidity, mortality and health seeking behaviour in a large cohort of young children from a randomized placebo-controlled trial on the effects of zinc supplementation on malaria (Müller et al. 2001). As it has been shown that the intervention influences diarrhoea (but not malaria) morbidity and probably all-cause mortality, the data reported here are not fully representative for the pattern of morbidity and mortality in the population studied. Moreover, the treatment-seeking behaviour may have been influenced by the presence of field staff in the villages and their advice to visit a health centre in case of illness. Although these effects are not likely to be large, they may have led to an underestimate of morbidity and mortality rates as well as to an overestimate of treatment-seeking at health centres/hospitals.

The great majority of disease episodes in young children of our study area was associated with fever and about half were attributed to falciparum malaria, which confirms the major impact of malaria in this age group in endemic areas (Greenwood et al. 1987a; Brinkmann & Brinkmann 1991; Snow et al. 1999). Fever and malaria

Table 4 Treatment-seeking behaviour during final disease and causes of death in 17 children of a cohort study in rural Burkina Faso

No.	Village	Sex	Treatment during FD	Dur FD (days)	Diagnosis	Date and age (mo) of death
1	S	F	None	5	Malaria	11/99 (13)
2	S	M	HH nine dbd (CQ, PAR), HH six dbd (TET), HC three dbd (PAR), one dbd (TRA)	9	Malaria	9/99 (14)
3	N	M	HH one dbd (CQ, TRA)	2	Malaria	8/99 (13)
4	T	F	None	1	Malaria	11/99 (21)
5	S	M	HH 21 dbd (PAR, CQ, TRA), HC 16 dbd (CQ, COT)	21	Malaria	10/99 (20)
6	N	F	None (died at hospital arrival)	1	Malaria	7/99 (21)
7	S	F	HH four dbd (CQ), HH two dbd (PAR, TRA)	4	Malaria	7/99 (29)
8	C	F	HC three dbd (PAR)	3	Diarrhoea Malnutrition	6/99 (11)
9	C	F	None	7	Diarrhoea Malnutrition	7/99 (13)
10	C	F	None	5	Diarrhoea	7/99 (16)
11	C	F	None	5	Diarrhoea Malnutrition	10/99 (20)
12	C	F	None	5	Diarrhoea	10/99 (28)
13	C	M	HC four dbd (ORS)	5	Diarrhoea Malnutrition	7/99 (30)
14	S	M	None	30	Anaemia Malnutrition	12/99 (32)
15	D	M	None	30	Malnutrition	11/99 (19)
16	S	M	HH five dbd (TRA)	5	Pneumonia	6/99 (28)
17	C	M	None	31	Hepatitis	11/99 (18)

FD, final disease; Dur, duration; mo, months; C, Cisse; N, Nokui; S, Solimana; T, Tebere; F, female; M, male; HH, household; HC, health centre; dbd, days before death; CQ, chloroquine; PAR, paracetamol; TET, tetracycline; COT, cotrimoxazole; ORS, oral rehydration solution; TRA, traditional treatment.

episodes were frequently accompanied by diarrhoea, vomiting and cough, which has also been recognized in other malaria endemic areas of SSA (Rooth & Björkman 1992; Müller et al. 1996; Rogier et al. 1999).

Most fever cases in study children received some form of treatment, with multiple treatment being common and most treatment taking place at the household/village level through left-over drugs from former disease episodes, drugs bought from shops or a minority of still functioning village health workers, and through treatment by traditional healers. Only few treatments took place at the health centre/hospital level, and the frequency of such visits was associated with subarea and distance to the health centre/hospital as well as with a more severe illness presentation. Treatment was usually with chloroquine, the official first-line treatment for uncomplicated malaria in Burkina Faso, often accompanied by antipyretics (mainly paracetamol) and traditional remedies. These findings support similar observations from other malaria endemic regions of SSA and point to the importance of accessibility to formal health services in rural SSA (De Francisco et al. 1994; McCombie 1994; Ahorlu et al. 1997; Baume et al. 2000; Théra et al. 2002). While most antibiotic treatment for young children was provided through the formal health sector, tetracycline treatment took place at household/village level. This observation is disturbing and calls for better education on the dangers of antibiotic treatments in general and tetracycline treatment in the case of children in particular, in respective communities.

A large proportion of deaths in study children was caused by malaria and diarrhoea, which supports the major importance of these two diseases in young children of rural SSA (Jaffar et al. 1997; Garenne et al. 2000). The observation of significant clustering of childhood mortality in a few villages of the CRSN study area has already been described (Sankoh et al. 2001). The pattern of cause-specific mortality in our cohort children and the lack of effective treatment in most deceased diarrhoea cases, together with the findings from a case-control study on risk factors for childhood mortality provide strong evidence for untreated diarrhoea with underlying malnutrition being responsible for the observed excess mortality in the village of Cisse (Ndah 2001). As a consequence of these findings, an intervention is under way to improve the water hygiene in the village of Cissé and a discussion on new strategies to reduce malnutrition in young children has been initiated at the national level.

Surprisingly, most of the deceased study children with a malaria diagnosis showed typical signs and symptoms of cerebral malaria before death. This finding is not in agreement with the opinion of severe anaemia being the most common cause of malaria deaths in areas of high transmission intensity but could probably reflect the influence of a more seasonal distribution of transmission (WHO 2000). However, although the validity of our post-mortem diagnosis can be considered much superior to classical verbal autopsy procedures because of the additional parasitological and clinical information available, this retrospective method is known for an overall low sensitivity and specificity in the diagnosis of malaria (Snow et al. 1992; Todd et al. 1994; Quigley et al. 1996). Finally, the small number of deaths in our cohort calls for some caution in the interpretation of findings.

It has been reported that certain illnesses are considered best treated by modern health services, while others are considered best treated by traditional methods, and often a mixture of both is sought (McCombie 1994). Severe manifestations of malaria like cerebral malaria and severe anaemia were often not associated with malaria by the people, and traditional healers were more likely to be consulted in such cases (McCombie 1994; Baume et al. 2000). However, these observations were neither supported by the health seeking behaviour in our cohort children with a postmortem diagnosis of cerebral malaria, nor by the findings from an exploratory anthropological study on malaria in the area (Okrah et al. 2002).

The observation that two of seven children with a malaria diagnosis had died within the first 24 h after onset of symptoms supports the evidence for a possible rapid development of malaria disease in young children (Greenwood et al. 1987a,b; Molyneux et al. 1989; Mabeza et al. 1995). Moreover, four of seven children with a malaria diagnosis died despite having received chloroquine treatment during their final illness. This is quite disturbing and could either be caused by an insufficient drug level (as a result of false dosage, low drug quality or vomiting/diarrhoea) and/or by the level of emerging chloroquine resistance in the area (Müller et al. 2003). Even more disturbing is the observation of a largely insufficient treatment at the peripheral health centres, with one of the deceased children having received only paracetamol, and one having received chloroquine again instead of an appropriate second-line treatment. This supports similar findings on the poor quality of malaria treatment in peripheral health services of Burkina Faso and elsewhere in SSA (Dürrheim et al. 1999; Baume et al. 2000; Krause & Sauerborn 2000; Font et al. 2001; Nsimba et al. 2002).

In conclusion, malaria is the major cause for morbidity and mortality of young children in the Nouna area of rural Burkina Faso. Multiple treatment at home is the most frequent response to febrile illness, and health care-seeking at formal health services depends on accessibility and disease severity. While diarrhoea mortality was associated with malnutrition and lack of treatment, malaria mortality was associated with a rapid development of severe disease, with symptoms of cerebral malaria, and with non-use of an appropriate second-line treatment. These findings call for more effective prevention and treatment of malaria, malnutrition and diarrhoea in the rural communities of SSA, as well as for better supervision of existing malaria treatment guidelines in formal health services.

Acknowledgement

The study was funded by the Deutsche Forschungsgemeinschaft (SFB 544, Control of Tropical Infectious Diseases).

References

Ahorlu CK, Dunyo SK, Afari EA, Koram KA & Nkrumah FK (1997) Malaria-related beliefs and behaviour in southern Ghana: implications for treatment, prevention and control. *Tropical Medicine and International Health* **2**, 488–499.

Baume C, Helitzer D & Kachur SP (2000) Patterns of care for childhood malaria in Zambia. *Social Science and Medicine* **51**, 1491–1503.

Brinkmann U & Brinkmann A (1991) Malaria and health in Africa: the present situation and epidemiological trends. *Tropical Medicine and Parasitology* **42**, 204–213.

Dabis F, Breman JG, Roisin AJ, Haba F & The ACSI CCCD Team (1989) Monitoring selective components of primary health care: methodology and community assessment of vaccination, diarrhoea and malaria practices in Conakry, Guinea. *Bulletin of the World Health Organization* **67**, 675–684.

De Francisco A, Armstrong-Schellenberg J, Hall AJ, Greenwood AM, Cham K & Greenwood BM (1994) Comparison of mortality between villages with and without Primary Health Care workers in Upper River Division, The Gambia. *Journal of Tropical Medicine and Hygiene* **97**, 69–74.

Deming M, Gayibor A, Murphy K, Jones T & Karsa T (1989) Home treatment of febrile children with antimalarial drugs in Togo. *Bulletin of the World Health Organisation* **67**, 695–700.

Dürrheim DN, Frieremans S, Kruger P, Mabuza A & de Bruyn JC (1999) Confidential inquiry into malaria deaths. *Bulletin of the World Health Organization* **77**, 263–266.

Font F, Alonso Gonzales M, Nathan R et al. (2001) Diagnostic accuracy and case management of clinical malaria in the primary health services of a rural area in south-eastern Tanzania. *Tropical Medicine and International Health* **6**, 423–428.

Garenne M, Kahn K, Tollmann St & Gear J (2000) Causes of death in a rural area of South Africa: an international perspective. *Journal of Tropical Paediatrics* **46**, 183–190.

Greenwood B (1989) Impact of culture and environmental changes on epidemiology and control of malaria and babesiosis: the microepidemiology of malaria and its importance to malaria control. *Transactions of the Royal Society of Tropical Medicine and Hygiene* **83** (Suppl.), 25–29.

Greenwood B, Bradley A, Greenwood A et al. (1987a) Mortality and morbidity from malaria among children in a rural area of The Gambia. *Transactions of the Royal Society of Tropical Medicine and Hygiene* **81**, 478–486.

Greenwood B, Greenwood A, Bradley AK, Tulloch S, Hayes R & Oldfield FSJ (1987b) Deaths in infancy and early childhood in a well-vaccinated, rural, West African population. *Annals of Tropical Paediatrics* **7**, 91–99.

Jaffar S, Leach A, Greenwood AM et al. (1997) Changes in the pattern of infant and childhood mortality in Upper River Division, The Gambia, from 1989 to 1993. *Tropical Medicine and International Health* **2**, 28–37.

Kouyaté B, Traoré C, Kielmann K & Müller O (2000) North and South: bridging the information gap. *Lancet* **356**, 1035.

Krause G & Sauerborn R (2000) Community-effectiveness of care – the example of malaria treatment in rural Burkina Faso. *Annals of Tropical Paediatrics* **7**, 99–106.

Mabeza GF, Moyo VM, Thumas P et al. (1995) Predictors of severity of illness on presentation in children with cerebral malaria. *Annals of Tropical Medicine and Parasitology* **89**, 221–228.

McCombie SC (1994) *Treatment-Seeking for Malaria: a Review and Suggestions for Future Research*. Resource Paper No. 2. (TDR/SER/RP/94.1) WHO, Geneva.

Molyneux CS, Mung'ala-Odera V, Harpham T & Snow RW (1999) Maternal responses to childhood fevers: a comparison of rural and urban residents in costal Kenya. *Tropical Medicine and International Health* **4**, 836–845.

Molyneux ME, Taylor TE, Wirima JJ & Harper G (1989) Clinical features and prognostic indicators in paediatric cerebral malaria: a study of 131 comatose Malawian children. *Quarterly Journal of Medicine* **71**, 441–459.

Müller O, Becher H, Baltussen A et al. (2001) Effect of zinc supplementation on malaria morbidity among West African children: a randomized double-blind placebo-controlled trial. *British Medical Journal* **322**, 1567–1572.

Müller O, Boele van Hensbroek M, Jaffar S et al. (1996) A randomized trial of chloroquine, amodiaquine, and pyrimethamine-sulfadoxine in Gambian children with uncomplicated malaria. *Tropical Medicine and International Health* **1**, 124–132.

Müller O, Traoré C & Kouyate B (2003) Clinical efficacy of chloroquine in young children with uncomplicated malaria – a community-based study in rural Burkina Faso. *Tropical Medicine and International Health* **8**, 202–203.

Ndah EA (2001) *Risk factors for childhood mortality in a rural area of Burkina Faso*. MSc Thesis. Department of Tropical Hygiene and Public Health, Ruprecht-Karls-University of Heidelberg.

Nshakira N, Kristensen M, Ssali F & Whyte SR (2002) Appropriate treatment of malaria? Use of antimalarial drugs for children's fevers in district medical units, drug shops and homes in eastern Uganda. *Tropical Medicine and International Health* **7**, 309–316.

© 2003 Blackwell Publishing Ltd

Nsimba SED, Massele AY, Eriksen J, Gustafsson LL, Tomson G & Warsame M (2002) Case management of malaria in under-fives at primary health care facilities in a Tanzanian district. *Tropical Medicine and International Health* **7**, 201–209.

Okrah J, Traoré C, Palé A, Sommerfeld J & Müller O (2002) Community factors associated with malaria prevention by mosquito nets: an exploratory study in rural Burkina Faso. *Tropical Medicine and International Health* **7**, 240–248.

Quigley MA, Armstrong Schellenberg JRM & Snow RW (1996) Algorithms for verbal autopsies: a validation study in Kenyan children. *Bulletin of the World Health Organization* **74**, 147–154.

Reuben R (1993) Women and malaria – special risks and appropriate control strategy. *Social Science and Medicine* **37**, 473–480.

Rogier C, Ly AB, Tall A, Cissé B & Trapé JF (1999) *Plasmodium falciparum* malaria in Dielmo, a holoendemic area in Senegal: no influence of acquired immunity on initial symptomatology and severity of malaria attacks. *American Journal of Tropical Medicine and Hygiene* **60**, 410–420.

Rooth I & Björkman A (1992) Fever episodes in a holoendemic malaria area of Tanzania: parasitological and clinical findings and diagnostic aspects related to malaria. *Transactions of the Royal Society of Tropical Medicine and Hygiene* **86**, 479–482.

Ruebush T, Kern M, Campbell C & Oloo A (1995) Self-treatment of malaria in a rural area of western Kenya. *Bulletin of the World Health Organization* **73**, 229–236.

Sankoh OA, Ye Y, Sauerborn R, Müller O & Becher H (2001) Clustering of childhood mortality in rural Burkina Faso. *International Journal of Epidemiology* **30**, 485–492.

Snow RW, Armstrong JRM, Forster D *et al.* (1992) Childhood deaths in Africa: uses and limitations of verbal autopsies. *Lancet* **340**, 351–355.

Snow RW, Craig M, Deichmann U & Marsh K (1999) Estimating mortality, morbidity and disability due to malaria among Africa's non-pregnant population. *Bulletin of the World Health Organization* **77**, 624–640.

Tanner M & Vlassoff C (1998) Treatment-seeking behaviour for malaria: a typology based on endemicity and gender. *Social Science and Medicine* **46**, 523–532.

Théra MA, D'Alessandro U, Thiéro M *et al.* (2002) Child malaria treatment practices among mothers in the district of Yanfolila, Sikasso region, Mali. *Tropical Medicine and International Health* **5**, 876–881.

Todd JE, de Francisco A, O'Dempsey TJD & Greenwood BM (1994) The limitations of verbal autopsy in a malaria-endemic region. *Annals of Tropical Paediatrics* **14**, 31–36.

Trape J (2001) The public health impact of chloroquine resistance in Africa. *American Journal of Tropical Medicine and Hygiene* **64** (Suppl.), 12–17.

WHO (1997) World malaria situation in 1994. *Weekly Epidemiological Record* **72**, 269–292.

WHO (2000) Severe falciparum malaria. *Transactions of the Royal Society of Tropical Medicine and Hygiene* **94** (Suppl.), 1–90.

Authors

Dr **Olaf Müller** (corresponding author) and **Prof. Heiko Becher**, Department of Tropical Hygiene and Public Health, Ruprecht-Karls-University, INF 324, 69120 Heidelberg, Germany. E-mail: heiko.becher@urz.uni-heidelberg.de; olaf.mueller@urz.uni-heidelberg.de
Dr **Corneille Traoré** and Dr **Bocar Kouyaté**, Centre de Recherche en Santé de Nouna, B. P. 34, Nouna, Burkina Faso.
E-mail: Corneille.traore@caramail.com; bocar.crsn@fasonet.bf

3.7 Risk factors of infant and child mortality in rural Burkina Faso

BECHER H, MÜLLER O, JAHN A, GBANGOU A, KYNAST-WOLF G, KOUYATE B

Bull WHO 82 (4): 265-274

Reprinted with permission from the World Health Organization.

Risk factors of infant and child mortality in rural Burkina Faso

Heiko Becher,[1] Olaf Müller,[1] Albrecht Jahn,[1] Adjima Gbangou,[2] Gisela Kynast-Wolf,[1] & Bocar Kouyaté[2]

Objective The aim of the study was to quantify the effect of risk factors for childhood mortality in a typical rural setting in sub-Saharan Africa.
Methods We performed a survival analysis of births within a population under demographic surveillance from 1992 to 1999 based on data from a demographic surveillance system in 39 villages around Nouna, western Burkina Faso, with a total population of about 30 000. All children born alive in the period 1 January 1993 to 31 December 1999 in the study area ($n = 10\ 122$) followed-up until 31 December 1999 were included. All-cause childhood mortality was used as outcome variable.
Findings Within the observation time, 1340 deaths were recorded. In a Cox regression model a simultaneous estimation of hazard rate ratios showed death of the mother and being a twin as the strongest risk factors for mortality. For both, the risk was most pronounced in infancy. Further factors associated with mortality include age of the mother, birth spacing, season of birth, village, ethnic group, and distance to the nearest health centre. Finally, there was an overall decrease in childhood mortality over the years 1993–99.
Conclusion The study supports the multi-causation of childhood deaths in rural West Africa during the 1990s and supports the overall trend, as observed in other studies, of decreasing childhood mortality in these populations. The observed correlation between the factors highlights the need for multivariate analysis to disentangle the separate effects. These findings illustrate the need for more comprehensive improvement of prenatal and postnatal care in rural sub-Saharan Africa.

Keywords Infant mortality; Maternal mortality; Twins; Age factors; Birth intervals; Ethnology; Seasons; Health services accessibility; Risk factors; Survival analysis; Burkina Faso (*source: MeSH, NLM*).

Mots clés Mortalité nourrisson; Mortalité maternelle; Jumeaux; Facteur âge; Intervalle entre naissances; Ethnologie; Accessibilité service santé; Saison; Facteur risque; Analyse survie; Burkina Faso (*source: MeSH, INSERM*).

Palabras clave Mortalidad infantil; Mortalidad materna; Gemelos; Factores de edad; Intervalo entre nacimientos; Etnología; Accesibilidad a los servicios de salud; Estaciones; Factores de riesgo; Análisis de supervivencia; Burkina Faso (*fuente: DeCS, BIREME*).

الكلمات المفتاحية: معدل وفيات الرضّع؛ معدل وفيات الأمومة؛ ولادة التوائم؛ عوامل العمر؛ الفترة بين الولادات؛ الإثنية؛ مواسم الولادة؛ الحصول على الخدمات الصحية؛ عوامل الاختطار؛ تحليل البقاء؛ بوركينا فاسو. (المصدر: رؤوس الموضوعات الطبية – إقليم شرق المتوسط).

Bulletin of the World Health Organization 2004;82:265-273.

Voir page 272 le résumé en français. En la página 272 figura un resumen en español.

يمكن الاطلاع على الملخص بالعربية في صفحة 272.

Introduction

A total of 10.5 million children under 5 years of age were estimated to have died worldwide in 1999, and the great majority of these deaths occurred in developing countries (*1*). Most childhood deaths have been attributed to diarrhoea, acute respiratory illness, malaria, measles, and malnutrition — conditions that are either preventable or treatable with low-cost interventions (*2*). The highest mortality rates worldwide are still in sub-Saharan Africa (SSA), where approximately 15% of newborn children are expected to die before reaching their fifth birthday (*1*).

Childhood mortality rates have declined considerably over the past few decades in most of SSA, but since the 1990s mortality rates have started to increase again in parts of the continent (*1*). This new trend has been attributed mainly to the effects of the AIDS epidemic and to the spread of chloroquine-resistant malaria (*3–5*).

In all of SSA except South Africa, reliable information on birth rates, death rates, and causes of deaths are lacking because of a poor public health infrastructure and non-existence of vital registration systems (*6*). Existing mortality estimates including approaches to identify relevant risk factors are thus based on data from Demographic and Health Surveys (DHSs), research sites with established Demographic Surveillance Systems (DSSs), and specific epidemiological studies (*4, 7–21*). Risk factors for childhood mortality can be grouped as follows: socioeconomic status, fertility behaviour, environmental health conditions, nutritional status and infant feeding, and the use of health services (*20*).

Here, we present findings from a comprehensive analysis of risk factors for mortality and their varying effects by age in a cohort of 10 122 liveborn children followed over a period of 7 years in a rural area of Burkina Faso, West Africa, and we compare these with results from the most recent DHS in Burkina Faso from 1998 to 1999 (*22*).

Study population and methods

Study area

The study was conducted in the research zone of the Centre de Recherche en Santé de Nouna (CRSN) in the Nouna Health District in north-western Burkina Faso (*23*). Today, the study

---

[1] University of Heidelberg, Department of Tropical Hygiene and Public Health, Im Neuenheimer Feld 324, 69120 Heidelberg, Germany. Correspondence should be sent to Dr Becher (email: heiko.becher@urz.uni-heidelberg.de).
[2] Centre de Recherche en Sante de Nouna, Burkina Faso, Africa.

Ref. No. **02-0243**
(*Submitted: 20 May 02 – Final revised version received: 26 August 03 – Accepted: 09 September 03*)

area comprises 41 villages and Nouna town. Subsistence farming is the main socioeconomic activity of the population. Formal health services in the CRSN study area comprise a hospital in Nouna town and four local health centres. Malaria, diarrhoea, and respiratory infections are major causes of childhood mortality. Malnutrition is highly prevalent in young children living in the study villages and has been associated with childhood mortality (24). Malaria transmission intensity is high but markedly seasonal (25).

Demographic Surveillance System

The database for this study is based on the DSS of the CRSN (21, 24, 26). A baseline census had been undertaken in 1992, and two control censuses were done in 1994 and 1998. During the time of the second control census a cross-sectional study of all mothers within the study region regarding maternity health issues was performed; all births and deaths were also recorded. The average population size in the study period was about 30 000 inhabitants. Registration of vital events was by trained field staff who routinely collected the relevant information from specific village informants. The interval for data collection varied between 1 and 3 months (21). The variables registered include births, deaths, pregnancies, and migration in and out of the household, as well as information on all the dates related to these events. The DSS database also contains several other tables of data on various topics such as household economics and maternal health.

Study population

All children born between 1 January 1993 and 31 December 1999 in 39 villages of the CRSN study area were included. We identified a total of 10 122 births, of which 1043 children were identified in a cross-sectional study on maternal health in 1998. Of these, 162 children were reported to have died either "within the first week" or "within week 2 to 4". For these children, we assigned arbitrary survival times of 2 and 15 days, respectively.

Statistical analysis

The main end-point for the analysis was overall survival. For the survival analysis, a proportional hazards model was used to investigate simultaneously the relative effect of demographic, ethnic, and reproductive factors on childhood survival rates (27, 28). The effects are given as hazard rate ratios. For each child, the observation time t was taken as the time from birth until death, the date of fifth birthday, or the date of 31 December 1999, whichever came first. For emigrated individuals the observation time was taken as the time from birth until the date of emigration. For all risk factors it may be assumed that the effect is different at infant and childhood age, therefore we used separate models. For infant age (<1 year) modelling, the observation time t was truncated at the first birthday. For childhood (age 1–5 years) mortality modelling, all children were included from their first birthday and the underlying time variable in the Cox model was set to (t–1). In the final model all variables that showed a significant impact in either of the two age groups were included. These are "year of birth", "sex", "ethnic group", "religion", "age of mother at birth of child", "season of birth", "twin birth", "birth order", "distance to health centre", "time to birth of next sibling", "time since last sibling was born and vital status of last sibling", and "vital status of mother".

The covariates "time to birth of next sibling" and "vital status of mother" entered the model as time-dependent covariates as follows: time to next sibling (birth spacing) — if a sibling was born before the respective child reached the age 18 months, the covariate was set to 1 from the date of birth of the next sibling; vital status of mother — if the mother died, the corresponding variable was set to 1 from the date of death.

For analysis we used the SAS-procedure PHREG (SAS Institute, Cary, NC, USA) (29), which allows the analysis of continuous and time-dependent covariates.

Results

Data description

Table 1 shows the distribution of variables by vital status. A total of 10 122 live births with 1340 deaths were analysed. The male/female ratio shows that the frequency of male births was slightly higher than that of female births (50.4% vs 49.3%; 0.3% with missing information; sex ratio 1.02). Birth frequency was not uniformly distributed over the observation time, and was significantly higher in 1997 compared with each of the other years. The median ages of mothers and fathers at birth of the child were 25 and 34 years, respectively. Dafing and Bwaba were the two most dominant ethnic groups, and Muslim was the dominant religion (60.2%). Table 2 shows the strong correlation between ethnic group and religion in the study population.

Only a small proportion of mothers and fathers were reported dead before the child reached 3 years of age, but there was no information on the vital status of a high proportion of fathers. The median time of birth spacing between siblings was 28 months, the frequency of twins was 3.0%, and the births were evenly distributed over the year). In all, 64.6 % of the children were living less than 10 km away from a health centre compared with 34.8 % living far away. The overall mean follow-up time for the children of the study was 2.6 years.

Survival analysis

Table 3 shows the results of the multivariate Cox model. Generally, the magnitude of effect for the factors considered here was stronger for infants (<1 year) than for children (1–5 years). In terms of hazard rate ratio, the strongest factor was the death of the mother. Although death of the mother is a rare event, among those 18 children whose mother died within their first year of life, 9 died within the follow-up period; the rate ratio for infants was 15.6 (95% confidence interval (CI) = 7.61–31.8) and 5.35 for children (95% CI = 1.69–16.9).

Twins also experienced an increased mortality risk. The rate ratio for the first 6 months of life was 4.33 (95% CI = 3.22–5.83) and about twofold for the following 6 months.

Overall, we observed a highly significant reduction in mortality over the observation period. This trend was observed both for infants and for children up to the age of 5 years. The effect, however, was much stronger for infants. There is some confounding with other factors in the full model. When considering year of birth separately, the yearly hazard ratio is 0.856, which yields a 61% reduction over the 7-year observation period. Although other data from Burkina Faso support the general trend, the magnitude of reduction found here is surprising and suggests an underreporting of infant deaths (see Discussion).

Ethnicity was shown to be strongly associated with infant mortality, with infants in Bwaba, Mossi, and Samo having a significantly lower mortality than those in the Dafing or Peulh

Table 1. **Distribution of demographic variables and risk factors of children born around Nouma, western Burkina Faso, 1993–99**

Characteristic	No. of children who died in first year of life[a]	No. of children who died in second, third, fourth, or fifth year of life[a]	No. of children alive at end of follow-up[a]	Total
Sex				
Male	351; 6.9	356; 7.0	4396; 86.1	5103
Female	297; 6.0	320; 6.4	4371; 87.6	4988
Unknown	16; 51.6	0; 0	15; 48.4	31
Year of birth				
1993	124; 10.0	159; 12.8	956; 77.2	1239
1994	134; 10.2	140; 10.6	1043; 79.2	1317
1995	111; 7.1	146; 9.4	1297; 83.5	1554
1996	92; 7.4	68; 5.5	1087; 87.2	1247
1997	90; 5.0	112; 6.2	1614; 88.9	1816
1998	48; 3.4	51; 3.6	1331; 93.1	1430
1999	65; 4.3	0; 0	1454; 95.7	1519
Age of mother at birth of child (years)				
<18	102; 11.4	68; 7.6	726; 81.0	896
18–35	400; 5.9	459; 6.8	5929; 87.3	6788
36+	85; 7.2	86; 7.3	1004; 85.4	1175
Unknown	77; 6.1	63; 5.0	1123; 88.9	1263
Age of father at birth of child (years)				
<20	6; 5.3	11; 9.7	96; 85.0	113
20–40	213; 5.4	366; 9.4	3331; 85.2	3910
41+	71; 4.8	142; 9.6	1265; 85.6	1478
Unknown	374; 8.1	157; 3.4	4090; 88.5	4621
Ethnic group				
Dafing	315; 7.8	288; 7.1	3437; 85.1	4040
Bwaba	149; 5.5	170; 6.3	2377; 88.2	2696
Mossi	75; 4.1	110; 6.0	1645; 89.9	1830
Peulh	94; 8.7	78; 7.2	910; 84.1	1082
Samo	10; 3.9	15; 5.8	232; 90.3	257
Others	5; 3.5	13; 9.1	125; 87.4	143
Unknown	16; 21.6	2; 2.7	56; 75.7	74
Religion				
Muslim	425; 7.0	434; 7.1	5238; 85.9	6097
Catholic	123; 4.8	142; 5.6	2292; 89.6	2557
Protestant	32; 6.1	33; 6.3	460; 87.6	525
Animiste/other	68; 7.9	64; 7.4	733; 84.7	865
Unknown	16; 20.5	3; 3.8	59; 75.6	78
Mother died before child reached 3 years				
No	614; 6.5	624; 6.6	8158; 86.8	9396
Yes	9; 21.4	6; 14.3	27; 64.3	42
Unknown	41; 6.0	46; 6.7	597; 87.3	684
Father died before child reached 3 years				
No	295; 5.3	525; 9.5	4714; 85.2	5534
Yes	2; 2.3	4; 4.6	81; 93.1	87
Unknown	367; 8.2	147; 3.3	3987; 88.6	4501
Spacing to next sibling				
No younger sibling or >36 months	298; 4.8	313; 5.0	5623; 90.2	6234
<18 months	133; 25.6	49; 9.4	337; 64.9	519
18–36 months	192; 7.2	268; 10.0	2225; 82.9	2685
Unknown	41; 6.0	46; 6.7	597; 87.3	684

(Table 1, cont.)

Characteristic	No. of children who died in first year of life[a]	No. of children who died in second, third, fourth, or fifth year of life[a]	No. of children alive at end of follow-up[a]	Total
Spacing to previous sibling				
No elder sibling or >36 months	322; 6.7	296; 6.2	4163; 87.1	4781
<18 months	40; 8.8	38; 8.4	377; 82.9	455
18–36 months	239; 6.1	277; 7.0	3428; 86.9	3944
Unknown	63; 6.7	65; 6.9	814; 86.4	942
Birth order				
First	209; 8.7	124; 5.2	2058; 86.1	2391
Second, third, or fourth	247; 5.7	302; 7.0	3747; 87.2	4296
Fifth or higher	167; 6.1	204; 7.4	2380; 86.5	2751
Unknown	41; 6.0	46; 6.7	597; 87.3	684
Twin birth				
Yes	59; 19.3	40; 13.1	206; 67.5	305
No	605; 6.2	636; 6.5	8576; 87.4	9817
Season of birth				
Dry	313; 5.6	407; 7.2	4901; 87.2	5621
Rainy	189; 6.5	192; 6.6	2533; 86.9	2914
Unknown	162; 10.2	77; 4.9	1348; 84.9	1587
Distance to health centre				
<10 km	384; 5.9	427; 6.5	5723; 87.6	6534
>10 km	267; 7.6	248; 7.0	3009; 85.4	3524
Unknown	13; 20.3	1; 1.6	50; 78.1	64
Total	**664**	**676**	**8782**	**10 122**

[a] Figures in italics are row percentages.

Table 2. **Distribution of ethnic group by religion**

Religion	Ethnic group						Total
	Dafing	Bwaba	Mossi	Peulh	Samo	Other	
Muslim	3467	58	1210	1078	181	103	6097
Catholic	356	1608	504	0	50	39	2557
Protestant	66	351	80	2	23	3	525
Natural religion[a]	144	666	31	2	3	2	848
Other/NA[b]	7	13	5	0	0	70	95
Total	4040	2696	1830	1082	257	217	10 122

[a] Indigenous beliefs.
[b] NA = information not available.

(rate ratios were close to 0.5). The mortality of infants from the two major religions, Muslim and Catholic, was similar when using the multivariate model. However, because there was a strong association between ethnic group and religion, these two variables must be considered jointly. Without ethnic group in the model, Muslims appear to have a highly significant increased risk compared with Catholics and Protestants.

The time between the birth of the child and the birth of the next younger or older sibling was associated with mortality. However, because mortality within family is correlated with birth spacing, our results must be considered with caution (see Discussion). For the next older sibling, this effect was apparent only for infants with a rate ratio (RR) of 1.36. Here, the vital status of the older sibling was of additional relevance. If it had died before age 1 or before the birth of the index child, this independently increased the risk by a factor of 1.45. This suggests a clustering effect of infant mortality within families. The effect of birth spacing to the next youngest child was obviously restricted to children older than 1 year. Here, we observed a very pronounced effect RR 1.54).

Both the age of the mother and birth order have a significant independent impact on mortality. These two variables are strongly correlated, and again, only a multivariate model allows the independent effect of either factor to be estimated. Both low age (<18 years) of mother and being the first child were found to be associated with an increased infant mortality

Table 3. **Rate ratios for infant and childhood survival, Nouna Demographic Surveillance System, Burkina Faso, using a proportional hazards regression model**

Variable	Infants (<1 year)			Children (1–5 years)		
	Rate ratio	P-value	95% CI[a]	Rate ratio	P-value	95% CI
Sex						
Female	1.0			1.0		
Male	1.12	0.16	0.96–1.30	1.07	0.41	0.92–1.24
Birth spacing to next youngest sibling						
Born after age 18 months or no younger sibling in follow-up period	(not applicable)			1.0		
Born before age 18 months				1.54	0.01	1.10–2.16
Birth spacing to next oldest sibling						
Next oldest sibling older than 18 months at birth of index child or no older sibling	1.0			1.0		
Born before older sibling reached age 18 months	1.36	0.05	0.99–1.87	1.16	0.33	0.86–1.57
Older sibling died before birth or before age 1 year						
No, or no older sibling	1.0			1.0		
Yes	1.45	0.02	1.06–1.96	1.11	0.44	0.85–1.45
Mother's vital status						
Alive	1.0			1.0		
Died	15.6	<0.0001	7.61–31.8	5.35	0.004	1.69–16.9
Single/twin						
Single	1.0			1.0		
Twin (0–<6 months)	4.33	<0.0001	3.22–5.83			
Twin (6–<12 months)	2.28	0.02	1.12–4.66			
Twin (12–60 months)				2.38	<0.0001	1.72–3.29
Year of birth (years)	0.80	<0.0001	0.77–0.84	0.95	0.07	0.90–1.00
Age of mother (years)						
<18	1.40	0.01	1.09–1.79	1.41	0.02	1.05–1.89
18–35	1.0			1.0		
≥36	1.29	0.07	0.98–1.70	1.05	0.71	0.80–1.38
NA[b]	0.80	0.23	0.55–1.16	0.58	0.03	0.35–0.95
Religion						
Muslim	1.0			1.0		
Catholic	1.03	0.85	0.79–1.34	0.73	0.02	0.56–0.95
Protestant	1.40	0.11	0.93–2.10	0.88	0.52	0.59–1.31
Natural or other/NA[b]	1.66	0.002	1.21–2.27	0.96	0.82	0.69–1.35
Ethnic group						
Dafing	1.0			1.0		
Bwaba	0.59	0.0003	0.45–0.79	1.02	0.90	0.77–1.36
Mossi	0.51	<0.0001	0.39–0.66	0.87	0.25	0.69–1.10
Peulh	1.14	0.26	0.90–1.45	0.99	0.92	0.77–1.27
Samo	0.52	0.04	0.28–0.98	0.75	0.29	0.45–1.27
Other/NA[b]	0.94	0.80	0.57–1.54	1.23	0.44	0.72–2.09
Distance to health centre						
<10 km	1.0			1.0		
>10 km	1.33	0.0006	1.13–1.57	1.11	0.22	0.94–1.30
Birth order						
First	1.32	0.01	1.07–1.64	0.80	0.07	0.63–1.02
Second, third, or fourth[c]	1.0			1.0		
Fifth or higher	1.10	0.39	0.89–1.37	1.03	0.78	0.85–1.25
Season of birth						
Dry	1.0			1.0		
Rainy	1.21	0.04	1.01–1.46	0.95	0.57	0.80–1.13

[a] CI = confidence interval.
[b] NA = information not available.
[c] Individuals with missing information in baseline category.

risk (RR 1.40, 95 % CI = 1.09–1.79 and RR 1.32, 95 % CI = 1.07–1.64, respectively). Low age of mother also remained a risk factor for ages 1–5 years. There was no risk observed with age of the father.

Being born during the rainy season was associated with a significantly higher risk of mortality during the first year of life compared with being born during the dry season (rate ratio 1.21, P = 0.04).

As a surrogate measure for the availability of formal health services, the distance to the nearest health centre was used as the only available variable. We found 33% significantly increased infant mortality if the nearest health centre was more than 10 km away.

Discussion

Infant and childhood mortality in sub-Saharan Africa

There are numerous studies on infant and childhood mortality risk factors in rural SSA, often based on DHSs — for example, for Burkina Faso (30), Ghana (31), Benin (32), or others. In the present study we used survival modelling techniques with time-dependent covariates based on longitudinal data from a DSS.

We showed a continuous reduction in childhood mortality rates over most of the study period, which confirms the overall trend in West Africa (1, 11, 16). Data for Burkina Faso report a decline from 122.2 per 1000 for 1985–89 to 93.7 per 100 for 1990–94 (30). It is unlikely that HIV/AIDS already plays a big role in childhood mortality in our study area, because clinical cases are still rare and because mortality in both fathers and mothers was still low compared with areas of high HIV/AIDS endemicity (4). Resistance to chloroquine, the main drug used for malaria treatment in the area, is still relatively low in this part of Burkina Faso (33). Nevertheless, the observed reduction in mortality in our data is surprisingly high. There is some confounding with the other factors considered, and if the time trend is analysed in a univariate model, then the yearly hazard RR for infants is 0.856, which yields a 61% reduction over a 6-year period. Such a large reduction could only be achieved by a drastic improvement of the health care system or living conditions in the study area, which did not take place. The implementation of a national vaccination programme in the study area on polio, measles, and vitamin A supplementation, as well as the increasing health system research activities at the CRSN since 1993, may have had some beneficial effect; however, we think that our results on time trends should be considered with caution. Improved field conditions have been implemented in 1999 after some problems in field management during 1996–98, and we conclude that underreporting of infant deaths in the years 1996–99 contributed to the observed reduction in mortality.

Major risk factors

Major risk factors for childhood mortality identified in our study are death of the mother and twin birth. Both are more pronounced in the first year of life. We considered the death of the mother only if it occurred within the observation time of the child. Therefore, the finding can be seen as a consequence of several factors such as reduced childcare, no breastfeeding, and improper bottle feeding, rather than an overall indication for a family specific mortality risk. Koblinski and colleagues (34) report that among infants who survive the death of the mother, fewer than 10% live beyond their first birthday. However, because these factors are not very frequent, they contribute only to a small proportion of all childhood deaths, despite the high relative risk. Other factors such as a birth spacing of less than 18 months, birth during the rainy season, and belonging to certain ethnic groups and religions were also associated with childhood mortality and account for a larger overall proportion of deaths.

We showed a marked age dependency of mortality risk in twins. The mortality risk was very high only during the first 6 months; thereafter it was still twice as high as that of singles. This finding confirms the particularly high mortality risk of twins and calls for special attention towards twins during their first year of life (19). Lower birth weight in twins and lower intensity of breastfeeding is likely to contribute to the observations.

The strong effect of the death of the mother before the first birthday of a child confirms the importance of the mother during the early life of a child in rural Africa (35). This effect is furthermore likely to explain a considerable proportion of childhood mortality in areas of high HIV/AIDS endemicity (36).

Sufficient birth spacing has been promoted through mother–child health programmes in many countries, as this is perceived to be beneficial for the health and well-being of both mother and children (12–14). Our data indicate that educating families on the importance of sufficient birth spacing would have a large impact in reducing childhood mortality in the still highly fertile populations of rural Africa (20). We found a 50% increased risk of death for a child (age 1–5 years) if the next sibling was born within 18 months. The effect of the birth spacing to the next oldest sibling is more complex since if this sibling has died early, the subsequent interval is usually shorter because of curtailment of lactation and because of a replacement effect — that is, the family has another child sooner to replace the one that has died. In our data we found a mean birth interval of 2.5 years if the older sibling is alive, and of 1.8 years if it died before age 1 year, a difference which is highly significant. The vital status of the older sibling also has an effect on the mortality of the child, with an independent rate ratio of 1.4 (95% CI = 1.1–2.0). This is likely to be a familial cluster effect and points to the effect of family specific factors such as nutrition and other lifestyle factors. This factor was investigated in the latest DHS in Burkina Faso of 1998/99 (22) and yielded similar results: for infants, the mortality ratio was 1.7 (154.6/91.1) for an interval less than 2 years compared with an interval of 2–3 years. For children over 1 year the corresponding ratio was 1.3.

Other variables analysed in the DHS in relation to childhood death are sex, age of the mother, birth order, and weight at birth. We do not have data on birth weight; however, the other variables showed very similar patterns. The age categories were slightly different: in the DHS young age at birth of the mother (<20 years) vs 20–29 years showed a 34% increased risk for infant death compared with a 40% increased risk for <18 years vs 18–35 years found in our data.

The Burkina Faso DHS analyses, however, are all univariate and thus do not account for confounding between the factors. For example, there is a strong correlation between birth order and age at birth of mother. In our study population, the univariate rate ratio of the first birth vs second to fourth birth is 1.56 (95% CI = 1.29–1.87), whereas in the full model adjusted for all covariates the independent effect under this model is only 1.32. We can therefore conclude that the risks as reported in the DHS must be treated with some caution because the confounding effects are not taken into account, and it is likely that a full multivariate analysis of the DHS data would yield lower RRs.

The sex ratio found in our data corresponds closely to the reported sex ratio (male/female) of 1.03 for Burkina Faso (37). Also, for blacks in the United States of America a ratio 1.03 was observed in the preceding years (38), which is significantly lower than in whites. We can therefore conclude that this finding does not suggest a selection bias.

In most of West Africa, the rainy season coincides with an increased incidence of malaria and other diseases and with a shortage of food. Thus, in the Gambia more children die during and shortly after the rainy season than in the rest of the year (15). However, the possible role of season of birth regarding respective short-term and long-term consequences for health and survival is controversial (39, 40). We found an association between being born in the rainy season and mortality, but only with mortality during the first year of life. Thus, our findings are not very different from the non-significant effect observed in the Gambia (40).

We observed a significant effect of distance to the nearest health centre on mortality for infants whose parents live more than 10 km away. The effect of this factor is somewhat stronger if considered separately for births occurring in the rainy season, where a greater distance to a health centre is more difficult to manage; however, this difference is not significant. We did not find an effect for children after their first birthday. This finding provides some evidence for the importance of having access to functioning health services in rural SSA. In the case of Burkina Faso, the uninterrupted availability of affordable quality drugs at all peripheral health centres over the past decade may possibly have a role in the observed effect on mortality.

Finally, the observed associations between childhood mortality and ethnicity and religion show the diversity of mortality risk factors in a given population, which are likely to be explained by several cultural, educational, socioeconomic, and environmental differences (10). Because religion and ethnic group are strongly correlated with each other, it is difficult to disentangle their effects with the data available. However, there was no difference between the two dominant religions, Muslim and Catholic, in the multivariate model with adjustment for ethnic groups. For these, strong differences were observed. The groups with low infant mortality (Bwaba, Mossi, and Samo) are those with the highest proportions of Christians. These groups also have a higher average social class. In a study in Ghana (31), the effect of ethnic group disappeared after controlling for socioeconomic variables. Because these variables are not available in our dataset, we cannot parallel this analysis.

Data quality and validity

The fact that we identified several births in a separate cross-sectional study that were not included in the DSS gives rise to the question of completeness of the database. Assuming that both surveys may be considered as independent, which is in our view a reasonable assumption, we estimated the number of missing children through common capture–recapture methods (41), which yielded 3.4% of all births. We consider it unlikely, however, that these are linked to specific risk factors under consideration here, therefore we see no reason for bias in the results (42).

We do not have an explanation for the differences in number of births in the different years. Although some random variation naturally occurs, the database contains a high peak for 1997 and a low peak in 1996. We cannot exclude with certainty an underreporting of births in one year; however, this does not easily explain the high peak in 1997. We checked whether some children born in 1996 were erroneously assigned a birth year 1997, but found no evidence for this. It also appeared that all villages in the study show a similar pattern. Therefore, we consider an unknown error in data collection procedure as the most probable explanation. To check whether this may have an impact on the overall results, we also analysed the data separately by year of birth. However, because the results were consistent, we believe that the data deficiencies had little effect on the overall analysis.

For the analysis, we used the Cox proportional hazards model, which is common for survival analysis and which easily allows a simultaneous analysis of time-dependent covariates. Because it can be assumed that the effect of most covariates is not constant, we chose to analyse infant and childhood (up to 5 years) age in separate models. An additional complication arises from the fact that the children are considered as independent observations, although there are several possible cluster effects within the data, the most relevant being clustering of deaths within the same household. Other sources of clustering effects such as the village also exist. To approach that, we did an analysis by randomly selecting one child per family and fitted the same model repeatedly. The results confirmed those from the full model. For example, the mean estimated RR for twins in the first 6 months, a variable on which the clustering effect is likely to be strong, from a small simulation with 10 randomly selected datasets is 4.31 compared with 4.33 from the full dataset. It is somewhat reassuring that no severe bias in the estimation has occurred .

Conclusion

Our study in a rural area of Burkina Faso confirms the importance of all five major risk groups for childhood mortality: socioeconomic status, fertility behaviour, environmental health conditions, nutritional status and infant feeding, and the use of health services. These findings call for a broader approach to future child health programmes to enable further reductions in childhood mortality in rural Africa. Such programmes need to include improvements of accessibility to formal health services, specific attention towards twins during their first year of life, emphasis on educating whole families in birth spacing, and efforts to improve the nutritional status of young children, as well as continuing with improvements in the control of malaria, diarrhoea, respiratory diseases, HIV/AIDS, and vaccine-preventable diseases. ■

Acknowledgements

We thank Dr Osman A. Sankoh for helpful comments and discussions, Dr Florant Somé for information on the ethnic groups in the study area, and Ms Gabriele Stieglbauer for efficient help with data management and programming.

Funding: This work was supported by the DFG (German Research Foundation) under the collaborative research grant (SFB) 544 "Kontrolle tropischer Infektionskrankheiten".

Conflicts of interest: none declared.

Résumé

Facteurs de risque de mortalité infanto-juvénile dans les régions rurales du Burkina Faso

Objectif L'étude avait pour but de quantifier l'effet des facteurs de risque de mortalité infanto-juvénile dans un contexte rural typique d'Afrique subsaharienne.

Méthodes Nous avons effectué une analyse de survie chez les enfants d'une population couverte par un système de surveillance démographique de 1992 à 1999, en utilisant les données de ce système pour 39 villages situés autour de Nouna, dans l'ouest du Burkina Faso. La population totale de la zone d'étude s'élevait à environ 30 000 personnes. Tous les enfants nés vivants pendant la période du 1er janvier 1993 au 31 décembre 1999 dans cette zone (n = 10 122) et suivis jusqu'au 31 décembre 1999 ont été inclus dans l'étude. La variable considérée était la mortalité toutes causes confondues chez l'enfant.

Résultats Au cours de la période d'observation, 1340 décès ont été enregistrés. L'utilisation d'un modèle de Cox pour obtenir une estimation simultanée du risque relatif associé à chaque facteur a montré que les facteurs de risque de mortalité les plus importants étaient la mort de la mère et le fait d'être issu d'une naissance gémellaire. Dans les deux cas, le risque était plus prononcé pendant la première enfance. Parmi les autres facteurs associés à la mortalité figuraient l'âge de la mère, l'intervalle entre les naissances, la saison de naissance, le village, le groupe ethnique et la distance au centre de santé le plus proche. On a enfin observé une diminution globale de la mortalité infanto-juvénile sur la période 1993-1999.

Conclusion L'étude confirme la multiplicité des causes de décès chez l'enfant dans les régions rurales d'Afrique de l'Ouest pendant les années 1990 et la tendance générale, déjà observée dans d'autres études, à une diminution de la mortalité infanto-juvénile dans ces populations. La corrélation observée montre qu'une analyse multivariée serait nécessaire pour distinguer les effets individuels de chaque facteur de risque. Ces résultats illustrent la nécessité d'améliorer de façon plus complète les soins pré- et postnatals dans les régions rurales d'Afrique subsaharienne.

Resumen

Factores de riesgo de mortalidad infantil y en la niñez en una zona rural de Burkina Faso

Objetivo El objetivo del estudio fue cuantificar el efecto de los factores de riesgo de mortalidad en la niñez en un entorno rural típico del África subsahariana.

Métodos Realizamos un análisis de supervivencia de los niños nacidos en una población sometida a vigilancia demográfica entre 1992 y 1999 basándonos en los datos de un sistema de vigilancia demográfica implantado en 39 aldeas cercanas a Nouna, en el oeste de Burkina Faso, con una población total de aproximadamente 30 000 habitantes. Se incluyó a todos los niños nacidos vivos durante el periodo del 1 de enero de 1993 al 31 de diciembre de 1999 en el área de estudio (n = 10 122) y sometidos a seguimiento hasta el 31 de diciembre de 1999. Como variable de resultado final se usó la mortalidad en la niñez por todas las causas.

Resultados Durante el periodo de observación se registraron 1340 defunciones. En un modelo de regresión de Cox, una estimación simultánea de las tasas de riesgo mostró que los factores de riesgo de mortalidad más importantes eran la muerte de la madre y el hecho de ser gemelo. Para ambos, el riesgo era máximo durante la lactancia. Otros factores asociados a la mortalidad fueron la edad de la madre, el tiempo transcurrido desde el último parto, la época del año en que tuvo lugar el nacimiento, la aldea, el grupo étnico y la distancia al centro de salud más cercano. Por último, se produjo una disminución general de la mortalidad en la niñez a lo largo de los años 1993–1999.

Conclusión El estudio respalda la idea de multicausalidad de las defunciones en la niñez en el África Occidental rural durante los años noventa, así como la tendencia general, observada en otros estudios, de disminución de la mortalidad en la niñez en esas poblaciones. La correlación observada entre los factores subraya la necesidad de realizar análisis multifactoriales para desimbricar los distintos efectos. Estos resultados ilustran la necesidad de una mejora más integrada de la atención prenatal y posnatal en el África subsahariana rural.

ملخص

عوامل الاختطار لوفيات الأطفال والرضَّع في أرياف بوركينا فاسو

ملخص: استهدفت هذه الدراسة قياس تأثير عوامل الاختطار على معدل وفيات الطفولة في منطقة ريفية نموذجية في جنوب الصحراء الأفريقية.

الطريقة: تم تحليل معدل بقيا المواليد في مجموعة سكانية من خلال ترصُّد ديموغرافي أُجري في الفترة من ١٩٩٢ إلى ١٩٩٩ واستند إلى معطيات ترصُّد ديموغرافي آخر نفذ في ٣٩ قرية محيطة بمدينة نونا الواقعة غرب بوركينا فاسو، والتي يبلغ عدد سكانها الإجمالي حوالي ٣٠ ألف نسمة. وشملت الدراسة جميع الأطفال الذين وُلدوا أحياء في منطقة الدراسة في الفترة من ١ كانون الثاني/يناير ١٩٩٣ إلى ٣١ كانون الأول/ديسمبر ١٩٩٩، والذين بلغ عددهم ١٠ ١٢٢ طفلاً. وتم استخدام مسببات وفيات الطفولة كمتغير ناتج.

الموجودات: تم تسجيل ١٣٤٠ وفاة في فترة الملاحظة. وبيَّن التقدير الفوري لنسب معدلات الخطر، الذي أُجري في إطار نموذج تحليل التحوف الإحصائي لكوكس أن وفاة الأم وولادة توائم هي أقوى عوامل الاختطار المسبِّبة للوفيات. وكان الاختطار أكثر وضوحاً في الرضَّع في كلتا الحالتين. وشملت عوامل الخطر الأخرى المقترنة بالوفيات: عمر الأم، والفترة بين الولادات، وموسم الولادة، والقرية، والمجموعة الإثنية، والبعد عن أقرب مركز صحي. ولوحظ أيضاً انخفاض شامل في وفيات الطفولة في السنوات من ١٩٩٣ إلى ١٩٩٩.

النتيجة: تعزِّز هذه الدراسة وجهة النظر التي تعزو وفيات الطفولة في أرياف غرب أفريقيا خلال عقد التسعينات إلى عدة مسببات، كما تعزِّز الاتجاه العام الملاحظ في دراسات أخرى، والمتمثل في انخفاض وفيات الطفولة في هذه المجموعات السكانية. ويؤكِّد الترابط الملاحظ بين هذه العوامل ضرورة تحليل متغيرات متعدِّدة للتعرُّف على تأثير كل منها على حدة. وتشير هذه النتائج إلى الحاجة لمزيد من التحسُّن الشامل في الرعاية السابقة للولادة والتالية للولادة في أرياف بلدان جنوب الصحراء الأفريقية.

References

1. Ahmad OB, Lopez AD, Inoue M. The decline in child mortality: a reappraisal. *Bulletin of the World Health Organization* 2000;78:1175-91.
2. Tulloch J. Integrated approach to child health in developing countries. *Lancet* 1999;354 Suppl 2:16-20.
3. Müller O, Garenne M. Childhood mortality in sub-Saharan Africa. *Lancet* 1999;353: 673.
4. Adetunji J. Trends in under-5 mortality rates and the HIV/AIDS epidemic. *Bulletin of the World Health Organization* 2000;78:1200-6.
5. Trape JF. The public health impact of chloroquine resistance in Africa. *American Journal of Tropical Medicine and Hygiene* 2001;64 Suppl:12-7.
6. Cooper RS, Osotimehin B, Kaufman JS, Forrester T. Disease burden in sub-Saharan Africa: What should we conclude in the absence of data? *Lancet* 1998;351:208-10.
7. Pickering H, Hayes RJ, Ngandu N, Smith PG. Social and environmental factors associated with the risk of child mortality in a peri-urban community in The Gambia. *Transactions of the Royal Society of Tropical Medicine and Hygiene* 1986;80:311-16.
8. Velema JP, Alihonou EM, Gandaho T, Hounye F. Childhood mortality among users and non-users of primary health care in a rural West African community. *International Journal of Epidemiology* 1991;20:474-9.
9. Hill A. Infant and child mortality: levels, trends, and data deficiencies. In: Feachem RG, Jameson DT, editors. *Disease and mortality in sub-Saharan Africa*. Oxford: Oxford University Press; 1991.
10. Blacker JGC. Infant and child mortality: development, environment, and custom. In: Feachem RG, Jameson DT, editors. *Disease and mortality in sub-Saharan Africa*. Oxford: Oxford University Press; 1991.
11. Pison G, Trape JF, Lefebvre M, Enel C. Rapid decline in child mortality in a rural area of Senegal. *International Journal of Epidemiology* 1993;22:72-80.
12. Binka FN, Maude GH, Gyapong M, Ross DA, Smith PG. Risk factors for child mortality in northern Ghana: a case-control study. *International Journal of Epidemiology* 1995;24:127-35.
13. Ronsmans C. Birth spacing and child survival in rural Senegal. *International Journal of Epidemiology* 1996;25:989-97.
14. Kuate Defo B. Effects of infant feeding practices and birth spacing on infant and child survival: a reassessment from retrospective and prospective data. *Journal of Biosocial Sciences* 1997;29:303-26.
15. Jaffar S, Leach A, Greenwood AM, Jepson A, Müller O, Ota MO, et al. Changes in the pattern of infant and childhood mortality in upper river division, The Gambia, from 1989 to 1993. *Tropical Medicine and International Health* 1997;2:28-37.
16. Hill AG, MacLeod WB, Sonko SS, Walraven G. Improvements in childhood mortality in The Gambia. *Lancet* 1999;352:1909.
17. Leach A, McArdle TF, Banya WA, Krubally O, Greenwood AM, Rands C, et al. Neonatal mortality in a rural area of The Gambia. *Annals of Tropical Paediatrics* 1999;19:33-43.
18. Garenne M, Kahn K, Tollmann S, Gear J. Causes of death in a rural area of South Africa: An international perspective. *Journal of Tropical Pediatrics* 2000;46:183-90.
19. Justesen A, Kunst A. Postneonatal and child mortality among twins in Southern Eastern Africa. *International Journal of Epidemiology* 2000;29:678-83.
20. Rutstein SO. Factors associated with trends in infant and child mortality in developing countries during the 1990s. *Bulletin of World Health Organization* 2000;78:1256-70.
21. Yé Y, Sanou A, Gbangou A, Kouyaté B. Nouna Demographic Surveillance System, Burkina Faso. In: INDEPTH, editor. *Health and demography in developing countries, Vol. 1: Population, health and survival in INDEPTH sites*. Ottawa, Canada: IDRC/CRDI; 2001.
22. Institut National de la Statistique et de la Démographie. *Enquête Démographique et de Santé, Burkina Faso 1998-1999*. Calverton (MA): Macro International.
23. Kouyate B, Traore C, Kielmann K, Müller O. North and South: bridging the Information gap. *Lancet* 2000;356:1034-35.
24. Sankoh OA, Ye Y, Sauerborn R Müller O, Becher H. Clustering of Childhood Mortality in Rural Burkina Faso. *International Journal of Epidemiology* 2001;30:485-92.
25. Müller O, Becher H, Baltussen A, Ye Y, Diallo A, Konate AT, et al. Effect of zinc supplementation on malaria morbidity among West African children: a randomized double-blind placebo-controlled trial. *BMJ* 2001;322:1-6.
26. Kynast-Wolf G, Sankoh OA, Kouyaté B, Becher H. Mortality patterns 1993-1998 in a rural areal of Burkina Faso, West Africa, based on the Nouna Demographic Surveillance System. *Tropical Medicine and International Health* 2002;7:349-56.
27. Klein JP, Moeschberger ML. *Survival analysis*. New York (NY): Springer; 1997.
28. Valsecchi MG, Silvestri D, Sasieni P. Evaluation of long-term survival: use of diagnostics and robust estimators with Cox's proportional hazards model. *Statistics in Medicine* 1996;15:2763-80.
29. SAS/STAT *Software changes & enhancements*. Cary (NC): SAS Institute; 1997.
30. Ouoba P. Mortality of children under five years of age. [Mortalité des enfants de moins de cinc ans]. In: *Enquete Demographique et de Sante, Burkina Faso*. Calverton (MD): Demographic Health Surveys; 1998:135-44. In French. Available from: URL: http://www.measuredhs.com/start.cfm
31. Gyimah SO. *Ethnicity and infant mortality in sub-Saharan Africa: The case of Ghana*. Discussion Paper No. 02-10. London, Canada, University of Western Ontario: Population Studies Centre; 2002. Available from: URL: http:www.ssc.uwo.ca/sociology/popstudies/dp/dp02-10.pdf
32. Mboup G. Mortality of children under five years of age. [Mortalité des enfants de moins de cinc ans. In: *Republique du Benin Enquete Demographique et de Sante, Benin*. Calverton (MD): Demographic Health Surveys; 2001:115-24. Available from: URL: http://www.measuredhs.com/start.cfm
33. Müller O, Traoré C, Kouyaté B. Clinical efficacy of chloroquine in young children with uncomplicated malaria — a community based study in rural Burkina Faso. *Tropical Medicine and International Health* 2003;8:202-3.
34. Koblinsky MA, Tinker A, Daly P. Programming for safe motherhood: a guide to action, *Health Policy and Planning* 1994;9:252-66.
35. *Mother-baby package: implementing safe motherhood in countries*. Geneva: World Health Organization; 1994.
36. Quinn TC. Global burden of the HIV pandemic. *Lancet* 1996;348:99-106.
37. CIA. *The World Factbook* 2002. Available from: URL: http://www.worldfactsnow.com/factbook/country/Burkina_Faso/
38. Center of Disease Control. *National Vital Statistics Report* 2001;49:41. Available from: URL: http://www.cdc.gov/nchs/fastats/pdf/nvsr49_01t13.pdf
39. Moore SE, Cole TJ, Poskitt EM, Sonko BJ, Whitehead RG, McGregor IA, et al. Season of birth predicts mortality in rural Gambia. *Nature* 1997;388:434.
40. Jaffar S, Leach A, Greenwood A, Greenwood B. Season of birth is not associated with delayed childhood mortality in Upper River Division, The Gambia. *Tropical Medicine and International Health* 2000;5:628-32.
41. Hook EB, Regal RR. Recommendations for presentation and evaluation of capture-recapture estimates in epidemiology. *Journal of Clinical Epidemiology* 1999;52:917-26.
42. Jaffar S, Leach A, Greenwood A, Greenwood B. Season of birth is not associated with delayed childhood mortality in Upper River Division, The Gambia. *Tropical Medicine and International Health* 2000;5:628-32.

4 Health systems research

4.1 Introduction

In a very broad sense, a **health system** is the organization by which an individual's health care is provided. From an economic perspective, healthcare may be viewed as just another product or service to be purchased by an individual, however, in that simple definition the huge amount of problems are not visible that arise in health system development in developing countries.

In a series of studies, performed jointly by members of the CRSN and the University of Heidelberg, health systems research in the Nouna DSS area forms another major research focus. One of the ultimate goals is to implement a health insurance for the Nouna population. This is a major undertaking which is not achievable within a short time frame. In the following chapters some relevant milestones are presented which will hopefully lead to this final goal.

4.2 Measuring the local burden of disease. A study of years of life lost in sub-Saharan Africa

Würthwein R, Gbangou A, Sauerborn R, Schmidt CM

Int J Epidemiol. 2001 30(3): 501-8

Reprinted with permission from Oxford University Press.

Measuring the local burden of disease. A study of years of life lost in sub-Saharan Africa

Ralph Würthwein,[a] Adjima Gbangou,[b] Rainer Sauerborn[c] and Christoph M Schmidt[a,d]

Background	An effective health policy necessitates a reliable characterization of the burden of disease (BOD) by cause. The Global Burden of Disease Study (GBDS) aims to deliver this information. For sub-Saharan Africa (SSA) in particular, the GBDS relies on extrapolations and expert guesses. Its results lack validation by locally measured epidemiological data.
Methods	This study presents locally measured BOD data for a health district in Burkina Faso and compares them to the results of the GBDS for SSA. As BOD indicator, standard years of life lost (age-weighted YLL, discounted with a discount rate of 3%) are used as proposed by the GBDS. To investigate the influence of different age and time preference weights on our results, the BOD pattern is again estimated using, first, YLL with no discounting and no age-weighting, and, second, mortality figures.
Results	Our data exhibit the same qualitative BOD pattern as the GBDS results regarding age and gender. We estimated that 53.9% of the BOD is carried by men, whereas the GBDS reported this share to be 53.2%. The ranking of diseases by BOD share, though, differs substantially. Malaria, diarrhoeal diseases and lower respiratory infections occupy the first three ranks in our study and in the GBDS, only differing in their respective order. Protein-energy malnutrition, bacterial meningitis and intestinal nematode infections occupy ranks 5, 6 and 7 in Nouna but ranks 15, 27 and 38 in the GBDS. The results are not sensitive to the different age and time preference weights used. Specifically, the choice of parameters matters less than the choice of indicator.
Conclusions	Local health policy should rather be based on local BOD measurement instead of relying on extrapolations that might not represent the true BOD structure by cause.
Keywords	Burden of disease, years of life lost, verbal autopsy, sub-Saharan Africa
Accepted	12 October 2000

An effective health policy necessitates a reliable characterization of the burden of disease (BOD) and its distribution by cause. The Global Burden of Disease Study[1] (GBDS) is a major step towards the development of such a rational information-based health policy. It provides a comprehensive assessment of epidemiological conditions and the disease burden for all regions of the world in an attempt at facilitating priority setting in health policy and research, and the development of cost-effective health interventions.

A fundamental problem for less developed regions, in particular those of sub-Saharan Africa (SSA), is the dearth of epidemiological and demographic data.[2] In the absence of routine vital event registration in most of this region, the GBDS extrapolated the epidemiological data that was available (mainly from a vital registration system in South Africa), using cause-of-death models and expert judgements.[3] These results await validation by thorough analyses of mortality and morbidity in SSA.

In this paper we present the results of a study measuring the BOD in a health district in rural Burkina Faso. In a study population of 31 000 people under demographic surveillance, deaths are recorded via a vital events registration system, and causes of death are assigned through verbal autopsy (VA). Our principal objective is the analysis of locally measured BOD by cause of death, age, and gender in direct comparison with

---

[a] Alfred Weber-Institute, University of Heidelberg, Germany.
[b] Centre de Recherche en Santé de Nouna (CRSN), Burkina Faso.
[c] Department of Tropical Hygiene and Public Health, Heidelberg, Germany.
[d] Centre for Economic Policy Research (CEPR), London, UK.

Correspondence: Christoph M Schmidt, Alfred Weber-Institute, Grabengasse 14, 69117 Heidelberg, Germany. E-mail: Schmidt@Uni-Hd.De

the GBDS results. A special emphasis is laid on the ranking of diseases by disease burden. We ask whether local health policy needs to be based on local BOD measurement. Furthermore, providing estimates based on two different indicators (YLL and deaths) and on two alternative YLL specifications concerning age-weighting and discounting, we investigate the robustness of our conclusions.

Study Population and Methods

Burkina Faso had an estimated population of approximately 10.7 millions in 1998.[4] This small West African state is divided into 11 administrative health regions, which comprise 53 health districts overall, each covering a population of 200 000–300 000 individuals. At least one health care facility in each district is a hospital with surgery capacities.[5] The districts themselves are again sub-divided in smaller areas of responsibility which are organized around either a hospital or a so-called CSPS (Centre de Santé et de Promotion Sociale), the basic health care facility in the Burkinian health system.

The Nouna health district, which is identical to the province of Kossi, covers 16 CSPS, one district hospital and a population of roughly 230 000 inhabitants.[6] In this district a demographic surveillance system (DSS) has been implemented, surveying the population of four CSPS with a study population of 31 280 inhabitants (mid-year population 1998). Periodically updated censuses (the first census was performed in 1992, a first control census in 1994, and a second control census in 1998) are supplemented by a vital events registration system, recording approximately every 3 months births, deaths and migrations. For each recorded death, the cause of death is determined through VA.[7–9] Age was assessed through identifying the date of birth. This was done either based on birth certificates (only in a relatively small number of cases), or using a 'local events calendar' which incorporates seasonal landmarks, feasts, political events, and village events (e.g. initiation rites, death of a village headman, famines, etc.).[10]

Some 4–16 weeks after a death is recorded, a structured questionnaire is administered to the best informed relative(s) of the deceased by lay people having a minimum education of 10 years of schooling. The review of the questionnaires is performed independently by two physicians. Three causes of death can be assigned to each case. An underlying cause has to be assigned, which is used as the cause of death in our study, since our results are aimed at informing health policy. In the case of malnutrition, for example, a child might die from a supervening acute disease, but to be successful, health policy must aim to improve nutrition instead of promoting intervention against the supervening disease. Additionally, one associated cause of death and one immediate cause of death can be assigned. If the two physicians do not agree on the underlying cause of death, a third physician is consulted as a referee. If his determination agrees with one of the initial diagnoses, the case is coded accordingly. If not, the case is coded as undetermined.

Of the 464 deaths analysed, 10 deaths (2.2%) were not classified according to the International Classification of Diseases, 10th Revision (ICD-10), and for 76 deaths (16.4%) a cause of death could not be ascertained. Instead of distributing the undetermined cases proportionately across the disease categories as was done in the GBDS, we left them in a separate residual category. A proportional redistribution of these cases would only overstate the precision of our estimates.

Numerous conceptually different measures have been proposed for measuring the BOD, for instance mortality rates, different forms of years of life lost[11,12] (YLL), and disability-adjusted life years (DALY),[13] with the latter comprising YLL as one of their major elements. We concentrate on standard YLL according to the methodology proposed in the GBDS. On the one hand, we want to ensure comparability, and on the other hand, deaths and remaining life expectancy can be measured relatively reliably by cause and typically contribute most to the overall BOD in SSA. The GBDS, for example, attributes 77% of overall BOD in SSA to YLL, whereas only 23% are attributed to years lived with disability, the morbidity measure of the GBDS.

For our analysis individual YLL were calculated for all recorded 464 deaths in the Nouna health district over a period of 17 months (November 1997 to March 1999), and cross-classified by age, gender, and cause of death. The measure is not standardized according to population size or age,[14,15] since our major objective is the characterization of the local burden of disease in Burkina Faso, not a cross-country comparison of standardized figures.

For each individual i, years of life lost due to premature death are calculated as

$$YLL_i(r,k) = \int_{x=a}^{x=a+L(a)} kxe^{-\beta x} \cdot e^{-r(x-a)} dx,$$

where a is the age of the individual, $L(a)$ is the remaining life expectancy at age a, r is the discount rate, and k and β are the parameters of the age-weighting function. In particular, $k = 1$ implies full age-weighting, and $k = 0$ no age-weighting. The YLL(0.03,1) are the benchmark mortality measure in the GBDS.

To test the possibility that the deviations of our results from the GBDS can be explained through mere sample variation, we applied a χ^2 goodness-of-fit test. The distribution of the null hypothesis is the multinomial distribution of deaths over distinct disease categories of the GBDS. The test statistic is

$$\chi^2 = \sum \frac{(O_j - E_j)^2}{E_j},$$

with $E_j = n*p_j$, where p_j is the expected probability of disease category j as published by the GBDS and n is the sample size. O_j is the number of deaths of category j that occur in the sample. The test is based on the distribution of deaths over distinct cause-of-death categories instead of YLL, since a test statistic computed with YLL would not be χ^2-distributed. The test is asymptotically valid if $E_i \geqslant 5 \; \forall \; i$. Categories with an expected occurrence of deaths of less than 5 were grouped together to fulfil this prerequisite.

Results

Appendix Table 1 documents YLL by cause of death, sex, and age group, using a format identical to the tables presented in the GBDS. The classification system is the one used in the GBDS, which can basically be translated into the ICD-10 system. Overall mortality is divided into three broad disease categories I (communicable, maternal, perinatal, and nutritional conditions),

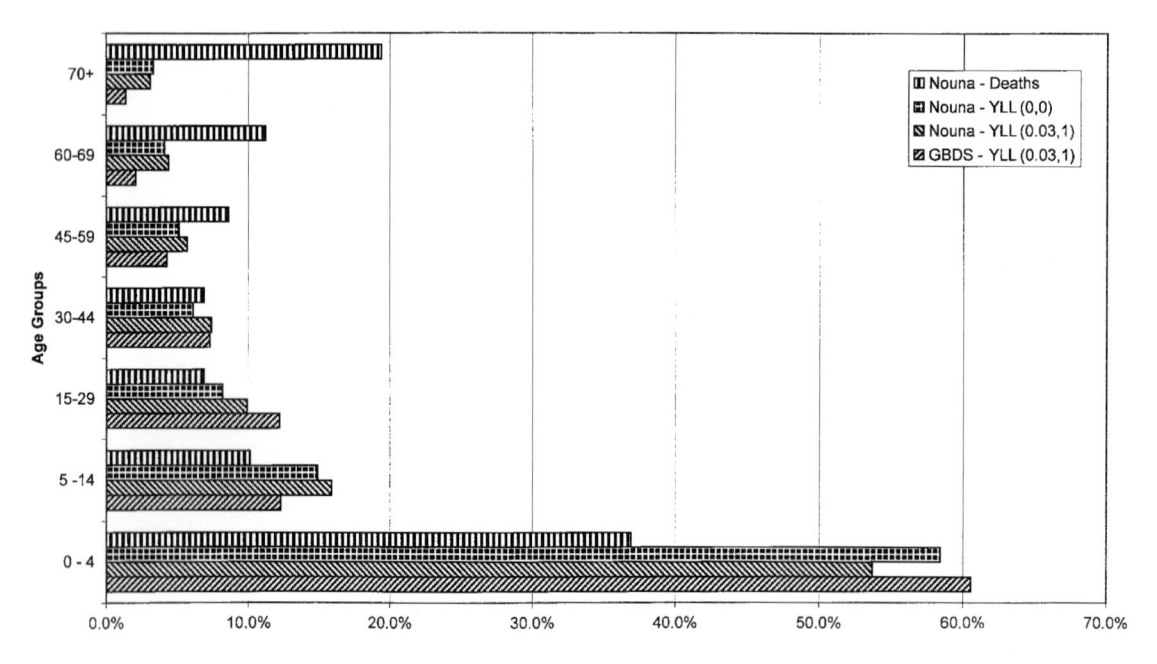

Figure 1 Distribution of burden of disease across age groups

II (non-communicable) and III (injuries). Their respective BOD shares are 90.0% for Nouna as compared to 76.7% for the GBDS for group I, 4.2% for group II compared to 12.9% and finally 5.8% and 10.5% for group III, respectively. (In this calculation we excluded YLL caused by war from the GBDS figures to ensure comparability in a case where the deviation can obviously and easily be reduced.)

The differences across gender between our results and the GBDS are minor. We estimated that 53.9% of the BOD is carried by men, whereas for SSA the GBDS reported this share to be 53.2%. However, 51.0% of the population in Nouna are men, as opposed to 49.4% in the GBDS. Therefore, in relative terms the burden of disease is slightly lower for men in Nouna.

Figure 1 displays the distribution of the results across age groups. The two bottom bars contrast the standard YLL(0.03,1) for Nouna with the GBDS results. Young age groups (up to 14 years of age) account for the overwhelming majority of estimated YLL both for Nouna and in the GDBS, however, their relative fraction is somewhat smaller in our Nouna study. The most striking difference occurs for small children (0–4 years), with the GBDS attributing almost 7 percentage points more to this age group (60.6% as compared to 53.7%). The two upper bars of Figure 1 are discussed below.

Table 1 provides a ranking of diseases by YLL that they have caused. For the GBDS, the ranking is also shown if the BOD is measured in DALY. In both our study and the GBDS the same three diseases occupied the first three places if measured in YLL, only varying in their specific rank. In our study population 27.7% of all estimated YLL were caused by malaria in contrast to 10.8% for SSA as given by the GBDS, where it only takes rank 3 (rank 4 in terms of DALY). In Nouna, malaria is followed by diarrhoeal diseases with a share of 20.5% of total disease burden, and by lower respiratory infections with a share of 11.7%. In the GBDS diarrhoeal diseases take rank 1 and lower respiratory infections take rank 2, in YLL as well as in DALY; in terms of DALY, unintentional injuries outrun malaria in taking rank 3.

An apparent feature of the data is that for the GBDS the BOD is much more evenly distributed across the diseases, whereas for Nouna more than half of the BOD measured in YLL was caused by the three major causes of death. Beyond rank three, substantial differences emerge. Three of the ten leading causes of YLL in the GBDS are not among the major ten causes of YLL in Nouna (intentional injuries, tuberculosis and malignant neoplasms), and the same holds for three of the ten leading causes of DALY (tuberculosis, neuro-psychiatric conditions, and maternal conditions). Protein-energy malnutrition occupies rank 5 in Nouna but only rank 15 in the GBDS, intestinal nematode infections are at rank 7 in Nouna but only at rank 38 in the GBDS. Meningitis is at rank 6 in Nouna in contrast to rank 27 for the GBDS.

A χ^2 goodness-of-fit test explores whether the differences in ranking between Nouna and the GBDS can be explained through mere sample variation, thus indicating whether, if we observed another sample, we would probably get the same ranking. The computed test statistic is $\chi^2 = 391$, while the critical value is $\chi^2_{(k=18,\ 0.995)} = 37.2$. The null hypothesis is rejected. There clearly seems to be a statistically significant different cause-of-death pattern in the health district of Nouna. To generate a hypothetical situation most favourable for the GBDS, in a sensitivity analysis we redistributed the residual cases according to the GBDS results and performed the appropriate χ^2 test once more. Our results are retained.

To analyse the sensitivity of our results to the particular choice of parameters and health-status indicators, we also calculated two alternative measures of the BOD: YLL(0,0) and

Table 1 Ranking of diseases by burden of disease caused

Diseases	GBD classification	Nouna Rank	Nouna % of total BOD	GBDS Rank	GBDS % of total BOD	Rank if measured in DALYs
Malaria	IA8	1	27.71	3	10.75	4
Diarrhoeal diseases	IA4	2	20.50	1	13.84	1
Lower respiratory infections	IB1	3	11.70	2	13.02	2
Unintentional injuries	IIIA	4	4.09	6	7.25	3
Protein-energy malnutrition	IE1	5	2.56	15	1.45	17
Bacterial meningitis	IA6	6	2.43	27	0.33	30
Intestinal nematode infections	IA14	7	2.22	38	0.03	34
Perinatal conditions	ID	8	1.82	5	7.56	6
Measles	IA5d	9	1.61	4	8.78	5
HIV	IA3	10	1.54	8	3.09	10
Intentional injuries*	IIIB	17	0.44	9	2.84	12
Tuberculosis	IA1	15	0.52	7	4.16	8
Malignant neoplasms	IIA	25	0.24	10	2.59	13
Neuro-psychiatric conditions	IIE	18	0.45	26	0.36	7
Maternal conditions	IC	13	0.60	11	2.44	9

Diseases are listed according to rank: first rank 1 to 10 for Nouna, then the rest of the top ten diseases for the GBDS that are missing under the top ten of Nouna.
* YLL from war have been excluded from the GBDS results.

the number of deaths. (Additional tables presenting the BOD in the same format as Appendix Table 1 but for deaths and YLL(0,0) can be downloaded at www.hyg.uni-heidelberg.de/ sfb544.) In principle, one could imagine that the parameter and indicator choice matters a lot, especially with respect to age, since the difference between YLL(0.03,1), YLL(0,0) and deaths is substantial across most of the age range (Figure 2).

Returning to Figure 1, the three upper bars compare the distribution of the three measures of BOD for Nouna across age groups. For the number of deaths, one can see the U-shaped pattern which is typical for developing regions. Burden of disease measured using crude deaths is concentrated in older age groups and in the age group 0–4 (infant and child mortality). In contrary, both YLL bars are constantly decreasing from younger to older age groups. The differences between YLL(0.03,1) and YLL(0,0) are less pronounced, with YLL(0,0) attributing a higher share of the BOD to the youngest age group (58.4% as opposed to 53.7%), and consequently lower shares to the remaining age groups.

With respect to gender, no substantial differences can be observed. While YLL(0.03,1) attribute 53.9% of the BOD to men, the corresponding figures are 53.5% for YLL(0,0) and 54.7% for deaths, respectively. This result confirms intuition, since it would be surprising if the particular choice of gender-insensitive indicators made a large difference.

Similar observations hold for the distribution across the three ICD-10 disease categories. Group I comprises 90.0% of the BOD measured using YLL(0.03,1), 90.8% using YLL(0,0), and 87.8% using deaths. For group II the shares are 4.2%, 3.9% and 6.6%, respectively, and for group III 5.8%, 5.3% and 5.6%. While YLL(0.03,1) and YLL(0,0) do not display perceptible differences, when using deaths as the indicator a relatively larger share of the BOD is attributed to non-communicable diseases. This is a reasonable result, since these diseases tend to be an important cause of death for older people.

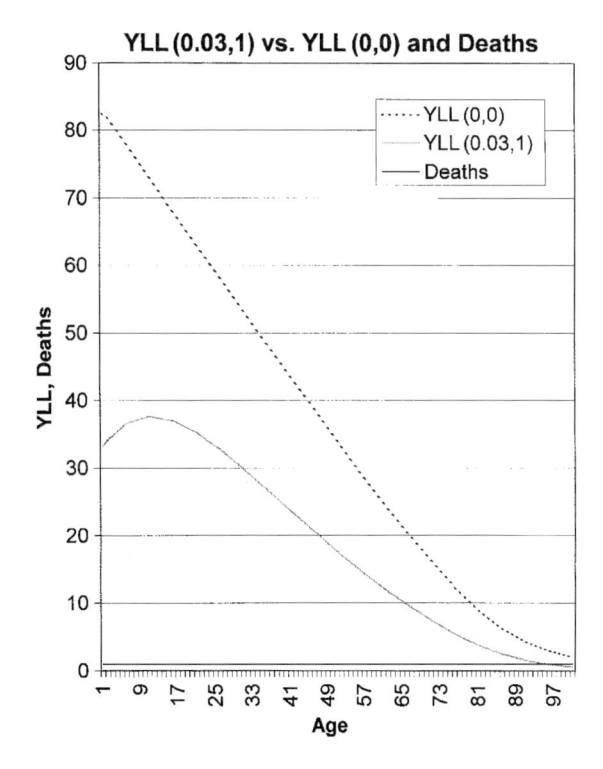

Figure 2 The graph shows the entries for females. A death of a woman dying at age 0 will be assigned 82.5 YLL(0,0) or 33.1 YLL (0.03,1) respectively. It will count as one if the number of deaths is used as the health-status indicator

Table 2 Ranking of diseases by burden of disease caused: YLL (0.03,1), YLL (0,0), or Deaths as Health-Status Indicators

Diseases	YLL(0.03,1)		YLL(0,0)		Deaths	
	Rank	in %	Rank	in %	Rank	in %
Malaria	1	27.71	1	28.01	1	25.86
Diarrhoeal diseases	2	20.50	2	21.13	2	19.18
Lower respiratory infections	3	11.70	3	11.98	3	12.07
Unintentional injuries	4	4.09	4	4.00	5	3.66
Protein-energy malnutrition	5	2.56	5	2.69	8	1.72
Bacterial meningitis	6	2.43	6	2.32	6	1.94
Intestinal nematode infections	7	2.22	8	2.02	4	3.88
Perinatal conditions	8	1.82	7	2.06	10	1.29
Measles	9	1.61	9	1.68	12	1.08
HIV	10	1.54	10	1.27	9	1.51
Inflammatory heart disease	11	1.30	11	1.26	6	1.94

Table 2 reports how the ranking of the leading causes of the BOD varies with the chosen health-status measure. There is almost no difference in ranking by cause of death whether or not age and time weighting is implemented. Only rank 7 and 8 change places, the rest retain their positions. Not only does the ranking stay almost the same, but also the shares of the total BOD differ only slightly. For rank 1, there is a difference of 1.1%, for rank 2 the difference is 3.0% and for rank 3 it is 2.3%. The highest proportional difference is for HIV (17.5%), but given its small share in total BOD (1.5% and 1.3%, respectively) even the largest relative difference among the ten major causes of death does not seem to be remarkable.

While the choice between YLL(0.03,1) and YLL(0,0) is apparently not instrumental, results change somewhat when we use deaths as the BOD indicator. The first three causes of death retain the same ranking, but there is less agreement between YLL and the number of deaths after rank 3.

Discussion

We have to acknowledge that with our approach we cannot really validate the GBDS study, since so far we cannot give explicit figures on the validity of our implemented VA system itself. However, the results we obtain raise serious doubt that for the health district we are looking at, the GBDS would be the right information base for a local health policy. Moreover, it is plausible to argue that this could very likely be true also for other regions of SSA.

In our analysis we operate with a limited sample size—we are distributing 464 deaths over more than 40 disease categories. This necessarily restricts our ability to accurately estimate the prevalence or incidence of single diseases, even though our number of reported cases is relatively high compared to other mortality studies in SSA.[8] For example, there are no reported deaths from tuberculosis in women below age 70. Findings like this are most probably merely a result of chance. For this reason, we will not discuss the detailed results (Appendix Table 1). Yet our data enable us to discuss the aggregate findings on the distribution of BOD by age and sex and to present a ranking of the most prevalent causes of death.

With respect to gender and age the Nouna results confirm more or less the general BOD structure reported by the GBDS for SSA as a whole, even if the GBDS seems to overstate the fraction of infant and child mortality compared to the Nouna results. The ranking of diseases by the share of disease burden, however, displays considerable differences. Basically, ranking, and thereby priority setting in health policy, depends on three things: the choice of indicator, the values incorporated in the indicator (age and time preferences) and the epidemiological data base that is used. Our results demonstrate a significant difference in ranking between the GBDS and Nouna, whereas the ranking by cause for Nouna shows little variation if a different indicator or different age and time weights are used.

Three competing explanations might be offered for the divergence between the Nouna and the GBDS data. First, instead of being an ideal weighted average of local BOD estimates over all regions of SSA, the GBDS results are an extrapolation of mortality data from a few parts of Africa, using cause-of-death models and a variety of expert judgements. Thus, while being a convincing pragmatic approach in the absence of local data, the GBDS might misrepresent the BOD structure of SSA as a whole. Only further local BOD analysis for other SSA regions would be able to validate the GBDS results as reliable mean estimations for SSA.

Second, measurement errors might have biased our estimates. For example, the large BOD shares attributed to the major diseases suggest that the medical doctors who reviewed the VA questionnaires might have tended to cluster deaths in the major categories they experienced in their daily work. While it seems unlikely that this problem could fully account for the observed differences to the GBDS, further validation studies of the VA method are warranted. In the literature the potential and limitations of VA methods are examined critically.[16–19] On balance, it is argued that the VA method is the best option in a situation where the majority of deaths occur without recourse to modern health care facilities.

Another measurement error problem could be the over-representation of the months November through March, since we used the whole available sample size of 17 months. To check whether this would affect our conclusions, we recalculated our results on a 12-month-basis (January to December 1998). The conclusions remain unchanged.

The third explanation for the divergence between the GBDS and our results could be that rural Burkina Faso might be very different from other parts of SSA. There is evidence that it is poorer and less developed than the average SSA country,[4] implying a relatively young population, fewer medical facilities, low vaccination coverage, a lower quality of housing, water supply and storage facilities, and generally a low level of hygiene. Not only will this have consequences for the high BOD share of disease category I (Nouna seems to lag behind in the epidemiological transition), but also for the high occurrence of protein-energy malnutrition and intestinal nematode infections.

Furthermore, Burkina Faso lies inside the meningitis belt, which is of course not the case for SSA as a whole, and it is a region of high malaria transmission. Malaria is probably endemic in most regions of SSA, but its endemicity varies widely. Chandramohan,[16] for example, reports the BOD shares of meningitis and malaria to be 11.4% and 8.9% in a region in Tanzania, 15.7% and 2.0% in Ethiopia, and 4.3% and 14.2% in Ghana, respectively.

Thus, even if the GBDS provided an accurate portrait of SSA as a whole, SSA would be quite heterogeneous in terms of BOD. Burkinian deviations from this typical BOD structure could not be an isolated phenomenon, but would have to be outweighed by countervailing deviations in other SSA regions. Overall, these arguments clearly underscore the need for local BOD measurement and priority setting. The available expert estimates from the GBDS are apparently not sufficient to provide a characterization of the BOD in SSA which is detailed and accurate enough to provide a basis for local health policy.

Acknowledgements

This research was supported by the Deutsche Forschungsgemeinschaft under the research grant Sonderforschungsbereich 544, Control of Tropical Infectious Diseases. We thank all the staff of the CRSN, the Ministry of Health of Burkina Faso, and the households surveyed for their valuable help and co-operation. We are grateful to Sarosh Kuruvilla, Frederick Mugisha and two anonymous referees for valuable comments and suggestions.

KEY MESSAGES

- This study presents locally measured burden of disease (BOD) data for a health district in Burkina Faso and compares them to the results of the Global Burden of Disease Study (GBDS) for sub-Saharan Africa (SSA).
- As BOD indicator, standard years of life lost are used.
- Regarding age and gender, our data exhibit the same qualitative BOD pattern as the GBDS results.
- The ranking of diseases by BOD share, a crucial information for the design of a national or local health policy, differs substantially.
- We conclude that local health policy should rather be based on local BOD measurement instead of relying on extrapolations that might not represent the true BOD structure by cause.

References

[1] Murray CCJL, Lopez AD (eds). *The Global Burden of Disease*. Boston, MA: Harvard University Press, 1996.

[2] Kaufman JS, Asuzu MC, Rotimi CN, Johnson OO, Owoaje EE, Cooper RS. The absence of adult mortality data for sub-Saharan Africa: a practical solution. *Bull World Health Organ* 1997;**75**:389–95.

[3] Murray CCJL, Lopez AD. Estimating causes of death: new methods and global and regional applications for 1990. In: Murray CCJL, Lopez AD (eds). *The Global Burden of Disease*. Boston, MA: Harvard University Press, 1996.

[4] World Bank (ed.). *African Development Indicators 2000*. Washington DC: World Bank, 2000.

[5] Burkina Faso Ministry of Health (ed.). *Statistiques Sanitaires 1996*. Ouagadougou, 1996.

[6] Burkina Faso Ministry of Health (ed.). *District Sanitaire de Nouna—Plan d'Action 1999*. Nouna, 1998.

[7] Anker M, Black RE, Coldham C *et al. A Standard Verbal Autopsy Method for Investigating Causes of Death in Infants and Children*. Geneva: World Health Organization, 1999.

[8] Chandramohan D, Maude GH, Rodrigues LC, Hayes RJ. Verbal autopsies for adult deaths: issues in their development and validation. *Int J Epidemiol* 1994;**23**:213–22.

[9] Bang AT, Bang RA, SEARCH Team. Diagnosis of causes of childhood deaths in developing countries by verbal autopsy: suggested criteria. *Bull World Health Organ* 1992;**70**:499–507.

[10] INDEPTH. *Demographic Surveillance Systems for Assessing Populations and their Health in Developing Countries*. INDEPTH, 2000.

[11] Gardner JW, Sanborn JS. Years of potential life lost (YPLL)—what does it measure? *Epidemiology* 1990;**1**:322–29.

[12] Lee WC. The meaning and the use of the cumulative rate of potential life lost. *Int J Epidemiol* 1998;**27**:1053–56.

[13] Murray CCJL. Rethinking DALYs. In: Murray CCJL, Lopez AD (eds). *The Global Burden of Disease*. Boston, MA: Harvard University Press, 1996.

[14] Sasieni PD, Adams J. Standardized lifetime risk. *Am J Epidemiol* 1999; **149**:869–75.

[15] Marlow AK. Potential years of life lost: what is the denominator? *Int J Epidemiol* 1995;**49**:320–22.

[16] Chandramohan D, Maude GH, Rodrigues LC, Hayes RJ. Verbal autopsies for adult deaths: their development and validation in a multicentre study. *Trop Med Int Health* 1998;**3**:436–46.

[17] Ronsmans C, Vanneste AM, Chakraborty J, Van Ginneken J. A comparison of three verbal autopsy methods to ascertain levels and causes of maternal deaths in Matlab, Bangladesh. *Int J Epidemiol* 1998;**27**: 660–66.

[18] World Health Organization. Measurement of overall and cause-specific mortality in infants and children: memorandum from a WHO/UNICEF meeting. *Bull World Health Organ* 1994;**72**:707–13.

[19] Snow RW, Armstrong JRM, Forster D *et al.* Childhood deaths in Africa: uses and limitations of verbal autopsies. *Lancet* 1992;**340**:351–55.

Appendix Table 1 YLL by age, sex and cause
464 Deaths (November 1997 – March 1999)

Cause	Total	Male	Female	Males 0–4	5–14	15–29	30–44	45–59	60–69	70+	Females 0–4	5–14	15–29	30–44	45–59	60–69	70+
Mid-year population 1998	31 287	15 884	15 403	2710	4890	3965	2118	1266	538	397	2613	4507	3655	2252	1416	561	399
All Causes*	10 949.9	5896.9	5053.0	3328.1	1070.2	273.5	444.5	318.4	254.1	208.1	2552.6	664.5	807.5	360.9	307.3	225.2	135.0
I. Communicable, maternal, peri-natal and nutritional conditions	8190.5	4557.4	3633.1	2883.3	663.2	169.0	374.6	183.0	142.4	142.0	1999.7	515.7	608.5	102.4	153.5	163.0	90.4
A. Infectious and parasitic diseases	6363.9	3568.0	2796.0	2165.0	625.7	169.0	278.7	117.2	117.8	94.7	1381.4	442.3	510.4	79.3	140.8	163.0	78.9
1. Tuberculosis	57.2	47.6	9.6	–	–	–	28.4	14.8	–	4.5	–	–	–	–	–	–	9.6
2. STDs excluding HIV	–	–	–	–	–	–	–	–	–	–	–	–	–	–	–	–	–
3. HIV	168.1	115.1	53.0	–	–	63.3	47.3	–	–	4.5	–	–	–	53.0	–	–	–
4. Diarrhoeal diseases	2244.4	1222.5	1021.9	930.5	147.5	–	22.1	64.1	32.6	25.6	552.7	183.6	133.8	–	77.8	51.8	22.2
5. Childhood-cluster diseases	242.9	136.1	106.8	136.1	–	–	–	–	–	–	69.4	37.4	–	–	–	–	–
a. Pertussis	34.0	34.0	–	34.0	–	–	–	–	–	–	–	–	–	–	–	–	–
b. Poliomyelitis	–	–	–	–	–	–	–	–	–	–	–	–	–	–	–	–	–
c. Diphtheria	–	–	–	–	–	–	–	–	–	–	–	–	–	–	–	–	–
d. Measles	176.0	69.2	106.8	69.2	–	–	–	–	–	–	69.4	37.4	–	–	–	–	–
e. Tetanus	33.0	33.0	–	33.0	–	–	–	–	–	–	–	–	–	–	–	–	–
6. Bacterial Meningitis	266.5	148.1	118.4	103.4	37.1	–	–	–	7.6	–	–	37.1	70.6	–	–	10.7	–
7. Hepatitis B and hepatitis C	65.3	33.6	31.6	–	–	–	26.5	–	7.1	–	–	–	31.6	–	–	–	–
8. Malaria	3033.9	1749.0	1284.9	994.9	441.1	105.6	78.2	38.3	35.9	54.9	724.6	147.4	274.3	26.2	–	79.4	33.0
9. Tropical-cluster diseases	–	–	–	–	–	–	–	–	–	–	–	–	–	–	–	–	–
10. Leprosy	–	–	–	–	–	–	–	–	–	–	–	–	–	–	–	–	–
11. Dengue	–	–	–	–	–	–	–	–	–	–	–	–	–	–	–	–	–
13. Trachoma**	–	–	–	–	–	–	–	–	–	–	–	–	–	–	–	–	–
14. Intestinal nematode infections	243.4	108.4	134.9	–	–	–	76.3	–	27.0	5.2	–	36.8	–	–	63.0	21.1	14.1
15. Other infectious and parasitic	42.3	7.6	34.7	–	–	–	–	–	7.6	–	34.7	–	–	–	–	–	–
B. Respiratory infections	1281.4	649.3	632.1	378.2	37.5	–	95.8	65.8	24.6	47.4	482.0	36.8	65.9	23.1	12.8	–	11.5
1. Lower respiratory infections	1281.4	649.3	632.1	378.2	37.5	–	95.8	65.8	24.6	47.4	482.0	36.8	65.9	23.1	12.8	–	11.5
2. Upper respiratory infections	–	–	–	–	–	–	–	–	–	–	–	–	–	–	–	–	–
C. Maternal conditions	32.2	–	32.2	–	–	–	–	–	–	–	–	–	32.2	–	–	–	–
D. Perinatal conditions	232.2	166.0	66.2	166.0	–	–	–	–	–	–	66.2	–	–	–	–	–	–
1. Low birth weight	66.0	66.0	–	66.0	–	–	–	–	–	–	–	–	–	–	–	–	–
4. Other perinatal conditions	166.1	100.0	66.2	100.0	–	–	–	–	–	–	66.2	–	–	–	–	–	–
E. Nutritional deficiencies	280.8	174.2	106.6	174.2	–	–	–	–	–	–	70.0	36.6	–	–	–	–	–
1. Protein-energy malnutrition	280.8	174.2	106.6	174.2	–	–	–	–	–	–	70.0	36.6	–	–	–	–	–

Cause	Total	Male	Female	Males 0-4	Males 5-14	Males 15-29	Males 30-44	Males 45-59	Males 60-69	Males 70+	Females 0-4	Females 5-14	Females 15-29	Females 30-44	Females 45-59	Females 60-69	Females 70+
II. Noncommunicable diseases	385.9	149.2	236.7	–	–	35.0	23.3	33.1	42.1	15.7	67.8	37.2	–	67.5	32.8	22.5	8.9
A. Malignant neoplasms	25.8	3.9	21.9	–	–	–	–	–	–	3.9	–	–	–	21.9	–	–	–
B. Other neoplasms	–	–	–	–	–	–	–	–	–	–	–	–	–	–	–	–	–
C. Diabetes mellitus	–	–	–	–	–	–	–	–	–	–	–	–	–	–	–	–	–
D. Endocrine disorders	–	–	–	–	–	–	–	–	–	–	–	–	–	–	–	–	–
E. Neuro-psychiatric conditions	49.3	7.6	41.7	–	–	–	–	–	7.6	–	–	37.2	–	–	–	–	4.4
F. Sense organ disease	–	–	–	–	–	–	–	–	–	–	–	–	–	–	–	–	–
G. Cardiovascular diseases	198.0	83.4	114.7	–	–	–	23.3	33.1	18.0	9.0	33.1	–	–	21.9	32.8	22.5	4.4
2. Ischaemic heart disease***	4.4	–	4.4	–	–	–	–	–	–	–	–	–	–	–	–	–	4.4
4. Inflammatory heart disease	142.0	31.7	110.2	–	–	–	–	17.1	9.5	5.2	33.1	–	–	21.9	32.8	22.5	–
5. Other cardiovascular	51.7	51.7	–	–	–	–	23.3	16.0	8.5	3.9	–	–	–	–	–	–	–
H. Respiratory diseases	–	–	–	–	–	–	–	–	–	–	–	–	–	–	–	–	–
I. Digestive diseases	51.2	16.5	34.7	–	–	–	–	–	16.5	–	34.7	–	–	–	–	–	–
2. Cirrhosis of the liver	16.5	16.5	–	–	–	–	–	–	16.5	–	–	–	–	–	–	–	–
4. Other digestive	34.7	–	34.7	–	–	–	–	–	–	–	34.7	–	–	–	–	–	–
J. Genito-urinary diseases	37.8	37.8	–	–	–	35.0	–	–	–	2.8	–	–	–	–	–	–	–
1. Nephritis and nephrosis	37.8	37.8	–	–	–	35.0	–	–	–	2.8	–	–	–	–	–	–	–
K. Skin diseases	–	–	–	–	–	–	–	–	–	–	–	–	–	–	–	–	–
L. Musculo-skeletal diseases	23.7	–	23.7	–	–	–	–	–	–	–	–	–	–	23.7	–	–	–
1. Rheumatoid arthritis	23.7	–	23.7	–	–	–	–	–	–	–	–	–	–	23.7	–	–	–
M. Congenital anomalies	–	–	–	–	–	–	–	–	–	–	–	–	–	–	–	–	–
N. Oral conditions	–	–	–	–	–	–	–	–	–	–	–	–	–	–	–	–	–
III. Injuries	522.3	363.6	158.7	69.2	258.7	–	25.9	–	–	9.9	35.3	–	–	56.2	49.8	11.7	5.7
A. Unintentional injuries	473.8	360.1	113.8	69.2	258.7	–	25.9	–	–	6.3	35.3	–	–	27.5	35.5	11.7	3.8
B. Intentional injuries	48.5	3.6	44.9	–	–	–	–	–	–	3.6	–	–	–	28.7	14.3	–	1.9
Causes not compatible to the GBDS classification system	199.0	83.5	115.5	33.0	37.5	–	–	–	9.5	3.6	34.1	–	32.2	29.3	12.8	–	7.1
Cause of death undetermined	1652.3	743.2	909.1	342.6	110.9	69.5	20.8	102.3	60.2	36.9	415.7	111.5	166.9	105.5	58.5	28.0	23.0

Notes:
* including YLL caused by undetermined cases or cases that were not classified according to the GBDS classification sytem.
** diseases like Japanese encephalitis that are not prevalent in the study region have been excluded from the table.
*** for disease category II and III, only subgroups with positive entries have been included.
The tables for YLL(0,0) and deaths can be downloaded at WWW.Hyg.Uni-Heidelberg.de/SFB544.

4.3 Examining out-of-pocket expenditure on health care in Nouna, Burkina Faso: implications for health policy

Mugisha F, Kouyate B, gbangou A, Sauerborn R.

Trop Med Int Health. 2002 7(2): 187-96

Reprinted with permission from Blackwell Publishers Ltd.

Examining out-of-pocket expenditure on health care in Nouna, Burkina Faso: implications for health policy

Frederick Mugisha[1], Bocar Kouyate[2], Adjima Gbangou[2] and Rainer Sauerborn[1]

1 Department of Tropical Hygiene and Public Health, Heidelberg University, Heidelberg, Germany
2 Centre de Recherche en Santé de Nouna (CRSN), Nouna District, Burkina Faso

Summary

OBJECTIVE   To examine household out-of-pocket expenditure on health care, particularly malaria treatment, in rural Burkina Faso.

METHOD   Comprehensive analysis of out-of-pocket expenditure on health care through a descriptive analysis and a second, multivariate analysis using the Tobit model with emphasis on malaria, based on 800 urban and rural households in Nouna health district.

RESULTS   Households will spend less on malaria, either in or outside the health facility, if given the choice to do so, because they feel confident to self-treat malaria. Seeking health care from a qualified health worker incurs more out-of-pocket expenditure than self-treatment and traditional healers, and if necessary, households sell off assets to offset the expenditure. More than 80% of household out-of-pocket expenditure is allocated to drugs.

CONCLUSION   This has policy implications for malaria control and the Roll Back Malaria Initiative. Communities need to be educated on the risks of malaria complications and the potential risk of inappropriate diagnosis and treatment. Drug or health services pricing policy needs to create an incentive to use the health services. In the fight against malaria, building alliances between households, traditional healers and health workers is essential.

keywords   out-of-pocket expenditure, malaria, Burkina Faso, household, age bias, gender bias

correspondence   Frederick Mugisha, Department of Tropical Hygiene and Public Health, Im Neuenheimer Feld 324, 69120 Heidelberg, Germany. Fax: +49 6221 56 5948; E-mail: frederick.mugisha@urz.uni-heidelberg.de

Introduction

Like most African countries, Burkina Faso introduced user fees as a mode of financing government health services within the framework of the Bamako Initiative. This was in response to the severe problems in financing health services in most of sub-Saharan Africa. Government health budgets declined in real terms in response to macroeconomic problems at the time while demand for health services increased, partly because of population growth and successful social mobilization. The Bamako Initiative was announced at a meeting of African Ministers of Health, sponsored by the World Health Organization (WHO) and United Nations Children Fund (UNICEF) in 1987. Its goal is 'universal accessibility to Primary Health Care (PHC). The attainment of this goal would be enhanced through a substantial decentralization of health decision making to the district level, community level management of PHC, user financing under community control and a realistic national drug policy and provision of basic essential drugs, leading to a self-sustaining PHC with emphasis on promoting the health of women and children (WHO 1988).'

User charges in government health services were considered feasible because when 'free' government services were rationed or of poor quality, people paid substantial amounts for health care in the private sector, often for inappropriate treatment or medicines. User fees were intended to redirect private expenditure towards more effective government health services and appropriate treatment, as retained fees would ensure regular drug availability and better quality.

Studies in Burkina Faso (Sauerborn et al. 1994) and elsewhere (Acharya et al. 1993; Pannarunothai & Mills

1997; Sen 1997; Fabricant *et al.* 1999) have shown that the introduction of fees resulted in deterring people, especially the poor and children, from using health care services. In contrast to this, a widely cited study from Cameroon found that the poor used more state-provided health care despite fee increases as a result of quality improvements (Litvack & Bodart 1993). Similarly, growing demand after introduction of cost recovery and better quality of care was found in a pilot study in Niger (Diop *et al.* 1995).

The impact of user fees is forcing some governments to rethink or to abolish the regime altogether. Uganda, for example, abolished them in March 2001 (Wendo 2001), although the experience so far has been that health facilities have been overwhelmed and shortage of drugs is now frequent (Kikonyogo 2001). Only in district, regional and national referral hospitals are patients given the option of paying and being served quickly or queuing for free services. The FY 2001 Foreign Operations Appropriations Bill allows the US to oppose any IMF, World Bank or regional development bank loan that calls for user fees or service charges from poor people for primary education or primary health care (US Congress 2000).

One of the effects of user fees, which has not attracted much attention, is the multiplier effect it has in worsening the disease burden of some illnesses, either by causing delays in treatment leading to complications, or by inappropriate self-diagnosis and treatment, which may increase drug resistance. Malaria is an excellent example: It can be treated in just 3 days, yet kills millions every year. While many factors are responsible, delays in diagnosis and treatment are the main reason for its high mortality and complications such as cerebral malaria, severe anaemia, jaundice, and renal failure. An estimated 80% of malaria-related deaths are caused by cerebral malaria (Kakkilaya 2001), hence early treatment is essential to successful control of malaria. Unfortunately patients postpone seeking care; partly because of the fear of paying user fees (Foster 1991) until such complications begin to manifest (Ebisawa *et al.* 1980). Secondly, to economize, patients may buy insufficient quantities of the drug, or share one dose between two or more people if more than one family member is sick (Foster 1991). This increasingly renders some largely affordable and effective drugs such as chloroquine (CQ) ineffective by building resistance. As a result some countries have had to abandon CQ as the first-line drug in favour of more expensive alternatives. Malawi, for example, replaced CQ with sulphadoxine-pyrimethamine (SP) in 1993 (Zoguereh & Delmont 2000), and Kenya is in the process to do the same (Shretta *et al.* 2000).

In this paper, we examine the burden of out-of-pocket expenditures on households in Nouna, Burkina Faso. To assess the impact of the likelihood of delaying treatment and possible drug resistance, we analyse the burden of out-of-pocket expenditure by disease or health condition, in relation to its components and to the strategies employed to offset the expenses. We describe the factors for differential burden among households with particular emphasis on malaria.

Data and sample

The data is based on a panel survey of 800 households in the district of Nouna, north-western Burkina Faso, conducted under the auspices of the Nouna Health Research Center as part of an ongoing project to evaluate health care interventions. The Demographic Surveillance System (DSS) in the area provided the sampling frame. Households were sampled in a two-stage cluster procedure, with each household having the same probability of being selected (Levy & Lemeshow 1999). At the first stage, we selected seven clusters in urban Nouna and 20 clusters in the 41 rural villages; at stage two, respondent households were selected in each cluster. The sample proportions of rural and urban households reflect their respective fractions in the DSS: We selected 480 of 4630 households in the 41 villages, and 320 of 2802 households in Nouna 320 (62% rural, 38% urban).

The survey questionnaire comprised of socioeconomic and morbidity modules. To capture seasonal variation, the morbidity module is used four times a year and the socioeconomic module twice a year. This paper draws on data collected in the first two survey rounds conducted during the dry (June) and rainy season (September) in 2000. Each adult responded to questions pertaining to him/herself and appropriate proxies were identified for children and individuals who could not answer for themselves. If a household member was absent, interviewers made three more attempts to see the adult in question.

The perception of illness rather than disease was used to analyse out-of-pocket expenditure in Burkina Faso for two reasons: first, it is the perception that determines whether an individual seeks self-treatment or any other type of health care provider (Coreil 1983). Secondly, the resulting expenditure depends to some extent on the perceived type and severity of illness. To allow the possibility of future comparison with other similar studies, the illnesses were translated and mapped according to the Global Burden of Disease Classification (Murray & Lopez 1996). We use the term 'disease' to denote a labelled diagnostic category, not as one that has been clinically determined.

Aggregate incomes were measured based upon local prices and quantities of agricultural products (animal and crops), regular cash incomes (salaries and pensions in some cases) and cash transfers, as the population is predominantly farmers who produce for home consumption and a little surplus for sale. Incomes were measured in two steps: first by summing up the value of sold animal products, crop products, cash earnings and transfers to the households; secondly, by subtracting expenditure on seeds, bought animals and cash transfers out of the households. If households bought animals and did not sell them in the reference period, this was considered savings and excluded. If the sale of crop products was bigger than the harvest, then the value of the sold crops replaced the value of the harvest. The value of animals, crops and material assets (plough, carts) was computed separately, similar to a procedure used to estimate incomes of rural communities in Sierra Leone (Fabricant *et al.* 1999), where a high correlation with wealth proxies, such as people's ranking of the rich individuals and families in the community, was found.

Statistical methods

We also present estimates based on the Tobit model for examining out-of-pocket expenditure on health care. We used the probit estimation to identify the role of malaria in treatment choice and the ordered probit estimation to determine the likelihood of an illness being severe. Not all out-of-pocket expenditure incurred was observed over the entire study period. Some episodes had not ended and for these, complete information was only available on independent variables (age, sex, and income) but not for the dependent variable (out-of-pocket expenditure on health care). We did know the minimum amount of out-of-pocket spent on health care. The Tobit model, the adjusted Tobit model and sample selection models (Scott Long 1997) apply to continuous but limited dependent variables such as out-of-pocket expenditure on health care used in econometric literature.

Tobit analysis is done separately for treatment within and outside health facilities using the following variables as independent: whether an illness is malaria or not, age, sex, value of material assets, value of agricultural produce, value of animals, payment arrangement, urban/rural and household size. Household income, which is the sum of individual incomes belonging to the household, did not affect the out-of-pocket expenditure and therefore was dropped from the analysis and replaced by individual components. All monetary values are in Burkina Faso currency CFA (1 USD 550 CFA, March 2001). Severity of the illness as perceived by the patients was considered endogenous and not used as a dependent variable.

Results

The role of malaria on treatment choice and severity is noteworthy. Malaria does not determine treatment choice using the probit estimation method. But people in the urban area and those with a high income (determined by the value of animals) were more likely to seek care from the health facilities, indicating ease of geographical and monetary access. Using the ordered probit estimation, malaria was less severe than other illnesses (-4.75, $P < 0.0001$) and illnesses reported by people in urban areas were less severe (-4.27), indicating again the problem of geographical access to health facilities for timely treatment. Nouna town is served by the district hospital while the rural areas have few first-line health facilities.

Out-of-pocket expenditure by illness

We examined the out-of-pocket expenditure according to illness and expenditure components (Table 1). *Hospitalization* is expenditure for a hospital bed and services but excluding drugs; *transport* includes all forms of transport; *stay* is expenditure on upkeep while seeking care; *consultation* is consultation fee, and *others* refers to any other expenditure including laboratory examinations.

Ranking of illness and out-of-pocket expenditure on health care provides insights into how differently the morbidity and economic burden attributable to different illnesses impact on the population. For example, a highly ranked illness caused by morbidity may be the one with the greatest out-of-pocket expenditure, which is the case with malaria (Table 1). Relative rankings show differential impact; oral conditions, for example, ranks 8th as a cause of morbidity, but 13th as a cause of out-of-pocket expenditure, implying that the population with this illness experienced a significantly lower burden because of out-of-pocket expenditure relative to morbidity.

Comparing malaria and other illnesses, Figure 1 shows the components of out-of-pocket expenditure on health care. Clearly drugs make up the greatest proportion: 90% in case of malaria, against 4% on transport, 3% on consultation, none on stay while seeking treatment and 1% on hospitalization. For other illnesses, 84% of the expenditure is on drugs, 3% on transport, 4% on consultation, 4% for stay while seeking treatment and 3% on hospitalization.

Out-of-pocket expenditure and reason by treatment choice

We also examined out-of-pocket expenditure by treatment choice, specifically to understand how

Table 1 Components of household out-of-pocket expenditure by disease, Nouna, Burkina Faso

Global burden of disease classification	Case	Case rank	Transport	Consultation	Drugs	Stay	Hospitalization	Others	Total cost	Rank
I. Communicable, maternal, perinatal and nutritional conditions										
A. Infectious and parasitic diseases										
4. Diarrhoeal diseases	39	5	6750	2850	95 295	2700	2650	100	110 345	3
8. Malaria	292	1	9510	8480	225 895	900	2300	4700	251 785	1
9. Tropical cluster diseases	16	10	–	–	24 250	4150	900	–	29 300	10
13. Trachoma	7	13	–	550	25 750	–	2500	–	28 800	11
15. Other infection and parasitic diseases	16	11	7970	650	41 655	31 000	23 000	–	104 275	5
B. Respiratory infections	39	6	1950	4210	23 785	150	–	–	30 095	9
C. Maternal conditions	2	18	–	–	9700	600	1500	–	11 800	15
E. Nutritional deficiencies	4	15	–	–	7400	–	–	–	7400	17
F. Other Group I diseases	42	4	950	4200	48 220	150	1000	–	54 520	7
II. Non-communicable diseases										
A. Malignant neoplasms										
9. Breast cancer	2	19	–	–	5000	–	–	–	5000	18
D. Endocrine disorders	2	20	–	–	500	–	–	–	500	20
E. Neuro-psychiatric conditions										
4. Epilepsy	10	12	–	750	10 485	1000	–	–	12 235	14
13. Other neuro-psychiatric	6	14	–	500	9000	–	–	75	9575	16
F. Sense organ disease										
2. Cataracts	4	16	–	500	17 750	500	–	–	18 750	12
G. Cardiovascular diseases										
5. Other cardiovascular	26	7	–	6900	27 935	–	500	2100	37 435	8
H. Respiratory diseases										
2. Asthma	3	17	–	–	1250	–	–	–	1250	19
L. Musculo-skeletal diseases										
3. Other musculo-skeletal	54	2	950	6330	89 115	4000	1500	2800	104 695	4
N. Oral conditions	21	8	–	–	16 700	–	–	–	16 700	13
O. Other Group II diseases	43	3	7000	3500	163 650	3200	2250	–	179 600	2
III. Injuries										
A. Unintentional injuries										
4. Fires	2	21	–	–	75	–	–	–	75	21
6. Other unintentional injuries	19	9	–	3600	80 175	–	–	300	84 075	6
Coding not compatible	101		1540	6250	109 040	400	1100	10 600	128 930	
Other diseases unclassified	5		2500	–	11 500	–	–	–	14 000	
Total	755		39 120	49 270	1 044 125	48 750	39 200	20 675	1 241 140	

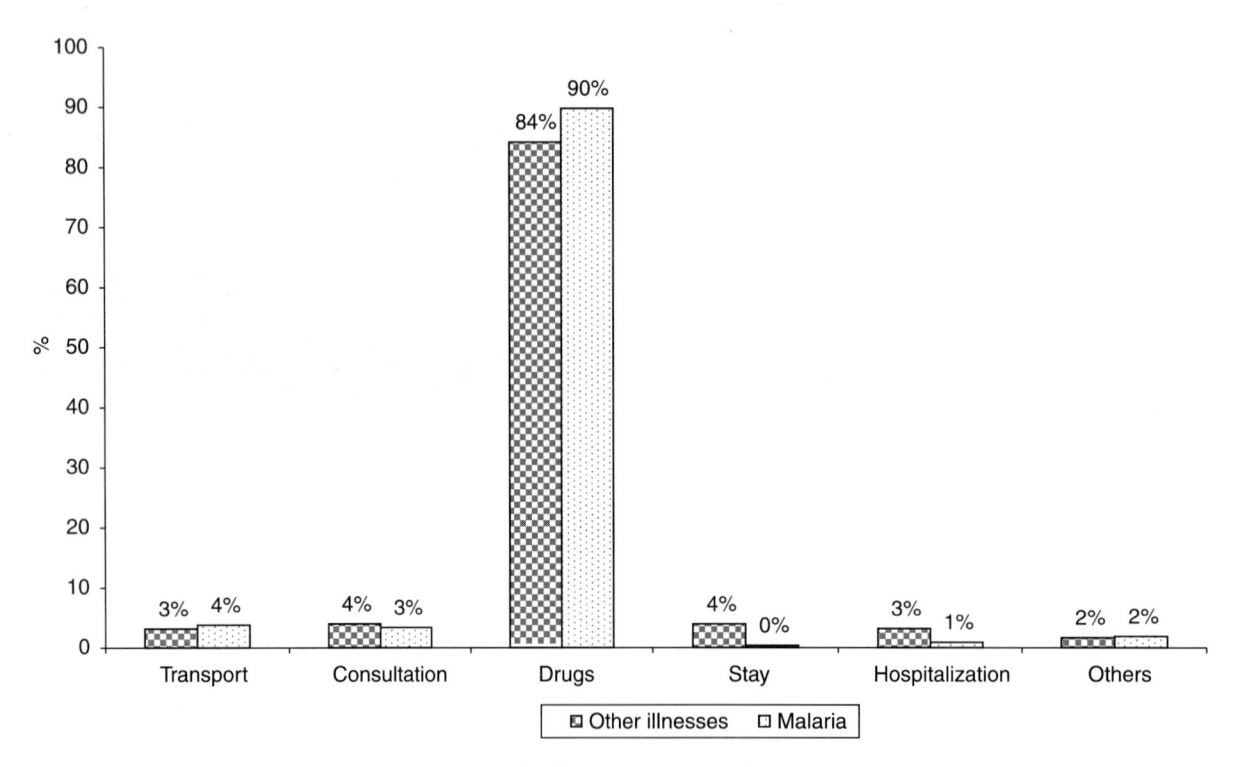

Figure 1 Components of out-of-pocket expenditure on health care in Nouna, Burkina Faso.

out-of-pocket expenditure varies with treatment choice and illness. A number of reasons were given for seeking self-treatment, trained health worker or traditional healers, most importantly lack of money, competence and severity of illness. These have policy implications for the control of malaria.

Figure 2 shows the reasons for choosing self-treatment, a trained health worker or a traditional healer and illustrates four points. On aggregate, as the illness becomes severe, patients choose to go to the health worker (see severity category) regardless of the illness in question. About 42.7% of malaria patients treat themselves because they feel competent to handle the situation, against 29.8% of patients with other illnesses. Regardless of the illness in question, a substantial number of patients chose self-treatment (81.2% for malaria, 64.3% for all other illnesses) – indicating a high preference for it, especially in cases of malaria. Traditional healers are rarely consulted for malaria treatment (0.9%) compared with other illnesses (17%). Much more out-of-pocket money was spent on treatment from health workers (748 540 CFA) than on self-treatment (373 340 CFA) or traditional healers (119 260 CFA).

Household strategies for mitigating the out-of-pocket e penditure burden

The strategies that households in Nouna use to mitigate out-of-pocket expenditure were pre-coded as (1) sold personal assets, (2) received free treatment, (3) received money as a gift, (4) borrowed money, (5) used cash, liquid savings and (6) worked for the money. But only four strategies were used, namely selling of personal assets, free treatment, money as a gift, and borrowing money. Table 2 shows that no households used cash or liquid savings. As expenditure on health rises, households sell assets to meet the cost. This observation is consistent for all illnesses but less so for malaria. More than three-quarters (78.9%) of households borrow money to pay for health care. This is slightly more for malaria. Free treatment and donations of money are very rare.

actors for differential out-of-pocket e penditure on health

We examined the factors for differential out-of-pocket expenditure using the Tobit estimation model separately for in and outside the health facility. The model estimates in Table 3 show differences for self-treatment and health

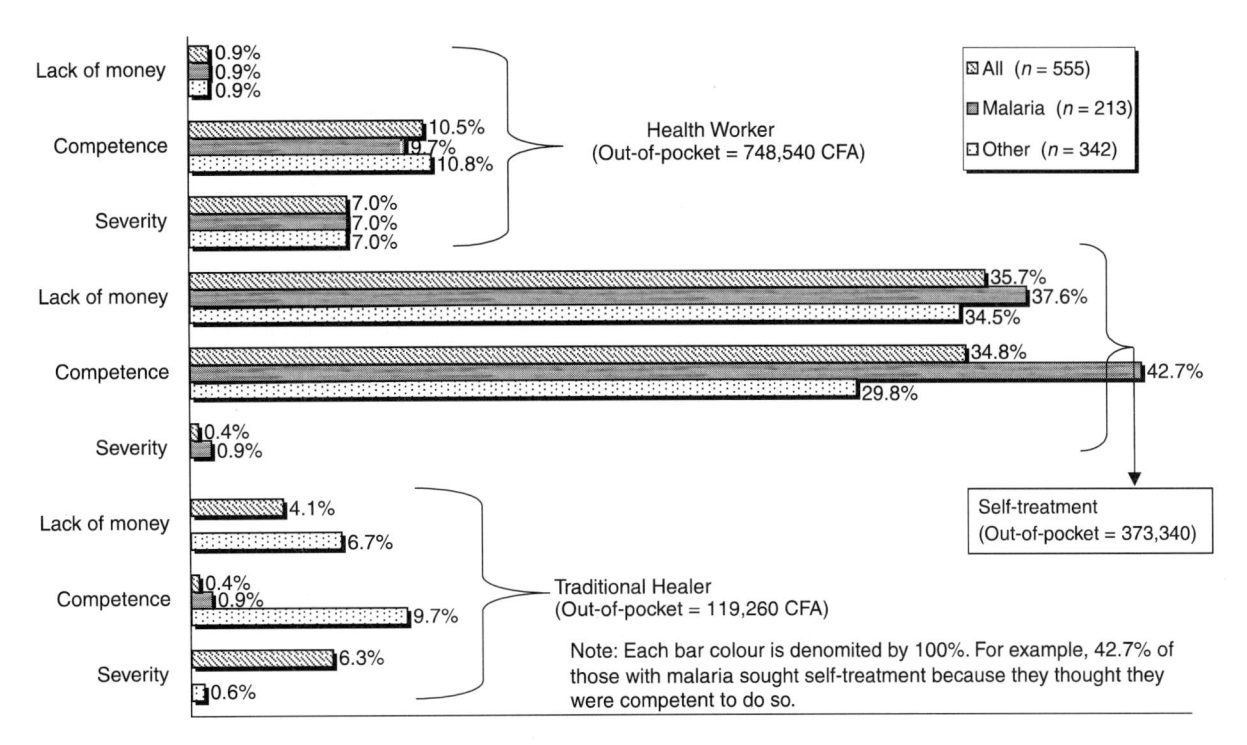

Figure 2 A comparison of treatment choice for malaria and other illness, Nouna Burkina Faso.

Table 2 Strategies for mitigating out-of-pocket expenditure on health in Nouna, Burkina Faso

Out-of-pocket expenditure	Mitigating household strategy				
	Selling of assets	Free treatment	Money as gift	Borrowed money	Total
Malaria					
Less, 800 CFA	6 (6.5)	0 (0)	1 (1.1)	86 (92.5)	93 (59.6)
Over, 800 CFA	9 (14.3)	1 (1.6)	(1.6)	52 (82.5)	63 (40.4)
Sub-total	15 (9.6)	1 (0.6)	2 (1.3)	138 (88.5)	156 (57.8)
All others					
Less, 800 CFA	4 (9.5)	1 (2.3)	3 (7.1)	34 (81.1)	42 (36.8)
Over, 800 CFA	19 (26.4)	6 (8.3)	6 (8.3)	41 (56.9)	72 (63.2)
Sub-total	23 (20.2)	7 (6.1)	9 (7.9)	75 (65.8)	114 (42.2)
Total	38 (14.1)	8 (3.0)	11 (4.1)	213 (78.9)	270 (100)

Values in parentheses are percentages.

facility treatment of malaria compared with all other illnesses, expenditure source or payment arrangement and value of material assets. Differences are observed for treatment in health facility only for age, sex and whether a household is urban or rural. There are significant differences in self-treatment only for payment arrangement and the value of animals.

It matters less whether treatment is sought from the health facility or self-treatment: less out-of-pocket money (significant at 1%) was spent on malaria compared with all other illnesses, 4503 CFA less for self-treatment and 8615 CFA less for the health facility. There are two possible explanations to this: first, the perception that malaria has been with the community for so long that it is perceived not as a threat but as an illness that can be treated with some tablets of CQ. This is corroborated by Figure 2, which shows that a large proportion of individuals chose self-treatment for malaria because they thought they were

Table 3 Model results of determinants of differential out-of-pocket expenditure on health, Nouna, Burkina Faso

Independent variable	Health facility			Self-treatment			Description of variables
	Coefficient	SE	t-Statistic	Coefficient	SE	t-Statistic	
Malaria	−8615.25	2036.85	−4.23	−4503.35	913.68	−4.93	1 – malaria; 0 – others
Payment arrangement	1075.42	2848.23	0.38	41801.53	3042.18	13.74	1 – sold assets; 0 – others
Age	123.26	46.75	2.64	16.13	20.77	0.78	Integer values
Sex	4168.22	2021.28	2.06*	339.89	934.43	0.36	1 – urban; 0 – rural
Urban	6747.98	2203.02	3.06	−1357.46	1061.75	−1.28	1 – male; 0 – female
Value of animals	<−0.01	<0.01	−1.93	<0.01	<0.01	−4.76	In CFA
Value of materials	<0.01	<0.01	2.03*	<0.01	<0.01	2.58*	In CFA
Value of crops	<−0.01	<0.01	−1.69	<0.01	<0.01	−1.48	In CFA
Household size	226.31	173.67	1.30	138.27	79.21	1.75	No. of people
Religion	−469.91	2060.69	−0.23	835.05	913.34	0.91	1 – muslim; 0 – others
Constant	2912.86	2790.04	1.04	4283.18	1433.34	2.99	
No. of observations	187			418			
Uncensored	96			251			
Right censored	91			167			
LR χ^2(10)	59.06			198.34			
Pseudo R^2	0.0269			0.0357			

* 5% Significant.
1% Significant.

competent. Secondly, the value of material assets owned is significant at 5% for both self-treatment and treatment in the health facility. As this is an indicator of income, one would expect that the higher the income, the more an individual household is likely to pay.

For self-treatment most people first borrow to offset expenditure, and then, as bills increase, resort to selling their assets (Table 2). The possible explanation for this is that households fear low bargaining power in the period of need and therefore prefer to borrow and offset the debt later, but as costs rise, their credit worthiness decreases, or nobody may be able to lend such an amount of money.

We found a significant difference in out-of-pocket expenditure for self-treatment associated with the value of animals: the greater their value, the less out-of-pocket money a household is likely to spend. At first this looks odd as animals are a proxy of wealth. But when looking at the culture of the community and economic activity, two issues become clear: animals, especially donkeys, are used for farming and it is essentially difficult to sell donkeys in the event of illness. Cattle are a way of life for some sections on the population, and they would rather die than sell their cattle.

People spent more out-of-pocket on treatment from the health worker than on self-treatment and traditional healers (not shown in the table). Using the probit analysis, the difference was significant at 1%. Treatment elsewhere may have been incomplete, and to complete the course may have required more expenditure. Health workers may be more expensive, incurring cost both for consultation and transport.

Being in the urban area determines how much a household pays for health care in the health facility rather than on self-treatment, possibly because of differences in income levels between urban and rural areas or geographical access to health facilities.

Finally, age and sex are significant regarding choosing treatment in health facilities vs. self-treatment. The older a person is, the more out-of-pocket she or he is likely to pay for health care. Sauerborn et al. (1996) found age to be one of the factors for differential out-of-pocket expenditure on health in the area. Households spend more on males than females. This is, however, only true for health facilities, not self-treatment.

Discussion

What implications do these results have for the global aim to Roll Back Malaria (RBM)? RBM comprises strategies to reduce access barriers to prompt and appropriate treatment, to sector-wide approaches and financing, to monitoring drug resistance and to improving quality of care at home. Our results have policy implications for these proposed strategies.

Less out-of-pocket is spent on malaria than other illnesses, yet it is the leading cause of morbidity and mortality in the population (Würtwein et al. 2000) regardless of treatment choice. Malaria may not be perceived as a threat any more (Sommerfeld et al. 2001), and people may consider themselves capable of diagnosing and treating malaria, and therefore prefer self-treatment to visiting public health facilities (Figure 2). This observation is worrying, and may have far-reaching implications for both policy and the future disease burden. In their study of perceived risk and vulnerability Sommerfeld et al. (2001) found that malaria ranked 10th in terms of being perceived as a threat, yet was the illness the community was most vulnerable to. People may not be able to diagnose and appropriately treat malaria. Studies elsewhere have shown that is the case; for example, only 20.1% of the mothers/guardians in Kibaha district of Tanzania knew the correct paediatric dose regime of CQ syrup, the most common medication (Nsimba et al. 1999). The policy concern is that communities need to be made aware of the risks of complicated malaria and the potential danger of inappropriate self-diagnosis and treatment.

Drugs make up about 90% of the total out-of-pocket expenditure for malaria and 84% for other illnesses, hence the likelihood of under dosing and consequent development of resistance is high (Shretta et al. 2000). One policy proposal would be to provide essential drugs free for those illnesses with the greatest burden, and to subsidize expenses for other treatment components for illnesses causing a lower burden.

Treatment choice and corresponding expenditure differences show that consistently more out-of-pocket expenditure was incurred in health facilities in comparison with self-treatment and traditional healers. About 98% of the respondents who cited lack of money as a reason for treatment choice chose either self-treatment or traditional healer. Other studies reveal a similar pattern, for example in Morocco, where those who visited public health facilities paid six times more than self-treaters (Hotchkiss & Gordillo 1999). The government could reduce the price of services, including drugs, to the level of other options, followed by mass information campaigns. The success of the Expanded Program on Immunization has largely depended on the availability of vaccines and awareness campaigns. The other option would be to make drugs for health conditions with the highest burden freely available.

A small proportion chose traditional healers, who are part of most communities in Africa, and whose role is likely to increase as economic conditions worsen. Arguably they can only treat a small portion of the illnesses in question successfully. It is not clear whether surveys capture all visits to traditional healers. Health policy should recognize and aim to integrate them in strategies to improve the health of the population.

Most households borrow to offset the out-of-pocket expenditure burden. This is in line with the theory that it is better to borrow than to liquidate ones assets as assets lose value when you are in need. Sauerborn (1994) found that 'loans were perceived as buffers between the time of need for cash and the time when households saw a possibility of paying back. Selling an animal under pressure would lead to a bad price. So it was more advantageous, even for the wealthy, to take a loan and take some time to sell the necessary number of animals at a time when prices would be favourable. The same was true for cereal crops'. However, as more out-of-pocket expenditure is incurred, it becomes increasingly difficult to secure a loan and people may have to resort to accepting a poor price.

Differential resource allocation within households has been reported in a number of studies (Chen et al. 1981) and these have largely shaped policy development and targeting of intervention policies (Sen 1984; Das Gupta 1987; Haddad & Reardon 1993). These studies have mainly investigated gender and age in allocation of resources, termed as gender and age bias, respectively. The results show that males are allocated considerably higher out-of-pocket expenditure on health than females while seeking treatment in the health facilities. This contrasts with studies in western Africa (Haddad & Reardon 1993) which did not find any gender difference but conforms to studies conducted in South Asia (Chen et al. 1981; Sen 1984; Das Gupta 1987) which found discrimination against females. A possible explanation is that the methods used in the analysis in the two studies referred to in West Africa could not detect the gender bias. Haddad used stratified outlay equivalent analysis on the International Food Policy Research Institute (IFPRI) data set in Burkina Faso, and could not find any differences in expenditure between boys and girls. Sauerborn et al. (1996) used analysis of variance and found that although the average health care expenditures for sick women was half that of sick men (480 CFA vs. 1160 CFA), the difference was not significant (P 0.06). In both cases above, one would suspect that there was no optimal use of the available data. In this paper, we attempted to make the best use of all available data by Tobit analysis, and did not find gender bias in out-of-pocket expenditure on health care, either.

As expected, age is statistically significant (Caldwell et al. 1983), but only for health facility treatment, not self-treatment (Sauerborn et al. 1996). Caldwell et al. found under representation of the young and old among patients, which they attribute to parent perceptions of childhood illnesses. Sauerborn *et al.* report differential health expenditure biased towards 11–59 year-olds based on case studies in age groups of 0–10, 11–59, and 60+ years.

Conclusion

Households will spend as little as possible on malaria because they feel confident to treat it themselves. Hence policies aimed at fighting the spread of malaria need to focus on at least three issues: educating population on the risks associated with malaria complications and the associated risk of inappropriate diagnosis and treatment; pricing of drugs and services to create an incentive to use the health services; and building alliances between households, traditional healers and medical health workers.

Acknowledgements

We thank Dong Hengjin of the Department of Tropical Hygiene and Public Health, Germany, Chutima Suraratdecha of International Health Policy Programme, Health Systems Research Institute, Thailand, and Hsu Ke of the Global Program on Evidence for Health Policy, World Health Organization, for their constructive comments on earlier drafts.

References

Acharya S, Carrin G & Herrin A (1993) *The Macroeconomy and Health Sector Financing in Nepal: a Medium-Term Perspective.* Macroeconomics, Health and Development Series No. 11. WHO, Geneva.

Caldwell JC, Reddy PH & Caldwell P (1983) The social component of mortality decline: an investigation in South India employing alternative methodologies. *Population Studies* 37, 185–206.

Chen L, Huq E & D'Souza S (1981) Sex bias in family allocation of health care in Bangladesh. *Population and Development Review* 7, 55–70.

Coreil J (1983) Allocation of family resources for health care in rural Haiti. *Social Science and Medicine* 17, 709–719.

Das Gupta M (1987) Selective discrimination against female children in rural Punjab, India. *Population and Development Review* 13, 77–100.

Diop F, Yazbeck A & Bitran R (1995) The impact of alternative cost recovery schemes on access and equity in Niger. *Health Policy and Planning* 10, 223–240.

Ebisawa I, Muto T, Tani S & Watanabe M (1980) Factors contributing to the prognosis of falciparum malaria. *Japanese Journal of E perimental Medicine* 50, 117–122.

Fabricant SJ, Kamara CW & Mills A (1999) Why the poor pay more: household curative expenditures in rural Sierra Leone. *International Journal of Health Planning and Management* 14, 179–199.

Foster SD (1991) Pricing, distribution, and use of antimalarial drugs. *Bulletin of the World Health Organization* 69, 349–363.

Haddad L & Reardon T (1993) Gender bias in the allocation of resources within the household in Burkina Faso: a disaggregated outlay equivalent analysis. *Journal of Development Studies* 29, 260–276.

Hotchkiss DR & Gordillo A (1999) Household health expenditures in Morocco: implications for health care reform. *International Journal of Health Planning and Management* 14, 201–217.

Kakkilaya BS (2001) *Malaria.* http://www.rationalmedicine.org/malaria.htm.

Kikonyogo N (2001) New malaria crisis in Rakai – scrapping of cost sharing had affected the hospital's plans for drug purchases. *The New Vision*, 8 October 2001, Kampala.

Levy PS & Lemeshow S (1999) *Sampling of Populations.* Wiley, New York.

Litvack JI & Bodart C (1993) User fees plus quality equals improved access to health care: results of a field experiment in Cameroon. *Social Science and Medicine* 37, 369–383.

Murray CJ & Lopez A (1996) *The Global Burden of Disease: a Comprehensive Assessment of Mortality and Disability from Diseases, Injuries, and Risk Factors in 1990 and Projected to 2020.* Havard School of Public Health, Boston, MA.

Nsimba S, Warsame M, Massele A & Mbatiya Z (1999) A household survey of source, availability, and use of antimalarials in a rural area of Tanzania. *Drug Information Journal* 33, 1025–1032.

Pannarunothai S & Mills A (1997) The poor pay more: health-related inequality in Thailand. *Social Science and Medicine* 44, 1781–1790.

Sauerborn R (1994) *Household Strategies to Cope with the Economic Cost of Illness: a Community Based Study in Burkina Faso.* Harvard School of Public Health, Boston, MA.

Sauerborn R, Nougtara A & Latimer E (1994) The elasticity of demand for health care in Burkina Faso: differences across age and income groups. *Health Policy and Planning* 9, 185–192.

Sauerborn R, Berman P & Nougtara A (1996) Age bias, but no gender bias, in the intra-household resource allocation for health care in rural Burkina Faso. *Health in Transition Reviews* 6, 131–145.

Scott Long J (1997) *Regression Models for Categorical and Limited Dependent Variables.* Sage Publications, Thousand Oaks, CA.

Sen AK (1984) Family and food: sex bias in poverty. In: *Resources, Values, and Development* (ed. AK Sen). Harvard University Press, Cambridge, MA.

Sen B (1997) *Health and Poverty in the Conte t of Country Development Strategy: a Case Study on Bangladesh.* Macroeconomics, Health and Development Series No. 26. WHO, Geneva.

Shretta R, Omumbo J, Rapuoda B & Snow RW (2000) Using evidence to change antimalarial drug policy in Kenya. *Tropical Medicine and International Health* 5, 755–764.

Sommerfeld J, Sanou M, Kouyate B & Sauerborn R (2001) Perceptions of risk, vulnerability and disease prevention in

Rural Burkina Faso: implications for community-based health care and insurance. *Journal of Human Organization* (in press).

US Congress (2000) *Making Appropriations for Foreign Operations, E port Financing, and Related Programs for the Fiscal ear Ending September 0, 2001 and for Other Purposes.* H.R. 4811, Washington.

Wendo C (2001) Government scraps cost-sharing. *The New Vision*, 18 February 2001.

WHO (1988) *Guidelines for Implementing the Bamako Initiative.* AFR/Rc38/Rev. 1. 1988. Regional Committee for Africa. Thirty-eighth Session, Brazzaville, 7–14 September.

Würtwein R, Gbangou A, Sauerborn R & Schmidt M (2000) *Measuring the Local Burden of Disease: a Study of ears of Life Lost in Rural Burkina Faso.* SFB Discussion Series, Berlin.

Zoguereh DD & Delmont J (2000) Antimalarial drugs and their directions for use in the African environment. *Sante* 10, 425–433.

4.4 Perceived quality of care of primary health care services in Burkina Faso

BALTUSSEN RM, YE Y, HADDAD S, SAUERBORN R.

Health Policy Plan. 2002; 17(1):42-8

Reprinted with permission from Oxford University Press.

Perceived quality of care of primary health care services in Burkina Faso

RMPM BALTUSSEN,[1,2] Y YÉ,[2] S HADDAD[3] AND RS SAUERBORN[1]

[1]Department of Tropical Hygiene and Public Health, Heidelberg, Germany, [2]Centre de Recherche en Santé de Nouna, Burkina Faso and [3]Groupe de Recherche Interdisciplinaire en Santé, Université de Montréal, Canada

Introduction: Patients' views are being given more and more importance in policy-making. Understanding populations' perceptions of quality of care is critical to developing measures to increase the utilization of primary health care services.
Objective: Documentation of user's opinion on the quality of care of primary health care services.
Methods: A 20-item scale, including four sub-scales related to health personnel practices and conduct, adequacy of resources and services, health care delivery, and financial and physical accessibility, was administered to 1081 users of 11 health care centres in the health district of Nouna, in rural Burkina Faso.
Results: The respondents were relatively positive on items related to health personnel practices and conduct and to health care delivery, but less so on items related to adequacy of resources and services and to financial and physical accessibility. In particular, the availability of drugs for all diseases on the spot, the adequacy of rooms and equipment in the facilities, the costs of care and the access to credit were valued poorly. Overall, the urban hospital was rated poorer than the average rural health care centre. Analysis of variance showed that, overall, health system characteristics explain 29% of all variation of the responses.
Conclusion: Improving drug availability and financial accessibility to health services have been identified as the two main priorities for health policy action. Policy-makers should respect these patient preferences to deliver effective improvement of the quality of care as a potential means to increase utilization of health care.

Key words: quality of care, primary health care, consumer perception, measurement

Introduction

In the past decade, increasing attention has been paid to quality of care as a means to enhance the effectiveness of health care systems in developing countries. In many developing countries, various actions have been taken to look into quality of primary health care, through either research and development (recently Bojalil et al. 1998; Brugha and Zwi 1998; Haddad et al. 1998a, b; Hotchkiss 1998; Newman et al. 1998; Archibong 1999; Noorali et al. 1999) or full-blown quality assurance (QA) (Chase and Carr-Hill 1994; Palestine National Health Authority 1994; Whittaker et al. 1998; Tassara 1999).

Typically, a distinction is made between observed quality of care and perceived quality of care (Palmer et al. 1991). The former, focusing merely on structural and process measures, relates to professionally defined standards of care, and refers to whether health care services adhere to these standards. The latter relates to the views of patients, which are attracting more and more importance (Donabedian 1980; WHO 1990). Patients' perception of quality of care is critical to understand the relationship between quality of care and utilization of health services, and increasingly it is treated as an outcome of health care delivery (Ross et al. 1993; Susman 1994; Reerink and Sauerborn 1996). Experiences in Bangladesh (Andaleep 1999), China (Yip et al. 1998), Nepal (Lafond 1995), Sri Lanka (Akin and Hutchinson 1999) and Vietnam (Guldner and Rifkin 1993) provide growing evidence that the perceived quality of care of health care services has a strong impact on utilization patterns.

This paper reports on the measurement of perceived quality of care of primary health care services in the health district of Nouna, Burkina Faso. Previous qualitative research on perceived quality of care in the same district showed that consumers were not satisfied with the health care services offered (Nikièma-Heinmüller and Borchert 1998). Government services are only consulted by 19% of the population, others choose home treatment (52%), traditional healers (17%) or local village health workers (5%) (Sauerborn et al. 1995). This translates in a utilization of government services as low as 0.17 consultations per capita in 1997 (DRS Cantaloup 1997). Understanding patients' perceptions on the quality of care of government facilities may allow policy-makers to improve this quality of care, and hence increase the services' utilization (Parker and Knippenberg 1991; Bitran 1995; Hotchkiss 1998). The present research acts as a baseline measurement for a Quality Assurance project started in 2000 in the health district of Nouna.

The measurement of perceived quality of care is still in its infancy, and its measurement tools are often not well described and/or validated (Bryce et al. 1992; Maynard-Tucker 1994; Newman et al. 1998), with a few exceptions. Recently, Andaleep (2001) has studied several dimensions of perceived quality of care in Bangladesh including responsiveness, assurance, communication, discipline and *baksheesh (*unofficial payments). He argues, arbitrarily, that these factors have a relatively greater influence on individuals' decisions regarding utilization compared with access and costs. Haddad et al. (1998b) developed and validated a scale in Guinea. This paper applies this instrument, adjusted for the specific context of Burkina Faso, and covers individual perceptions on health personnel practices and conduct, adequacy of resources and services, health care delivery, and financial and physical accessibility of care. This comprehensive approach allows us to assess the relative importance of determinants of quality of care that affect utilization patterns.

The aim of this paper is to inform policy-makers about the strengths and weaknesses of the quality of government primary health care services, as perceived by users, which can help define starting points to improve quality of care. Moreover, the present paper aims to contribute to the further development of an analytical framework for the measurement of perceived quality of care.

Methods

The study population

Data were collected on 1081 visitors of one urban hospital and 10 rural health care centres in the district of Nouna, in north-west Burkina Faso. The rural health centres provide basic outpatient services and include a dispensary and maternity unit staffed by a certified nurse and a trained midwife. The urban district hospital, with some 100 beds with surgical facilities, is the first referral level for the rural health centres and has a physician on staff. Visitors to the health facilities were approached as they left the facilities evaluated. They were included in the study, and an appointment was made for an interview at home, if their reason for the visit included a consultation with the staff. During the interview, a questionnaire was administered to the patients themselves or, in the case of children younger than 15 years, to the accompanying adult. The response rate to the interview questions was 96%. In addition to the items dealing with quality, the questionnaire included questions on respondents' socio-demographic characteristics. The majority of the respondents were female (57%), and 82% of the respondents were uneducated. The average age was 34 years.

Questionnaire

The instrument for quality assessment was based on an instrument developed and validated earlier for documenting quality of care in Guinea (Haddad et al. 1998b). The results of an exploratory study in Nouna district in Burkina Faso were used to assess whether the same items, as selected in the Guinea study, were also relevant for Burkina Faso

Table 1. Results of factor analysis[a]

Items	Factors				Communalities after extraction
	1	2	3	4	
Health personnel practices and conduct					
Compassion, support for patients	**0.76**	−0.02	−0.01	0.03	0.63
Respect for patients	**0.75**	0.05	−0.10	−0.01	0.62
Reception of patients	**0.75**	−0.07	−0.01	0.07	0.51
Honesty	**0.67**	0.10	−0.06	0.02	0.36
Follow up	**0.67**	−0.04	0.15	−0.05	0.44
Good clinical examination	**0.61**	0.11	0.20	−0.08	0.50
Adequacy of resources and services					
Adequacy of medical equipment	−0.03	**0.83**	0.06	−0.02	0.49
Adequacy of rooms	0.09	**0.76**	0.10	−0.15	0.57
Adequacy of doctors for women	−0.08	**0.68**	0.05	0.11	0.58
Number of good doctors	0.00	**0.68**	−0.02	0.13	0.56
Availability of drugs for all diseases on the spot	0.19	**0.46**	−0.11	0.14	0.49
Health care delivery					
Good diagnosis	0.01	0.09	**0.78**	−0.04	0.26
Prescription of drugs by doctors	0.00	0.12	**0.77**	−0.04	0.58
Quality of drugs	0.10	−0.10	**0.47**	0.34	0.63
Recovery, cure	0.21	−0.04	**0.32**	0.31	0.17
Financial and physical accessibility of care					
Payment arrangements	0.07	0.13	−0.09	**0.73**	0.53
Adequacy of costs	0.16	0.05	−0.11	**0.70**	0.51
Ease of obtaining drugs	0.02	−0.04	0.22	**0.64**	0.69
Distance	−0.11	0.06	0.02	**0.41**	0.60
Allowing sufficient time for patients	0.27	0.08	−0.01	**0.31**	0.36
% of variance explained by the factor after rotation	29%	9%	7%	6%	

[a] Principal component analysis with four factor extraction. Factor coefficients after oblimin with kaiser normalization.

Table 2. Description and reliability analysis of subscales and total score

	Subscale				
	Health personnel practices and conduct	Adequacy of resources and services	Health care delivery	Financial and physical accessibility	Perceived quality (total score)
No. of items	6	5	4	5	20
Possible range	−12 to +12	−10 to +10	−8 to +8	−10 to +10	−40 to +40
Mean	6.43	0.37	4.23	1.64	12.80
Median	7	1	4	2	13
Standard deviation	3.13	3.91	1.88	3.27	9.20
Cronbach's alpha	0.78	0.79	0.55	0.62	0.86

(Nikièma-Heinmuller and Borchert 1998). This study consisted of 20 focus groups in five villages, and aimed to identify the criteria lay people use to judge quality of care. The exercise resulted in a selection of a large number of items that were found to be important determinants of quality of care. There was a complete overlap with the pool of 20 items as defined by Haddad et al. Regrouping led to a questionnaire including 23 items.

The items were translated into the four main local languages (Bwamou, Djoula, Marka, Mooré) using the method of back-translation. It was then pre-tested on 25 people to allow for adjustment of wording. For each question, respondents could express one of five opinions: very unfavourable (−2), unfavourable (−1), neutral (0), favourable (+1) and very favourable (+2). The respondents were asked to express their opinion about the services in general, not on the one specific consultation after which they were approached by the research team. An unweighted aggregation procedure was used to calculate summary scores.

Results

Scale properties

On the basis of item analysis, 20 items were selected (Table 1). Factor analysis, to break down the items into homogeneous sub-scales, resulted in an item grouping which is coherent with the quality dimensions as proposed by various authors such as Donabedian (1980). Consequently this grouping has been used for the definition of four sub-scales (Table 1). The first sub-scale consists of six items related to the practices and conduct of the health personnel: patient follow-up, clinical examination, the reception of the patient, compassion, respect, time spent, and honesty of the staff. The second sub-scale includes five items related to the adequacy of resources and services in the facility, i.e. adequacy of the number of doctors, adequacy of doctors for women's treatment, adequacy of equipment, adequacy of rooms and availability of drugs. The third sub-scale includes four items including measures of health care delivery, i.e. prescription, quality of drugs, diagnosis and care outcomes. The fourth sub-scale includes five items related to the financial and physical accessibility of health care, i.e. the adequacy of fees, the possibility of making special payment arrangements, distance, the ease of obtaining drugs and the time devoted by the doctor.[1]

The results show that the respondents were favourable regarding the dimensions, 'health personnel practices and conduct' and 'health care delivery', but less so regarding 'adequacy of resources and services' and 'financial and physical accessibility'. The total score and the scores for three out of four sub-scales show mean scores that are larger than the median scores, indicating a skewed distribution which is often the case in studies on people's satisfaction or perceptions on the quality of care (Haddad et al. 1998b) (Table 2). The reliability of the scores, as indicated by the Cronbach's alpha values, ranges from 0.55 for the sub-scale health care delivery, to 0.86 for the total score. Modest reliability scores for the sub-scales health care delivery and accessibility can be explained by the limited number of items and the relative heterogeneous character of this sub-scale, and is not uncommon in opinion interviews (Haddad et al. 1998b).

Subgroup analysis

The impact of individual and system characteristics on the various scores are presented in Table 3. The results show that health personnel practices and conduct are perceived as poorer by relatively young people and those with at least primary education; the perceived adequacy of resources and services is judged poorer by relatively old people, females, those with at least primary education, and by those who live where the centre is located. Males and those with at least primary education rated health care delivery lower; respondents who live in another village than where the centre is located and with at least primary education rated financial and physical accessibility lower. Overall, the quality was judged lower by those with at least primary education.

Perceived quality of the health centres

To determine which centres differ in terms of perceived quality of care, we performed post-hoc tests, using a procedure (Tukey's honestly significant difference test) that allows for adjustment of the observed significance level for multiple comparisons. For the total score as well as for the

Table 3. Factors related to perceived quality: multivariate response model[a]

Independent variable	Dependent variable (scale)											
	Health personnel practices and conduct			Adequacy of resources and services			Health care delivery			Financial and physical accessibility			Perceived quality (total score)		
	B[b]	95%	CI	B	95%	CI	B	95%	CI	B	95%	CI	B	95%	CI
Intercept	**4.86**[c]	4.11	5.62	**−1.04**	−1.90	−0.18	**4.10**	3.62	4.57	−0.62	−1.38	0.14	**7.30**	5.24	9.36
Age ≤ 25	**−0.73**	−1.14	−0.32	**0.68**	0.21	1.15	−0.04	−0.30	0.22	0.21	−0.21	0.62	0.11	−1.02	1.24
Woman	0.05	−0.34	0.43	**−0.46**	−0.90	−0.02	**0.22**	−0.02	0.46	−0.26	−0.65	0.12	−0.46	−1.51	0.60
No education	**0.58**	0.10	1.05	**1.09**	0.54	1.63	**0.36**	0.06	0.66	**0.62**	0.13	1.10	**2.64**	1.33	3.95
Live where the centre is located	0.02	−0.36	0.40	**−0.54**	−0.98	−0.11	0.15	−0.09	0.38	**1.28**	0.90	1.66	0.90	−0.14	1.94
Centre (Ref = Urban hospital)															
Rural health centre #1															
#2	**1.99**	1.16	2.81	**4.80**	3.86	5.74	**0.61**	0.09	1.12	**3.57**	2.74	4.41	**10.97**	8.71	13.22
#3	**1.59**	0.78	2.40	**−0.98**	−1.90	−0.06	**−0.75**	−1.26	−0.24	**−1.27**	−2.08	−0.45	−1.41	−3.62	0.81
#4	**1.82**	0.99	2.64	**1.13**	0.19	2.07	−0.24	−0.76	0.28	**1.18**	0.34	2.01	**3.88**	1.62	6.15
#5	**2.75**	1.96	3.54	**3.60**	2.70	4.50	**0.85**	0.35	1.34	**4.50**	3.71	5.30	**11.71**	9.55	13.86
#6	**2.08**	1.28	2.88	**2.28**	1.37	3.19	−0.14	−0.64	0.36	0.21	−0.60	1.02	**4.43**	2.24	6.62
#7	0.35	−0.49	1.19	0.22	−0.73	1.18	**−1.08**	−1.61	−0.55	**2.21**	1.37	3.06	1.71	−0.59	4.01
#8	0.75	−0.13	1.63	**−2.06**	−3.06	−1.06	**−0.97**	−1.53	−0.42	0.44	−0.45	1.33	**−1.84**	−4.25	0.56
#9	−0.50	−1.22	0.23	**−1.87**	−2.70	−1.05	**−0.73**	−1.18	−0.27	0.53	−0.20	1.26	**−2.57**	−4.55	−0.58
#10	**4.19**	3.38	5.00	**2.19**	1.27	3.11	−0.06	−0.56	0.45	**1.08**	0.26	1.89	**7.40**	5.19	9.61
	−0.32	−1.19	0.55	0.49	−0.50	1.49	**−0.88**	−1.42	−0.33	0.52	−0.37	1.40	−0.19	−2.58	2.20
Variance explained (R^2)	21.9%			33.4%			11.4%			25.9%			30.6%		
Eta^2 (health centres)	20.0%			30.4%			10.6%			23.6%			29.1%		

[a] The associations were studied using multivariate response models which allow the simultaneous inclusion of various dependent variables in regression analyses, and improves the quality of estimators.
[b] The B values given have a direct interpretation: e.g. −0.73 for age ≤25 years on Health Personnel Practices & Conduct means that the younger patients give a score 0.73 lower than other patients, after adjusting for other variables such as gender, educational status, place of residence, and centre.
[c] Values printed in bold are significant at $p < 0.05$.

Perceived quality of care in Burkina Faso

four sub-scales, the perceptions on the quality of care often differ significantly between one health centre and the others (Table 3). In other words, the measures of perceived quality discriminate strongly between the different health centres.

The adjusted R^2 value, representing the percentage of variance explained by the various models, is larger than 20% for four of the five models. The health centres explain much of this variance.[2] This indicates, *in our model*, a high impact of health care system characteristics on the valuation of quality of care, relative to that of socio-demographic characteristics.

Discussion

This paper examines the quality of care of primary health care facilities in a rural region of Burkina Faso. There is a tendency for respondents to respond favourably to questions, as is systematically noted in research on perceived quality or satisfaction (Bitran 1995; Wouters 1995; Haddad et al. 1998b; Newman et al. 1998). This implies that results should be interpreted carefully and in a relative rather than an absolute sense. Despite this tendency, respondents' opinions are not very favourable in this study, as has also been shown by other studies in the same region (Nikièma-Heinmüller and Borchert 1998).

Respondents in various health centres (including the urban hospital) were relatively negative on items related to health personnel practices and conduct. The behaviour of health personnel has also been found to depress patient satisfaction in other studies (Abu-Zaid and Dan 1985; Waddington and Enyimayew 1989, 1990; Bichman et al. 1991; Haddad et al. 1995). The problem, however, rarely receives attention by health planners who seem to focus more on the technical aspects of quality (Bichman et al. 1991; Jarrett and Ofusu-Amaah 1992; Haddad and Fournier 1995). Consequently, the importance of interpersonal skills has been largely overlooked, an important quality aspect which in certain settings had been found to be mutually reinforcing the technical quality component (Gilson et al. 1994). Improving the attitudes of health personnel towards patients seems, therefore, a promising way to enhance perceived quality of care. The overall positive attitude of the respondents to health care delivery seems to conflict with earlier research in the same district which has shown inadequate physical examination, diagnosis and prescription by personnel (Krause et al. 1998a, b, 1999). Patients appear not to notice poor compliance rates with respect to these issues (Bitran 1995; Wouters 1995).

The quality of 'adequacy of resources and services' was valued as relatively poor. Respondents especially criticized the absence of drugs for all diseases on the spot. Many studies have shown that drug supply is a very important determinant of the utilization of health services (Abu-Zaid and Dann 1985; Waddington and Eniymayew 1989, 1990; Parker and Knippenberg 1991; Litvack and Bodart 1993; Bitran 1995; Haddad and Fournier 1995). These findings suggest that appropriate drug policies are likely to be among the single most important policy actions that could improve quality of health care.

Respondents judged the financial and physical accessibility of care relatively poorly. In particular, the high costs of care and the lack of access to credit were factors that considerably hampered perceived quality of care. They are closely linked to the existing fee-for-service payment scheme, which has been introduced as part of the Bamako Initiative. The identification of 'financial and physical accessibility' as a distinct dimension of quality of care is an important asset of this study. This adds to earlier empirical (Haddad et al. 1998b) and theoretical (Donabedian 1980) work which relates quality of care to the traditional factors mentioned above, 'health personnel practices and conduct', 'adequacy of resources and services' and 'health care delivery'.

The findings of this study have demonstrated the feasibility of conducting a detailed assessment of indicators of perceived quality across a variety of health centres. Socio-demographic characteristics had only limited impact on the respondents' perceptions on quality of care: in all sub-scales and the total score, they contributed less than 10% to the explained variance. The study was able to detect some significant impacts of respondents' age, sex, educational status and place of residence on their perceptions, but these were relative small. Moreover, since the population is relatively homogeneous in terms of these variables (obviously except for age and sex), the overall impact of these variables is also small. The role of socio-demographic variable effects on people's satisfaction has been widely studied (Hall et al. 1987) and is still controversial (Haddad et al. 1992). This study has shown that the observed variation in the perceived quality of care is largely explained by health centres' variations: the health centre variable contributed always more than 90% to the explained variance. Overall, more than 30% of all variation in respondents' perceptions was explained by both socio-demographic and health system variables, a proportion which can be considered as satisfactory in social science research (Kennedy 1998). Adding more items to the measurement scale would increase its explanatory power but also decrease its practicality. Moreover, respondents seem to discriminate well between the various dimensions of quality of care. Also, it has demonstrated that the population makes sensitively different judgements on the different health centres. This means that, even when at first sight the responses are generally positive, they are at the same time sensitive and discriminative and therefore potentially very useful for quality evaluations (Ross-Davies and Ware 1988; Haddad et al. 1992).

The scale by Haddad et al. (1998b) appeared an appropriate instrument to assess patient perceptions on quality of care with precision, and can be usefully applied to acquire further understanding of quality of care in other countries too. In the case of Burkina Faso, improving drug availability and accessibility to health services have been identified as the two main priorities for health policy action. Policy-makers should respect these patient preferences to deliver effective improvement in the quality of care and thereby increase utilization of health care.

Endnotes

[1] With the exception of two items, all subscales show communalities higher than 0.30. More than half (50.5%) of the 20 items-space variance is explained by a four-factor extraction.

[2] This is indicated by the Eta^2, which is larger than 0.20 for four of the five models.

References

Abu-Zaid HA, Dann WM. 1985. Health services utilisation and cost in Ismailia, Egypt. *Social Science and Medicine* **15b**: 451–61.

Akin J, Hutchinson P. 1999. Health-care facility choice and the phenomenon of bypassing. *Health Policy and Planning* **14**: 135–51.

Andaleeb SS. 1999. Public and private hospitals in Bangladesh: service quality and predictors of hospital choice. *Health Policy and Planning* **14**: 135–51.

Andaleeb SS. 2001. Service quality perceptions and patient satisfaction: a study of hospitals in a developing country. *Social Science and Medicine* **52**: 1359–70.

Archibong UE. 1999 Evaluating the impact of primary nursing practice on the quality of nursing care: a Nigerian study. *Journal of Advances in Nursing* **29**: 680–9.

Bichman W, Diesfeld HJ, Aagboton Y, Gbaguidi EAC, Simhauser U. 1991. District health systems: users' preferences for services in Benin. *Health Policy and Planning* **6**: 361–70.

Bitran R. 1995. Efficiency and quality in the public and private sectors in Senegal. *Health Policy and Planning* **10**: 271–83.

Bojalil R, Guiscafre H, Espinosa P et al. 1998. The quality of private and public primary health care management of children with diarrhoea and acute respiratory infections in Tlaxcala, Mexico. *Health Policy and Planning* **13**: 323–31.

Bryce J, Toole MJ, Waldman RJ, Voigt A. 1992. Assessing the quality of facility-based child survival services. *Health Policy and Planning* **7**: 155–63.

Chase E, Carr-Hill R. 1994. The dangers of managerial perversion: quality assurance in primary health care. *Health Policy and Planning* **9**: 267–78.

Donabedian A. 1980. *The definition of quality and approaches to its assessment.* Vol 1. Ann Arbor: Health Administration Press.

DRS Cantaloup. 1997. Burkina Faso: Ministry of Health.

Gilson L, Aliolio M, Heggenhougen K. 1994. Community satisfaction with primary health care services: an evaluation undertaken in the Morogoro region of Tanzania. *Social Science and Medicine* **39**: 767–80.

Guldner M, Rifkin S. 1993. *Sustainability in the health sector, Part 1: Vietnam case study.* London: Save the Children Fund.

Haddad S, Potvin L, Pineault R. 1992. Les études de satisfaction mesurent-elles des attributs des patients ou les caractéristiques des services qui leur sont fournis? (Do satisfaction studies measure attributes of patients or the characteristics of services provided?) In: Chytil MK, Duru G, Van Eimeren W, Flagle CD (eds). *Health Systems, the Challenge of Change.* Fifth International Conference on Health System Science, Prague, July 1992. Omnipress Publisher: pp. 1169–73.

Haddad S, Fournier P. 1995. Quality, costs and utilization of health services in developing countries. A longitudinal study in Zaire. *Social Science and Medicine* **40**: 743–53.

Haddad S, Fournier P, Machouf N, Yatara F. 1998a. What does quality mean to lay people? Community perceptions of primary health care services in Guinea. *Social Science and Medicine* **47**: 381–94.

Haddad S, Fournier P, Potvin L. 1998b. Measuring lay people's perceptions of the quality of primary health care services in developing countries. Validation of a 20-item scale. *International Journal for Quality in Health Care* **10**: 93–104.

Hall JA, Roter DL, Katz NR. 1987. Task vs. socio-emotional behaviours in physicians. *Medical Care* **25**: 399–412.

Hotchkiss DR. 1998. The trade-off between price and quality of services in the Philippines. *Social Science and Medicine* **46**: 227–42.

Jarret SW, Ofusu-Amaah S. 1992. Strengthening health services for MHC in Africa: the first four years of the 'Bamako Initiative'. *Health Policy and Planning* **7**: 164–72.

Kennedy P. 1988. *A guide to econometrics.* Cambridge: The MIT Press.

Krause G, Benzler J, Heinmuller R et al. 1998a. Performance of village pharmacies and patient compliance after implementation of an essential drug program in rural Burkina Faso, West Africa. *Health Policy and Planning* **13**: 159–66.

Krause G, Schleiermacher D, Borchert M et al. 1998b. Diagnostic quality in rural health centres in Burkina Faso. *Tropical Medicine and International Health* **3**: 962–74.

Krause G, Borchert M, Benzler J et al. 1999. Rationality of drug prescriptions in rural health centres in Burkina Faso, West Africa. *Health Policy and Planning* **14**: 288–91.

Lafond AK. 1995. Improving the quality of investment in health: Lessons on sustainability. *Health Policy and Planning* **10**: 63–76.

Litvack JL, Bodart C. 1993. User fees plus quality equals improved access to health care: results of a field experiment in Cameroon. *Social Science and Medicine* **37**: 369–83.

Maynard-Tucker G. 1994. Indigenous perceptions and quality of family planning in Haiti. *Health Policy and Planning* **10**: 306–17.

Newman RD, Gloyd S, Nyangezi JM, Machobo F, Muiser J. 1998. Satisfaction with outpatient health services in Manica Province, Mozambique. *Health Policy and Planning* **13**: 174–80.

Nikièma-Heinmüller B, Borchert M. 1998. Appréciation de la qualité des soins par la population dans un district sanitaire du milieu rural au Burkina Faso (Appraisal of the quality of care by the population in a rural health care district in Burkina Faso). Nouna, Burkina Faso: PRAPASS.

Noorali R, Luby S, Rahbar MH. 1999. Does use of a government service depend on distance from the health facility? *Health Policy and Planning* **14**: 191–7.

Palestine National Health Authority/Ministry of Health and Palestine Council of Health, Quality of Health Care Unit. 1994. *The strategic plan for quality for health care in Palestine.* Gaza City and Jerusalem: Ministry of Health.

Palmer RH, Donabedian A, Povar GJ. 1991. *Striving for quality in health care: an inquiry into policy and practice.* Washington, DC: Health Administration Press.

Parker D, Knippenberg R. 1991. *Community cost-sharing and participation: a review of the issues.* Bamako Initiative Technical Report Series 9. New York: UNICEF.

Reerink IH, Sauerborn R. 1996. Quality of care in primary health care settings in developing countries: recent experiences and future directions. *International Journal of Quality of Health Care* **8**: 131–9.

Ross-Davies A, Ware J. 1988. Involving consumers in quality of care assessment. *Health Affairs* **7**: 33–48.

Ross CK, Steward CA, Sinacore JM. 1993. The importance of patient preferences in the measurement of health care satisfaction. *Medical Care* **25**: 1138–49.

Sauerborn R, Ibrango I, Nougtara A et al. 1995. The economic costs of illness for rural households in Burkina Faso. *Tropical Medicine and Parasitology* **46**: 54–60.

Susman JL. 1994. Assessing consumer expectations and patient satisfaction. *Archives of Family Medicine* **3**: 945–6.

Tassara GG. 1999. Making a commitment to quality: development of the quality assurance programme in Chile, 1991–1999. *International Journal of Quality in Health Care* **11**: 443–5.

Waddington CJ, Enyimayew KA. 1990. A price to pay, part 2: the impact of user charges in the Volta region, Ghana. *International Journal of Health Planning and Management* **5**: 287–312.

Waddington CJ, Enyimayew KA. 1989. A price to pay: the impact of user charges in Ashanti-Akin district, Ghana. *International Journal of Health Planning and Management* **4**: 17–47.

Whittaker S, Burns D, Doyle V, Lynam PF. 1998. Introducing quality assurance to health service delivery–some approaches from South Africa, Ghana and Kenya. *International Journal of Quality in Health Care* **10**: 263–7.

WHO. 1990. *Measuring consumer satisfaction with health care*. Copenhagen: WHO Regional Office for Europe.

Wouters A. 1995. Improving quality through cost recovery in Niger. *Health Policy and Planning* **10**: 257–70.

Yip W, Wang H, Liu Y. 1998. Determinants of patient choice of medical provider: a case study in rural China. *Health Policy and Planning* **13**: 311–22.

Biographies

Rob Baltussen is an economist and has a Ph.D. in Health Economics from Maastricht University (The Netherlands). At the time of the study, he had an appointment as associate researcher at the Department of Tropical Hygiene and Public Health of the University of Heidelberg, and was based at the Centre de Recherche en Santé de Nouna in Burkina Faso. Currently, he works at the Global Programme on Evidence for Health Policy (GPE) of the World Health Organization in Geneva, Switzerland. His research interests include cost-effectiveness analysis, the measurement of disability weights for the calculation of DALYs, and the quality of primary health care services.

Yazoumé Yé is a geographer by training and works as associate researcher/database manager at the Centre de Recherche en Santé de Nouna in Burkina Faso. His current work includes the development of a demographic database in Burkina Faso and the institutionalization of demographic surveillance in Africa. His research interests are in the field of quality of care, in which he also worked as a consultant at e.g. WHO.

Slim Haddad, MD, Ph.D. is Associate Professor at the Department of Health Administration, University of Montreal. His research interests are in the areas of health policies evaluation (reform and financing of health care systems, effects of structural adjustment reforms), the determinants of the utilization of health care services (notably, financial accessibility, prices, and quality of services) and the evaluation of the quality of health care services (provider and lay people's perspectives).

Rainer Sauerborn, MD, Ph.D., is a paediatrician by training. He received his doctoral degree in public health from Harvard University. Since 1996 he has had the chair of Tropical Hygiene and Public Health at the University of Heidelberg, Germany. His research interests include the evaluation of measures to improve the quality of care, community-based insurance and the economic evaluation of public health interventions delivered at the community level.

Correspondence: RMPM Baltussen, Global Programme on Evidence for Health Policy, World Health Organization, CH-1211 Geneva 27, Switzerland. Email: baltussenr@who.int

4.5 Informal risk-sharing arrangements (IRSAs) in rural Burkina Faso: lessons for the development of community-based insurance (CBI)

SOMMERFELD J, SANON M, KOUYATE B, SAUERBORN R

Int. J Health Plann Mgmt 2002; 17: 147-63

Reprinted with permission from John Wiley & Sons Ltd.

Informal risk-sharing arrangements (IRSAs) in rural Burkina Faso: lessons for the development of community-based insurance (CBI)

Johannes Sommerfeld[1], Mamadou Sanon[2], Bocar A. Kouyate[2] and Rainer Sauerborn[1]*

[1]*Ruprecht-Karls University of Heidelberg, Medical Faculty, Department of Tropical Hygiene and Public Health (ATHOEG), Heidelberg, Germany*
[2]*Centre de Recherche en Santé de Nouna (CRSN), Nouna, Burkina Faso*

SUMMARY

In resource-poor environments, community-based insurance (CBI) is increasingly being propagated as a strategy to improve access of poor rural populations to modern health care. It has been repeatedly hypothesized that CBI schemes need to be grounded in national as well as local traditions of solidarity. This paper presents a typology of informal risk sharing arrangements (IRSAs) in a rural area of North-Western Burkina Faso and discusses their *modus operandi* as well as the underlying concepts of solidarity and reciprocity. The research was explicitly multi-disciplinary, combining anthropological and economic as well as qualitative and quantitative data collection methods. Focus group and interview data were complemented by a census of existing IRSAs. In addition to presenting the main features of existing institutions, the paper discusses whether IRSAs can serve as entry points for CBI schemes. In spite of the fact that existing IRSAs fulfil important solidarity functions in the rural Burkinian context, we conclude that they cannot serve as institutional models for more formalized CBI schemes. Community participation in a future CBI scheme will need to tap into existing notions of solidarity and mutuality. The CBI scheme itself, however, needs to be newly tailored. Copyright © 2002 John Wiley & Sons, Ltd.

KEY WORDS: community-based insurance (CBI); risk sharing; solidarity; reciprocity; Burkina Faso

INTRODUCTION

In recent years, community-based health insurance (CBI) has been propagated as an option to extend access to health care of poor rural populations in countries lacking

---

*Correspondence to: Professor R. Sauerborn, Department of Tropical Hygiene and Public Health, Ruprecht-Karls University of Heidelberg, Im Neuenheimer Feld 324, 69121 Heidelberg, Germany. E-mail: rainer.sauerborn@urz.uni-heidelberg.de

Contract/grant sponsor: German Association for Scientific Research.

Copyright © 2002 John Wiley & Sons, Ltd.

formal insurance markets (Aldermann and Parson, 1992; Atim, 1998 and 1999; Bennett *et al.*, 1998; Criel, 1998; Dror and Jacquier, 1999). In contemporary Burkina Faso, a landlocked country in the West African Sahel, low access to health care is a serious impediment to the effectiveness of modern health care intervention (Krause and Sauerborn, 2000; Barlow and Diop, 1995). In Kossi Province, the site of the present study, there are only 0.3 visits per capita and per year to modern health services. The financial costs involved in seeking such care and their timing at the time of need have been identified as major factors contributing to low access (Sauerborn *et al.*, 1994, 1996a).

The formal sector of the Burkinan economy comprises only 5% of the population. Social insurance for the formal sector has been limited until now to government employees, company employees and a few families living in relative economic prosperity. Some mutual health organizations, with varying success, have recently emerged (Fonteneau, 1999) without, however, providing coverage to a significant proportion of the rural population.

Households in Burkina Faso spend 6.4% of their annual expenditure on health care (Sauerborn *et al.*, 1994). The average household expenditure involved with an outpatient consultation at the local dispensary is 1432 FCFA (Sauerborn *et al.*, 1996a). The percentage of the sick seeking care in formal health services is 17.5%, while 15.4% see a traditional healer and 4.6% a local community health worker. There are very few private sector providers and these are located in the district town of Nouna. The largest share of illness episodes is treated at home (Sauerborn *et al.*, 1996b).

Fee-for-service payment is still the predominant mode of health care financing of a large majority of the population in the non-formal sectors of the economy. The Burkinian Ministry of Health has opted to follow the Bamako Initiative, with the introduction of user fees. In the study area, user fees lead to a decrease in the utilization of formal health services: the percentage of those who reported an illness episode in the preceding month and sought care at the formal health facilities dropped from 25.6% in 1993 (before the introduction of fees) to 18.7% in 1994 and 11.7% in 1995.

Burkina Faso's Ministry of Health has recently called for promoting solidarity-based modes of health care financing to increase the financial accessibility of health services in order to overcome the limitations of the existing system (Burkina Faso, 2000). The objective was to increase access to services and not to generate resources for the government, since funds would be retained and managed at the community or district levels. In June 1999, a national seminar was held to foster the creation of mutual health organizations in Burkina Faso (Concertation, 2000).

Social insurance schemes, regardless of their design, reflect the history and cultural notions of solidarity and reciprocity norms of societies in which they develop (Normand and Weber, 1994). A crucial question, therefore, is whether an insurance scheme developed in one society can be applied in another. In other words the question remains whether CBI schemes are socially and culturally feasible, tapping into established notions of solidarity and reciprocity, and adapted to informal sector economies in rural Africa (Sanou, 2000).

There is now an increasing awareness that CBI schemes need to be grounded in national values of solidarity and reciprocity (Criel *et al.*, 1998; Criel, 1998; Vuarin, 1996). One of the underlying questions is whether CBI schemes can be built upon existing risk sharing arrangements and notions of solidarity. Solidarity is a common feature of 'traditional' rural communities, who have always shared the economic risks of unpredictable and cost-intensive life-events, such as deaths, accidents and weddings (Creese and Bennett, 1997).

In rural economies of the developing world, voluntary arrangement of transactions based on long term mutual reciprocity, e.g. gifts, favours, work assistance, charity, etc, have, for a long time, been described by anthropologists and economists alike. These informal transactions have in many areas been replaced or complemented by semi-modern formal institutions such as credit cooperatives, Rotating Savings and Credit Associations (ROSCAs) and informal credit and insurance arrangements (Besley, 1995; Coate and Ravallion, 1993).

A considerable body of literature, both from anthropology and economics has shown that informal risk-sharing arrangements (IRSAs) are still very frequent in developing countries (Elwert, 1980; Fafchamps and Lund, 1999; Fafchamps, 1999a,b; Platteau, 1991; Platteau, 1997). A number of authors, however, have argued that traditional risk sharing institutions are in the process of demise in the process of individualization and formalization of transactions, as a result of increasing monetarization (Zimmerman and Carter, 1999; Reardon *et al.*, 1989). In addition, the modern concept of insurance is said to be mis- or non-understood in so-called traditional societies where, as Platteau (1997) has argued, solidarity is based on notions of balanced rather than conditional reciprocity.

The present study was carried out in 1998–2000 in Kossi Province, in the North-Western part of Burkina Faso, as an integral part of a larger research project entitled 'The Scientific Basis of Community-Based Insurance,' conducted conjointly by the Nouna Center for Health Research (CRSN) and the Department of Tropical Hygiene and Public Health (ATHOEG) of Heidelberg University. The research intended to assess the scope and prevalence of existing IRSAs in rural Burkina Faso and to evaluate their potential role in CBI. The research was explicitly multi-disciplinary, bringing together the qualitative ethnographic interest of anthropology and the more quantifying research paradigm of economics.

RESEARCH CONTEXT

IRSAs in West Africa and Burkina Faso

Informal or 'traditional' risk sharing institutions and solidarity mechanisms in West Africa have, for a long time, attracted the curiosity of anthropologists and economists. Rural economies in West Africa have established a number of social and economic mechanisms in order to cope with the financial consequences of economic random shocks (e.g. Fiske, 1990; Nguyen, 1998; Elwert, 1980). A great number of traditional solidarity networks can be identified from the literature, e.g. clan relationships, burial societies, cooperative labour exchange pools, cooperative work groups, fire associations, sea rescue associations, special fund societies, Rotating

Credit and Savings Associations (ROSCAs), beer societies, group borrowing schemes, credit cooperatives and regional associations (Were, 1999).

Research on Burkinian IRSAs needs to be contextualized in research on related social networks and structures. A number of investigators, from different disciplines, have, for example, shown the adaptability of informal, 'traditional' structures in Burkina Faso to social, economic and ecological change (Ahiadeke, 1996; Batterbury, 1994; Howorth and O'Keefe, 1999; Reardon and Matlon, 1989; Sakurai and Reardon, 1997). Not only is rural Burkina Faso strongly shaped by these institutions; solidarity is a crucial element of their *modus operandi* (Lédea Ouedraogo, 1990).

Burkinian households pursue informal and voluntary risk sharing strategies such as food and gift exchange, monetary as well as non-monetary credit (Fonteneau, 1999; Sakurai and Reardon, 1997). Ellsworth (1988), in a study of non-market exchanges among farmers in Burkina Faso, found that 28% to 33% of income is contributed to networks of family, friends and kin, i.e. personal insurance networks, whereas on average 24% of income is received from these networks. Ellsworth concludes that these transactions fulfil the function of an insurance as contributions appear to be non-random and benefits to be random. In the rural context of Burkina Faso, semi-modern institutions typically provide credit, mutual assistance and training, most commonly in the form of informal rotating savings and credit associations (ROSCAS), known in francophone West Africa as *tontines*.

As to the risks that are shared, such arrangements are set up to help members to cope with 'high risk/low probability' expenditures, such as for funerals or marriages as well as with 'low risk/high probability' expenditures, such as the purchase of agricultural equipment. Evidence suggests that informal credit, asset sales and gifts serve as insurance substitutes in agrarian economies such as the Burkinian (Eswaran and Kotwal, 1989; Kimball, 1988; Ellsworth, 1988). In rural Burkina Faso, economic *ex ante* risk strategies include the colonization of previously uninhabited savanna areas, traditional practices such as burning field vegetation and pastures to get rid of snakes and rodents. *Ex post* strategies among Burkinian farmers are documented as well. They include sales of livestock (poultry, dairy cattle, drought animals such as bullocks and pack animals such as donkeys) and other assets (hand plow, carts, or other farm tools and vehicles such as bicycles or mopeds). *Ex post* strategies further include precautionary non-monetary saving, i.e. stocking food crops such as millet or cash crops such as sesame or rice.

Mutual health institutions and insurance in Burkina Faso

Burkina Faso's mutual health movement is still in an embryonic stage (Fonteneau, 1999). Recently, a number of mutual health institutions have emerged, among them the *Mutuelle Laafi Tembo* in Ouagadougou, the *Mutuelle Laafi la Boumbou* de Guilla (Kaya), the *Mutuelle Boud Nooma de Sanrogho* (Kaya), the *Association Solidarité Santé* and the *Mutuelle Dakwena*, both in Bobo-Dioulasso. Supported by *World Solidarity* (WSM) and *Alliance Nationale des Mutualités Chrétiennes de Belgique* (ANMC), in 1998, a Burkinian branch of the Africa-wide support programme for mutual health institutions, the *Programme d'Appui aux Mutuelles de Santé en Afrique* (PROMUSAF/BF) has been established. In 2000, a Network of Mutual Health

Associations (*Reseau d'Appui aux Mutuelles de Santé*, RAMS) was created. A new formal law governing mutual health institutions is currently being conceived. This development has been strongly supported by the international donor community, e.g. ILO's ACOPAM programme and the American, Belgian and French development services.

Up until now, in Burkina Faso formal insurance institutions were limited to urban centres. In recent years, however, a number of commercial and state-owned insurance companies such as *FONCIAS,* the *Union des Assurances du Burkina* (UAB), the *Société Nationale d'Assurance et de Réassurance* (SONAR), the *Générale des Assurances and the COLINA* have emerged, offering life, health and vehicle insurance and reinsurance. In addition, social security insurance is provided to salaried and state employees (*salariés* and *fonctionnaires*) through the *Caisse Nationale de Sécurité Sociale* (CNSS) and the *Caisse Autonome de Retrait des Fonctionnaires* (CARFO).

METHODOLOGY

Study site

The research was focused on the research zone targeted by the CRSN for longitudinal health research, i.e. 40 villages spread out over a surface of 7154 square kilometers around the provincial capital of Nouna. The population is about 55 000, the age distribution of the population reflects the typical high mortality high fertility pattern of SubSaharan countries with 17.5% of the population under 5 years. The research zone is an area with five major ethnic groups now cohabitating in the area, i.e. the Bwaba (*Bobo Oulé*), the Moose (*Mossi*), the Marka (*Dafing*), the Samo and the Peulh (*Fulani*). Every group has its peculiar socioeconomic organization and its own language. Christianity coexists with Islam and traditional African belief systems. People use djoula as the *lingua franca* and language of commercial communication. Due to increasing population pressures within Burkina Faso, there is heavy migration into this still relatively sparsely populated region. In addition, there is widespread temporary out-migration of male adults into the neighbouring Côte d'Ivoire and national urban centres for agricultural as well as non-agricultural employment. As migrants are able to support their relatives and friends, these migration patterns play an important role for non-formal solidarity.

Agriculture and pastoralism are the main economic activities of the rural population. Sorghum, millet, maize and beans are the main crops for subsistence whereas cotton, sesame and peanuts are grown as cash crops. The season drives the agricultural calendar and household economics: the harvest time both for cash and food crops is in October/November, peak household income is in February, at which time household will be asked to pay their premiums (Sauerborn *et al.*, 1996b). In terms of health risks, infectious diseases dominate, with malaria and acute respiratory infections and diarrhoea being the biggest contributors to the local burden of disease (Würthwein *et al.*, 2001).

The provincial town of Nouna, the capital of the Kossi Province, is supplied by electricity and running water. Nouna is an important regional market place, and has a number of administrative services as well as a branch of a national bank. The research zone of the Nouna Health Research Centre (CRSN) comprises 40 villages and the provincial town of Nouna itself. In this zone, there is no formal insurance operating except a branch of CNSS serving some 400 salaried employees and their dependants throughout the Kossi Province. The population is served by four health centres and a medical centre in the town of Nouna. All health facilities are owned by the Ministry of Health and run by civil servants. There are virtually no private providers of Western-type care, except in the district capital. As a result of national efforts to decentralize the health sector, in 1994, administrative committees (*Comité de gestion*, COGES) were set up to ensure an efficient functioning of health institutions, and to promote community participation regarding health activities.

Methods

We surveyed a total of 40 communities. The mean population size of the communities was 883 (range 156–2909). Only two communities had a primary care health facility (CSPS); all others were at a distance of 2–27 km (mean 10.4 km) to the next primary care centre. Sixteen of the 40 (40.0%) had primary schools.

A variety of qualitative as well as quantitative research methods were employed. An initial exploratory phase involved document review, unstructured and semi-structured individual interviews as well as key informant interviews ($n = 25$) with members of the district health management team, representatives of local associations, community nurses, and local religious and political leaders to elucidate risk sharing practices in the traditional, non-formal system in the five ethnic groups living in the research zone. After the exploratory research phase, six villages and two semi-urban areas were purposively selected among the communities of the research zone to represent the socio-cultural and geographical diversity to the greatest extent possible. These villages show considerable heterogeneity in terms of ethnic composition, population size, proximity to roads and the provincial town of Nouna, and, to some degree, ecological and socio-economic situation. In these selected communities and in the town of Nouna, a total number of 37 focus group discussions were held using a pre-established set of core discussion topics and involving a wide spectrum of population segments in terms of age, gender and occupation. In order to avoid gender bias in data collection, we conducted group interviews with men and women separately. Also, we independently conducted group discussions with young and elderly people, farmers, cattle raisers, state employees and merchants. Most group interviews were tape recorded with the permission of the group participants and later transcribed and translated into French. Our textual data were analysed using ATLAS/ti 4.1. software (ATLAS/ti 1997).

Qualitative data analysis led to the development of a typology of informal and semi-formal risk sharing arrangements (IRSAs) in the area. The typology was integrated into an inventory which consequently was used by field research personnel of CRSN to assess the prevalence of risk sharing practices and institutions in the research zone.

RESULTS

A preliminary study of existing community-based risk sharing schemes in the project region (Fon, 1997) identified a variety of community-based institutions involved in risk-sharing. Forms of risk-sharing included credit saving funds, solidarity funds and rotating work assignments. Although none of these existing institutions constitutes by definition a health insurance scheme, assistance is provided to members through collective as well as individual donations, assisting hospitalized group members with loans for little or no interest.

Most of our focus group respondents were unaware of the existence of commercial insurance. Most scholarized individuals ('*intellectuels*') and many former and current migrants, however, had heard about car insurance, which is mandatory for vehicle owners in Burkina Faso. Such insurance was rarely fully understood in all its legal and procedural ramifications and considered highly profit-oriented. Only very few people expressed confidence in such a for-profit-enterprise.

Typology and frequency of existing informal risk sharing arrangements (IRSA)

Data from individual interviews and focus groups resulted in a preliminary list of existing informal and semi-formal institutions in the research zone. After intensive elucidation of their internal functioning we were able to group them into the following six different IRSA types. Data from the inventory on 'traditional' risk sharing schemes are summarized in Table 1.

Solidarity networks based on kinship, neighbourhood, ethnicity or profession

Individuals and groups of people linked by kinship or place of origin, by neighbourhood, ethnic group or profession belong to widespread social networks which generate and share resources in times of need, e.g. in the case of illness. Examples include financial solidarity within an extended family network, intra-community solidarity among families, neighbours and friends, and social funds among colleagues. For example, the catechists of the provincial parish have organized a solidarity

Table 1. Traditional solidarity and risk sharing arrangements in 40 village communities of the study area.

Solidarity networks	
Kin-based	*****
Neighbourhood	***
Ethnicity	**
Profession	*
Rotating Labour Arrangements	
Social network labour parties	37/40 (92.5%)
Age group labour parties	32/40 (80.0%)
Women's labour groups	24/49 (60.0%)
Collective work parties	
Village wide work parties	34/49 (85.0%)
Labour assistance to old and sick	36/40 (90.0%)
Labour assistance to father-in-law	38/40 (95.0%)
Labour assistance to village head	8/40 (20.0%)
Obligatory employment of a person in need	29/49 (72.5%)
Remunerated group labour	39/40 (97.5%)

*Indicates relative importance.

fund which is deducted from their annual allowance and serves, among other purposes, to cover unforeseen medical expenditures.

Rotating labour arrangements

Rotating labour arrangements (ROLAs) exist in all five socio-cultural settings as a form of non-monetarized solidarity mechanism based on balanced reciprocity. Affinity is the driving force behind this institution, mostly regardless of ethnic, religious, kin-based or gender-based considerations. In an arrangement commonly called *tchibla* in Djoula, two or more individuals, most often of the same gender and linked by proximity and affinity, or families agree to help each other in a rotative manner by pooling their labour force. These temporary groupings come together for agricultural tasks and the construction and renovation of houses. In the past 2 years this solidarity mechanism has been witnessed in 37 of 40 (85.0%) villages. A similar pattern called *gnogon demen* uniting persons of the same age group, however, is receding with the disappearance of a number of initiation rites. It was reported to be practised in 32 of 40 (80.0%) communities. In addition, rotative work parties among women, i.e. to crush shea (*karité*) nuts or pack down the soil to level floors as well as roofs of houses are reported in only 24 of 40 (60.0%) of communities.

Collective work parties

A number of temporary labour arrangements call upon widely shared notions of collectivity and solidarity. However, they were not necessarily based on reciprocal obligations. Village-wide work parties (*faso bara*, litt.: the work of the father land) are organized by the traditional village head (*dugutigi*), the village elder (*tchékòròba*) or the village administrator (*délégué*). The work arrangements constitute a moral obligation for community members to assist in community-wide activities such as the construction or renovation of schools, churches, mosques, health centres and administrative buildings. They also mobilize communities for road construction and renovation work or, among the Fulani, for cattle immunization campaigns. Thirty-nine of 40 villages (97.5%) had witnessed such practices in the previous 2 years. Another non-reciprocal solidarity mechanism implies that a community group assists an old or sick person in time-sensitive agricultural tasks, for example, harvesting or weeding. Commonly called assistance (*demen*) or 'helping each other' (*gnogon demen*), this kind of solidarity has been witnessed in most communities, however, is diminishing in number and importance, reportedly due to 'increasing egoism'.

A further important and widely practised social institution is *bran ki*, a work party for a future father-in-law. As marriages have a crucial social and religious importance and tie together large extended family networks, the entire community is mobilized to help the future husband to till the fields of his father-in-law. In the case where the fields are far away, old people may choose to delegate their contribution to young members of their families. This work pattern has been witnessed, in the past 2 years, by 38 of 40 (95.0%) villages. Work parties for the traditional village head have largely disappeared. While this has reportedly never existed in 17 communities, in 19 communities is has not been witnessed for at least 10 years. Only eight (20.0%) of the 40 villages reportedly have witnessed this activity in the past 2 years, largely as a sign of respect to their village head. In all other communities this kind of labour arrangement is more and more relegated to the past as a restricting and somewhat repressive obligation.

Two of the informal labour-based risk sharing schemes are monetarized. Groups of mostly younger people increasingly offer their collective labour force against monetary remuneration in order to finance group activities and provide, from the capital of the group, credit to its associated members. Such remunerated work groups have been reported from all but one community (97.5%). Traditionally, the request to work against remuneration of a poor person in despair cannot be refused. This institution has been reported from 29 of 40 communities (72.5%).

Semi-modern institutions

Table 2 summarizes results from the inventory on semi-formal institutions and the domains of their risk sharing. We found a total of 87 production groups, ten associations and 29 rotating savings and credit associations (*tontines*) in the area.

A variety of community-based production groups have emerged as a result of national economic and development activities. These production groups are commonly called *groupements villageois* or, in official terminology, pre-cooperative groups (*groupements précoopératifs*). They are ruled, like cooperatives, by national law No. 014/99/AN issued in 1999 regulating cooperative societies and groups in Burkina Faso. Such groups can be either constituted exclusively by men (*groupements villageois hommes*, GVH), by women (*groupements villageois femmes*, GVF) or, rarely, they are of mixed composition. Some of them are specialized in cotton production (*groupements des producteurs de coton*, GPC), and some in cattle breeding (*groupement des éleveurs*). On average, such groups have a mean membership of 20 individuals and have existed for 11.1 years (range 1–25 years). They rarely have regular financial contributions (*cotisations*). Mostly linked to cash crop production, i.e. mainly of cotton and sesame, these institutions serve exclusively economic needs, i.e. to allow peasants have access to the formal credit markets. Written agreements usually link members of the production group with regional marketing boards, i.e. for cotton (SOFITEX), sesame (TROPEX), often in conjunction with banks (CNCA, CRPA) to receive a credit against the assured purchase of the group's harvest yields. Surplus from successful economic operations is put into a solidarity fund from which certain expenses of members may be paid or credits with or without interest may be allocated.

Table 2 shows the extent of solidarity-based risk sharing practices for five major life events (birth, baptism, wedding, disease, funeral) reported for the past 2 years, by representatives of these production groups. Whereas financial risk sharing, i.e. gift giving (G), credit provision without interest (C) and credit provision with interest (CI) plays a negligable role in birth, baptisms, weddings, credit provision without interest has been reported for disease and funeral costs by five of 26 male production groups whereas a total of seven of 18 female groups (38.8%) and 13 of 33 (39.4%) of cotton production groups report credit provision in times of illness. Credit provision

Table 2. Semi-formal risk sharing arrangements in 40 villages of the CRSN study area (June 2000)

	#	Years	Members	Fin Volume	Birth G	Birth C	Birth Cl	Baptism G	Baptism C	Baptism Cl	Wedding G	Wedding C	Wedding Cl	Disease G	Disease C	Disease Cl	Funeral G	Funeral C	Funeral Cl
Production groups																			
GVH	26	11.0	24 (9–63)	93 684 (0–370 000)	0	1	1	0	1	1	0	2	1	1	5	1	1	5	1
GVF	18	5.2	22 (10–55)	41 468 (0–150 000)	1	1	1	2	2	1	2	1	1	1	3	4	4	0	1
Gvmixte	1	3.0	65	50 000	0	0	0	0	0	0	0	1	0	0	1	0	0	0	0
GPC	33	5.6	26 (11–62)	44 393 (0–200 000)	1	1	0	0	1	0	1	3	1	1	12	1	1	7	2
ROSCAs																			
Tontines	30	3.1	19 (10–40)	98 (17 500–445 425)	0	0	5	1	0	3	0	0	1	0	3	11	1	4	4
Associative institutions																			
Associations	10	10.8	26 (15–45)	12 711 (0–25 000)	1	0	0	1	0	0	2	0	0	2	1	0	2	1	0
Unions	0	0	0																
Federations	0	0	0																
Mutual institutions	0	0	0																

in times of illness is more extended than for funeral costs. This insight, however, must be tempered by the fact that credit provision was shown to be highly skewed to wealthy community members who could offer substantial collateral in the form of animals. In addition, credit was mainly provided in catastrophic, life-threatening events such as maternal haemorrhage (Sauerborn et al., 1996b). The credit system does therefore not remove the need for an alternative financing system.

In spite of the fact that most village production groups are formally accredited with the office of the provinces' high commissioner and officially bound by national laws and have internal regulations, most of them, however, have limited administrative capacities or are often ill-functioning due to disagreements among members. In the 1980s, the Burkinian government decided to strengthen the administrative capacity of cotton production groups by establishing Savings and Credit Cooperatives (*Coopératives d'Epargne et de Credit*, COOPEC). The initiative failed and the state decided to transfer the remaining funds into a bank. Groups constituted by women (GVF) are said to be better performing, mainly due to a more disciplined and prompt repayment of credits. While the group's debts are collectively shared, credits are often unequally distributed to serve individual needs. Consequently, the group's joint guarantee (*caution solidaire*) towards its creditor is a major contributor to widespread disenchantement with village production groups.

Rotating Saving and Credit Associations (ROSCA)

Following Ardener (1964) these can be defined as informal associations of people who make regular monetary or non-monetary contributions to a fund which is given to each contributor in rotation. In Burkina Faso, Rotating Saving and Credit Arrangements (ROSCA) are generally known as *tontine* or *pari* (from the French word *parier*, to bet). In the study area many *tontines* are self-managed by individuals linked by neighbourship, religious confession or shared ethnic affiliation. The monetary contributions are usually small (50–100 F CFA per week = US$0.07–0.15) and the rotation sequence may last from 1 week up to 6 months. After several months, the money accrued may be allocated either as capital to serve as investment for commercial activities or used to buy for the members goods such as dishes or loincloth. Usually, deductions are made from the common fund towards a loan fund or a contingency fund from which important risk sharing activities may be financed.

In recent years, a number of monetarized ROSCAs have been initiated throughout the province with the financial and technical assistance of a local association, the *Association de Tontines de Nouna* (ATN). As the weekly contribution rarely exceeds 100 FCFA, the financial volume of the association's micro-*tontines* is limited. Besides providing a non-market mechanism for savings and credit, *tontines* serve important social functions such as mutual visits, common festivities and sharing of the joy and sorrow among members. These functions are particularly of importance in non-monetary *tontines*. These are self-managed and mostly constituted by women. Members contribute in kind, e.g. soap, and allocate the 'fund' to a member who is celebrating an important life event such as the delivery of a newborn, a baptism or a wedding.

The 30 ROSCAs identified are of recent origin—they have been in existence for a mean of 3.1 years and had on average 19 members (range 10–40). As institutions promoting savings among their members, ROSCAs have the highest financial volume with an average of 44393 CFA in their fund. The purpose of ROSCAs is reflected in their risk sharing practices with respect to the five selected life events. Whereas financial gifts are almost never provided, ROSCAs serve as important institutions for accessing credit. However, most of the provided credit is interest-based. Interestingly, illness figures predominate relative to funeral cost, refuting the hypothesis that rural populations care more about funeral costs than about illness costs in their financial risk sharing. Fourteen of 30 ROSCAs (46.6%) reported credit provision for covering illness costs of one of their members. Eleven of the fourteen reported that credits would be provided with interest.

Associative institutions

Associative institutions are groups of people that come together with a common purpose. These institutions include associations, unions and, at a national level, federations. These institutions often serve as an institutional platform for local development initiatives. Solidarity is a crucial side function of the group's interest in serving shared objectives as reflected in their sometimes illustrate names: *mugnu kadi* ('it is good to have self-control'), *ben kadi* ('understanding is good'), *sabari kadi* ('forgiveness is good'). Associations seeking official recognition by the high commissioners' office are bound by the national law governing associations.

Of the 38 officially recognized associations in the Province, 20 have their registered office in Nouna town; none is registered in one of the 42 villages of the study area. In the study area associations are largely unrecognized by government authorities. Their founders and members are largely untrained. With 44393 CFA, the financial volume of these institutions is limited. Some, but not all, associations collect regular financial contributions from their members. The common fund is supplied by common economic activities such as the selling of cash crops harvested from collective fields, the buying and reselling of food crops such as millet or offering to the market the membership's labour force against payment (*tchibla*). Some associations get considerable credits at local banks.

NOTIONS OF SOLIDARITY AND RECIPROCITY

Solidarity in non-monetarized IRSA's is characterized by friendly social relationships among families, clans, friends, peers or neighbours that are mobilized for the purpose of assistance to an individual in times of need or distress. Solidarity is based on the assumption, a loan is a given (*djuru don leyi djuru sara ye; le prêt égale le rendu*) thus implying a certain expectation of reciprocity. Interestingly, the Djoula term for loan is *djuru* or string. Credit is considered a string or link based on an obligation between two individuals. The obligation is exclusively moral and rarely legally enforced. Sometimes, it is even relegated to the divine by saying to the debtor *nyi to ni allah ye* (I leave you with God).

SOLIDARITY

Solidarity in times of ill-health

A consideration of CBI implies the relative position, in society's valuation, of states of ill-health. In a majority of our focus group discussions sickness, contrary to death, was considered an individual 'problem'. Local aetiological discourse holds that it is not the individual person who gets a sickness; it is the sickness that gets (literally 'catches') the individual. Furthermore, a person needs a lot of strength to combat illness. Whereas a death case links lineages, sickness is considered an individual affair. Furthermore, sickness episodes are never considered a solely natural affair. They may be considered repercussions of wrongful or sinful personal behaviour (alcoholism, smoking, etc.) and thus non-market insurance would mean that people would have the liberty to be financially reimbursed for their own 'mistakes', in insurance terminology, societal rules prevent moral hazard. In other words, the rural population, in fact, tries to avoid 'thinking' disease. Contributing financial resources to prevent disease or costs to future disease, may be regarded as attracting 'bad fate against oneself' (*ka wère wère wèle i ma*).

In the case of sickness, asset sale is an important health financing strategy. Even the least privileged will own a chicken to sell. Relatives are the first resort in terms of financial arrangements. This resort is, in many cases, limited to providing immediate food support, i.e. delivering soup or fruit to the diseased patient. Giving money to buy medicines would be seen as meaning that a person does not have enough money to pay for his or her own needs.

DISCUSSION AND CONCLUSIONS

Solidarity is a crucial feature of the Burkinian social fabric in spite of a growing trend for individualism and monetarization. Without contributing to, and tapping into a varied set of solidarity mechanisms, the individual would face social and economic deprivation in the harsh economic and ecological conditions of the Sahel. Solidarity fulfils important functions. It allows people to situate themselves in extended social networks providing them with a sense of belonging and support. Deprived of social security as offered by the nation state, solidarity allows rural Burkinian farmers to participate in extended risk sharing networks that often transcend ethnic boundaries.

To what extent is such solidarity and risk sharing identical with insurance? In the research zone, the principle of insurance is perceived as foresight expressed by the saying *sini nyé sigi* (what I provide for tomorrow), the central popular notion for savings. There is a probability notion implied which can be used for the promotion of CBI. Mutual help would be a more appropriate term (*nyogon demen*, literally: to help together). CBI could, therefore, be popularized by the construct *nyogon demen bana ko la* (mutual aid for health).

In any society, the 'mutualization' of risk is the result of associative experiences of collectivities. In Burkina Faso, the associative movement (village production groups) have experienced serious organizational and financial deficits. Whereas national agrarian politics in the 1980s favoured village-wide production groups, just recently the advantages of small structures have been rediscovered.

A great variety of risk sharing institutions exist in the study area. Our ethnographic data suggest that informal, non-monetarized, so-called 'traditional' risk sharing arrangements, contrary to assumptions in the literature, are very prevalent and evidently not prone to immediate disappearance. They transport important solidarity notions inherent in the Burkinian society. Our data suggest that not all of the solidarity expressed in traditional arrangements is based on the idea of mutual reciprocity. Some arrangements are even altruistic.

Increasing monetarization of the Burkinian non-formal economy brings with it a tendency for collective group work to rise in size and in importance. Monetarization brings about egoism, even at the level of the extended family. This tendency will most likely affect future institutionalized risk sharing schemes. Proximity is a crucial and essential structural element of African institutions. As there is widespread mistrust of anonymous and bureaucratic institutions, one can, however, posit that the more institutionalized groups there are, the less effective they risk becoming. The specificity of African societies need, to be taken into account when promoting institutional development in rural African areas (Beauchamp, 1993–94). Before new mutual health institutions can be successful, they need to be grounded in local values of solidarity and reciprocity.

To be functional, CBI schemes need to be tailored around a number of presuppositions. There needs to be, in the community, a collective interest in financial precautions to ward off income shocks due to illness. More than that, communities need to have a positive attitude towards precautionary approaches for future ill-health (Sommerfeld et al., 2001). In addition, there needs to be awareness that certain health problems warrant insurance which relates to common attitudes towards, and perceptions of, health risks. Shared norms of solidarity and reciprocity can largely increase the trust in a pooling scheme. Finally, the ability to pay (ATP) and willingness-to-pay (WTP) are necessary in order to create trust in service providers. A study has just been completed to assess the amount people are willing to pay for CBI and the factors influencing this. The results will be published elsewhere.

New mutual health organizations in the rural Sahel face a number of challenges. The administrative set-up needs to fulfil popular expectations regarding leadership and transparency. New innovative ways to promote an administration based on proximity need to be conceived. Administrative skills, particularly, financial management skills, need to be strengthened. A benefit package based on issues of financial sustainability and popular expectation needs to be defined. Enrolment, modalities and the level of fee payment, membership administration and reimbursement procedures need to be developed and systematized. Potential sources for moral hazard need to be identified. The greatest challenge will be to bridge the need for proximity with the health care financing need to pool resources. One possibility to preserve the benefits of small size and proximity, yet avoiding the risks of bankrupcy inherent in small groups, would be to create a public re-insurance scheme covering high cost/low volume risks (cf. Dror, 2001).

Finally, nation states are called upon to provide clear-cut legal frameworks for mutual health organizations. Burkina Faso needs to provide a legal framework for the rapidly emerging mutual health organizations. To be successful as stimulators of local development, CBI schemes need to enrol marginalized and disadvantaged populations into national development processes. In Burkina Faso, the law on community associations (decree No 92-376/PRES dated 31 December 1992 putting into effect Law No 10/92/ADP dated 14 December 1992) provides sufficient legal framework to implement a community-based insurance scheme except that it does not provide any structure for social (i.e. public) re-insurance. The Burkinian government should assume two roles; providing a legal framework both for CBIs and re-insurance for small scale IRAs so that they can take on health care expenditures as additional item to share risks.

ACKNOWLEDGEMENTS

The research underlying this manuscript was sponsored by the German Association for Scientific Research (Deutsche Forschungsgemeinschaft, DFG) as part of the Special Research Area (Sonderforschungsbereich, SFB 544) 'Control of Tropical Infectious Diseases' of Heidelberg University.

REFERENCES

Ahiadeke C. 1996. Agrarian structure and social organization in a risk-prone environment: a comparison of the Birifor, Dagara, and the Lobi people of Burkina Faso. Population and environment: a. *J Interdisc Stud* **17**: 323–342.

Alderman H, Paxson CH. 1992. *Do the Poor Insure? A Synthesis of the Literature on Risk and Consumption in Developing Countries.* Policy Research Working Paper 16. World Bank: Washington, DC.

Ardener S. 1964. The comparative study of rotating credit associations. *J Roy Anthro Inst Great Britain Ireland* **94**: 201–229.

Atim C. 1998. *Contributions of Mutual Health Organizations to Financing, Delivery and Access to Health Care.* Partnerships for Health Reform: Bethesda, MD.

Atim C. 1999. Social movements and health insurance: a critical evaluation of voluntary, non-profit insurance schemes with case studies from Ghana and Cameroon. *Soc Sci Med* **48**: 881–896.

ATLAS/ti. 1997. *Visual Qualitative Data Analysis-Management-Model Building.* Release 4.1. Scientific Software Development: Berlin (http: //www.atlasti.de).

Barlow R, Diop F. 1995. Increasing the utilization of cost-effective health services through changes in demand. *Hlth Pol Plann* **15**: 284–295.

Batterbury S. 1994. Soil and water conservation in Burkina Faso: the role of community organizations. *Appropriate Technol* **21**(3): 6–9.

Beauchamp C. 1993–94. La question coopérative en Afrique Noire. *Coopératives et Développement* **25**: 27–43.

Bennett S, Creese A, Monasch R. 1998. *Health Insurance Schemes for People Outside Formal Sector Employment.* World Health Organisation, Division of Analysis, Research and Assessment (ARA). WHO: Geneva.

Besley T. 1995. Nonmarket institutions for credit and risk sharing in low-income countries. *J Econ Persp* **9**: 115–127.

Burkina Faso Ministry of Health. 2000. Ministère de la Santé. *Projet de Document de Politique Sanitaire Nationale (PSN).* Unpublished document ST/PSN-PNDS, Ministry of Health Ouagadougou, Burkina Faso.

Coate S, Ravallion M. 1993. Reciprocity without commitment: characterization and performance of informal insurance arrangements. *J Dev Econ* **40**: 1–24.

Concertation. 2000. Concertation entre les acteurs du développement des mutuelles de santé en Afrique de l'Ouest et du Centre. *Courrier de la Concertation*. No. 2, April 2000. http://www.concertation.org/docs/lettreinfo/HTML/LettreInfo_1.html.

Creese A, Bennett S. 1997. Rural risk-sharing strategies. In *Innovations in Health Care Financing: Proceedings of a World Bank Conference*, Schieber GJ (ed.). World Bank: Washington, DC; 163–182.

Criel B. 1998. District-based health insurance in sub-Saharan Africa. Part I: from theory to practice. *Stud Hlth Serv Pol* **9**.

Criel B, Van Dormael M, Lefèvre P, Menase U, Van Lerberghe W. 1998. Voluntary health insurance in Bwamanda, Democratic Republic of Congo. An exploration of its meanings to the community. *Trop Med Int Hlth* **3**: 640–653.

Diop F, Yazbeck A, Bitran R. 1995. The impact of alternative cost recovery schemes on access and equity in Niger. *Hlth Pol Plann* **10**: 223–240.

Dror DM. 2001. Reinsurance of health insurance for the informal sector. *Bull World Hlth Org* **79**: 672–678.

Dror DM, Jacquier C. 1999. Micro-insurance: extending health insurance to the excluded. *Int Soc Sec Rev* **52**: 71–97.

Ellsworth L. 1988. Mutual insurance and non-market transactions among farmers in Burkina Faso. PhD thesis, University of Wisconsin-Madison, USA.

Elwert G. 1980. Die Elemente der traditionellen Solidarität. *Kölner Zeitschr Soz Sozialpsych* **32**: 681–701.

Eswaran M, Kotwal A. 1989. Credit as insurance in agrarian economics. *J Dev Econ* **31**: 37–53.

Fafchamps M, Lund S. 1999. Risk-sharing networks in rural Philippines. http://www.economics.ox.ac.uk/faculty/members/marcei.fafchamps.

Fafchamps M. 1999a. Risk sharing and quasi-credit. *J Int Trade Econ Dev* **8**: 257–278.

Fafchamps M. 1999b. *Rural Poverty, Risk and Development*. Economic and Social Development Paper No. 144. Food and Agriculture Organization (FAO). FAO: Geneva.

Fiske P. 1990. Relativity within Moose ('Mossi') culture: four incommensurable models for social relationships. *Ethos* **18**: 180–204.

Fon P. 1997. *Community Based Risk Sharing in a Rural District of Burkina Faso*. M.Sc. thesis, Heidelberg University.

Fonteneau B. 1999. *L'Émergence de Pratiques d'Économie Sociale en Matière de Financement de la Santé au Burkina Faso*. Hoger Instituut voor de Arbeed: Université Catholique de Leuven.

Howorth C, O'Keefe P. 1999. Farmers do it better: local management of change in Southern Burkina Faso. *Land Degrad Develop* **10**: 93–109.

Krause G, Sauerborn R. 2000. Community-effectiveness of care—the example of malaria treatment in rural Burkina Faso. *Annals Trop Pediatr* **7**: 99–106.

Kimball MS. 1988. Farmers' cooperatives as behaviour towards risk. *Am Econ Rev* **78**: 224–232.

Ledea Ouedraogo B. 1990. *Entraide Villageoise et Développement: Groupements Paysans au Burkina Faso*. L'Harmattan: Paris.

Nguyen T-D-P G. 1998. *Food Insecurity and the Evolution of Indigenous Risk-Sharing Institutions in the Sahel*. PhD. The Ohio State University: Ann Arbor (UMI 9822353).

Normand C, Weber A. 1994. *Social Health Insurance: A Guidebook for Planning*. World Health Organization, International Labour Office: Geneva.

Platteau J-P. 1991. Traditional systems of social security and hunger insurance: past achievements and modern challenges. In *Social Security in Developing Countries*, Ahmad E, Drèze J, Hills J, Sen AK (eds). Clarendon: Oxford; 112–170.

Platteau J-P. 1997. Mutual insurance as an elusive concept in traditional rural communities. *J Dev Studies* **33**: 764–796.

Reardon T, Matlon P. 1989. Seasonal food insecurity and vulnerability in drought-affected regions of Burkina Faso. In *Seasonal Variability in Third World Agriculture: The Consequences for Food Security*, Sahn DE (ed.). The Johns Hopkins University Press: Baltimore and London; 118–136.

Sakurai T, Reardon T. 1997. Potential demand for drought insurance in Burkina Faso and its determinants. *Am J Agr Econ* **79**: 1193–1207.

Sanou B. 2000. La mutuelle de santé de Bobo-Dioulasso: Un projet, une matrice culturelle. http://www.concertation.org/Docs/Documents/DiscoursComm_3161243383_6949.html.

Sauerborn R, Nougtara A, Latimer E. 1994. The elasticity of demand for health care in Burkina Faso: differences across age and income groups. *Health Policy Planning* **9**: 185–192.

Sauerborn R, Nougtara A, Hien M, Diesfeld HJ. 1996a. Seasonal variations of the household costs of illness in Burkina Faso. *Social Sci Med* **43**: 281–290.

Sauerborn R, Adams E, Hien M. 1996b. Household strategies to cope with the direct and indirect costs of illness. *Social Sci Med* **43**: 291–301.

Sommerfeld J, Sanon M, Kouyaté B, Sauerborn R. 2002. Perceptions of Risk, Vulnerability and Disease Prevention in Rural Burkina Faso: implications for Community-based Health Care and Insurance. *Human Organisation* **60**(2): 139–146.

Vuarin R. 1996. Quelles solidarités sociales peut-on mobiliser pour faire face au coût de la maladie? In *Se Soigner au Mali: Une Contribution des Sciences Sociales: Douze Expériences de Terrain*. Brunet-Jailly J (ed.). Éditions Karthala, Éditions de l'ORSTOM: Paris; 299–316.

Were J. 1999. *Traditional Risk-Sharing Schemes: The Potential for Community-Based Health Insurance in Africa?* Unpublished manuscript. University of Heidelberg, Department of Tropical Hygiene and Public Health.

Zimmerman FJ, Carter MR. 1999. A dynamic option value for institutional change: marketable property rights in the Sahel. *Am J Agr Econ* **81**: 467–478.

4.6 Obtaining disability weights in rural Burkina Faso using a culturally adapted visual analogue scale

BALTUSSEN R, SANON M, SOMMERFELD J, WÜRTHWEIN R.

Health Econ. 2002; 11: 155-163

Reprinted with permission from John Wiley & Sons Ltd.

Obtaining disability weights in rural Burkina Faso using a culturally adapted visual analogue scale

R.M.P.M. Baltussen[a,b,*], M. Sanon[b], J. Sommerfeld[a] and R. Würthwein[c]
[a] Department of Tropical Hygiene and Public Health, University of Heidelberg, Germany
[b] Centre de Recherche en Santé de Nouna, Burkina Faso
[c] Alfred Weber-Institute, University of Heidelberg, Germany

Summary

Burden of disease (BOD) estimates used to foster local health policy require disability weights which represent local preferences for different health states. The global burden of disease (GBD) study presumes that disability weights are universal and equal across countries and cultures, but this is questionable. This indicates the need to measure local disability weights across nations and/or cultures. We developed a culturally adapted version of the visual analogue scale (VAS) for a setting in rural Burkina Faso. Using an anthropologic approach, BOD-relevant health states were translated into culturally meaningful disability scenarios. The scaling procedure was adapted using a locally relevant scale. Nine hypothetical health states were evaluated by seven panels of in total 39 lay individuals and 17 health professionals. Results show that health professionals' rankings and valuations of health states matched those of lay people to a certain extent. In comparison to that of the lay people, health professionals rated seven out of nine health states as slightly to moderately less severe. The instrument scored well on inter-panel and test–retest reliability and construct validity. Our research shows the feasibility of eliciting disability weights in a rural African setting using a culturally adapted VAS. Moreover, the results of the present study suggest that it might be possible to use health professionals' preferences on disability weights as a proxy for lay people's preferences. Copyright © 2002 John Wiley & Sons, Ltd.

Keywords   disability weights; DALY; burden of disease; valuation methods; cross-cultural adaptation

Introduction

Burden of disease (BOD) estimates used to foster local health policy require disability weights that represent local preferences for different health states. However, the global burden of disease (GBD) study presumes that disability weights are universal and equal across countries and cultures [1]. In a recent commentary, James and Foster [2] argue that health is so influenced by culture and economic differences that agreement on universal disability weights may prove to be impossible. Furthermore, a recent study among health professionals in 14 countries ranking a set of 17 health states with regard to their severity concluded that the resulting rank order differences are large enough to shed doubt on the assumption of universality of disability weights [3]. This indicates the need for measuring local disability weights across nations and/or cultures.

The question arises as to whether existing valuation instruments can be used to elicit such

*Correspondence to: GPE/EQC, World Health Organization, 20 Avenue Appia, CH-1211 Geneva 27, Switzerland. Tel.: +41 22 791 3825; fax: +41 22 791 4328; e-mail: baltussenr@who.int

Copyright © 2002 John Wiley & Sons, Ltd.

Received 23 June 2000
Accepted 14 May 2001

locally meaningful disability weights [4]. The authors of the GBD study, Murray and Lopez, argue that utility measurement techniques such as time-trade-off (TTO), standard gamble (SG), and person-trade-off (PTO) are cognitively demanding and become increasingly difficult to use with less educated individuals: *'If large scale empirical assessments in many different countries to inform health state valuations for the GBD are to be achieved, instruments that are reliable and valid for populations with widely varying educational attainments need to be developed'* [5]. In this paper, we agree with this point of view and argue that there is a need for locally meaningful valuation instruments, i.e. to evaluate BOD-relevant disease states by culturally appropriate instruments, including meaningful health state and disability scenarios and feasible scaling procedures [6]. However, little research has been done in developing countries on the development of such instruments [7–10]. The present paper asks whether a health state valuation instrument can be developed that produces meaningful disability weights for population groups with lower levels of formal education attainment as, in our case, that of rural Burkina Faso. We introduce a culturally adapted Visual Analogue Scale (VAS), and evaluate the instrument using the psychometric concepts of practicality, reliability and validity [11]. We suggest that this instrument could be applied to elicit disability weights for BOD studies on a broader scale.

Furthermore, this paper debates as to whose health states preferences should be considered. Should one consider community (lay people's) values, given the premise that the issue at stake refers to the allocation of societal resources, or should one, like it has been done in the GBD study[1], merely apply those of health professionals, since they have a better understanding of a wide range of health states? Williams [12] warns that the GBD study should *'make it possible to bring lay opinion to bear on matters that are dangerous to leave to experts'*. Health professionals' valuations may diverge as they might give too much weight to functional status and inadequately take into account more subtle and subjective influences of an illness. Moreover, they may not constitute a representative cross-section of the general public with regard to age, income, and socio-economic status [13]. In this paper, we ask as to whether health professionals' valuations can be used as a proxy for those of the community.

Utility measures to evaluate disability weights

Among utility measures, the SG, TTO and VAS have been used most often in health economics research in Western settings. They all measure preferences for health states on a scale from 0 (death) to 1 (full health) [14]. The SG asks the respondent to make a hypothetical choice between the certainty of continued life in the health state of interest and a gamble between varying probabilities of death and full health. The TTO presents the respondent with the task of determining what amount of time they would be willing to give up to be in a better versus a poorer health state. The VAS requires respondents to assign a number to each health state, usually on a scale from 0 (least desirable health state) to 100 (most desirable health state). Visual aids such as a 'feeling thermometer' are used to support this task.

A recent critical commentary raised doubts about the cross-cultural applicability of utility measures [2]. Although universal utility measures would be highly desirable, they may be regarded as cultural artifacts themselves as they transport Western values, notions of time, and concepts of science [15, 16]. Knowledge and attitudinal surveys such as health valuation surveys appear to be particularly prone to cultural reinterpretation of survey questions by respondents and thus to contextual bias [17]. For example, Yu *et al.* [18] showed great discrepancies in responses to different scales across various cultures and concluded that attitude measures such as the Likert scale and semantic differential scales are 'culture-specific, emic instruments' which largely depend upon a subject's interpretation of the measures. Utility measures based on statistical or objective probability introduce subjective or personal considerations of uncertainty and risk that are highly culture-bound.

In populations with low levels of formal education, another problem may arise from using numbers and thus reducing or transforming 'lived' experience, knowledge, and attitude into a single numerical value. A quantified valuation is never a 'value-free' act, and is based on lay or folk interpretations of numbers, statistics and probabilities, in other words, a lay epidemiology [19]. The question, therefore, is how far a population's relative degree of numeracy is developed, i.e. how far people are able to think in numbers and use them.

Another concern addresses the acceptability of methods to a particular culture under study. Of particular interest is the question of whether discrete choice instruments are acceptable in a respective culture and whether respondents are used to discrete choice responding. Varying culture-specific norms of self-disclosure and respondent burden may affect the measurement and thus produce variation in response [20].

Prior formative research focused on the feasibility of administering the SG, TTO and VAS in a rural Burkinian context [6]. In the SG exercise, respondents appeared to have difficulties in understanding the concept of risk taking, and often related 'risk' to destiny. By believing that man's fate ultimately lies 'in the hands of God', respondents were expressing excessive 'risks' or 'no risk' at all. Furthermore, both in the SG and TTO method, the respondents' behavior was strongly influenced by family interest and social values. In the TTO exercise, for example, respondents were not willing to trade-off life years if they still had to care for family members, but were eager to trade-off life years when they felt they were a burden on the family. It was concluded that one should be very cautious when applying SG and TTO for the purpose of obtaining health state valuations in the context of rural Burkina Faso. Regarding the VAS, it was observed that respondents seemed to easily rank order health states but tended to maintain identical proportions between the valuations of the health states concerned. The valuation of one's own health state by the VAS showed a relative low test–retest reliability of 0.64.

These observations led us to the development of a culturally adapted VAS – an alternative instrument to measure health states in a setting where the level of formal education is low – that seems more capable of expressing the beliefs and values of the community and transforming those into numerical values.

Methods

The country and study population

Burkina Faso is a land-locked country, situated at the border of the Sahel region in West Africa, with a population of 10. 7 million inhabitants as of 1998 [21], representing a multi-cultural and multi-linguistic setting, characterized by a strong oral culture. In spite of a state education system, there is a high level of formal illiteracy. Because of the (French) colonial history, there is a coexistence of African and Western values. The GDP per capita is estimated to be $150 per year, and more than 95% of the population live on subsistence farming. The high levels of infant and child mortality (219 per 1000 and 105 per 1000, respectively) [22] reflect large unmet needs. Our study was performed in the research area of the Nouna Health Research Center in the North-West of Burkina Faso. In this region, malaria, diarrhea and respiratory diseases are estimated to be the most important contributors to the total numbers of years of life lost [23].

Study procedure

Nine hypothetical health states were selected. Four of these health states were adapted from the 22 indicator conditions of the GBD study. The nine health states include asthma, back pain, blindness, deafness, diabetes, heart problems, paraplegia, major depression, and severe mental disorder. Formative anthropological research led to the development of cultural and linguistic equivalents of these health states, including definitions of locally meaningful disability scenarios (Table 1). Ultimately, these health state descriptions reflected perceived illness rather than bio-medically defined disease notions. The health states were illustrated using locally designed images.

Our scaling procedure retains the simplicity of the traditional VAS in which valuations are clearly visualized but replaces the difficult part of metric scaling – a concept unknown to most residents in rural Burkina Faso. Instead, it applies a culturally more adequate approach of representing valuations by physical units. The instrument expresses the degree of disability of a health state in terms of numbers of physical units (in our case 6 cm long wooden blocks), with 0 units representing the best health state imaginable, and 10 units representing the worst health state imaginable (Figure 1). Because of the explicit comparative nature of the exercise, one might hypothesize that this approach possesses interval properties. A further advantage is that the respondents are less intuited to retain identical proportions between the evaluated health states than in the traditional VAS, because the various states are not valued on one and the same visual scale.

Table 1. Nine hypothetical health states as explained to our study's respondents

Health state	Local expression	Description
Asthma	Sinsan	The individual has difficulty breathing and experiences moments when he/she does not get enough air, especially when lying down. The individual works normally when he or she is having no episodes. The individual is frightened that one day his breathing will stop and that he/she will die.
Back pain	Ko dimi	The individual has problems getting up in the morning because his back feels stiff. When the individual wants to lift something, he/she feels strain at waist-level. The individual has many problems working in the field because he or she has to rest every now and then. Females have difficulties preparing food or sweeping the courtyard.
Deafness	Bobo	The individual does not hear well. Only when somebody shouts very loud can the individual hear.
Diabetes (type I)	Sukaro bana	The individual eats and drinks often. The individual urinates often, up to 4 times per night. The individual has problems with his feet. The individual needs to go to the hospital once per week for an injection. The individual often feels tired and cannot work well for that reason.
Heart problems	Dusu kun dimi	The individual experiences pain in the chest with sensations like needle-sticks. The individual has difficulty breathing when walking or working. The individual cannot work properly in the field or, in the case of a woman, doing activities in the household like sweeping the courtyard or preparing food. The individual is afraid of dying because of these problems.
Paraplegia	Muruku bana	The individual cannot walk because his legs are paralyzed. The individual can do some domestic activities. The individual does not have a wheelchair to move around.
Major depression	Nimisa gwèlen	The individual experiences loss of interest or pleasure in nearly all activities. The individual is introverted, and has difficulties thinking and concentrating. The individual also experiences a loss of appetite.
Severe mental disorder	Fatoya	The individual shows strange behavior and often talks with people who can only be seen by him. The individual does many things in the wrong order.
Blindness	Fientoya	The individual is unable to distinguish the fingers of a hand at the distance of 3 m. The individual cannot see well at dusk. During the day, the individual can work well in the fields, but he/she cannot see far.

For the valuation exercise, the respondents were instructed to (i) consider the disability for some sort of 'average' case, i.e. a person of 40 years of age in a family with children; (ii) consider the person living in that health state during the period of one year; (iii) consider the prognosis of the health state to be unknown; and (iv) evaluate the disability regarding productive, religious, and social activities. Each valuation exercise was conducted in two steps. In the first step, the valuation procedure was performed on an individual basis. In the second step, the principle of elaboration [24] was applied, and respondents shared their valuations in a group and were encouraged to discuss these to arrive at well-thought valuations that better represent their preferences. The aim of the group session was not the development of group consensus but rather the encouragement of reflection. To test the impact of this 'elaboration', respondents' valuations before and after the group discussion were recorded. In addition to the valuation exercise, respondents were asked to rank the health states in terms of disability. To assess the test–retest reliability, the same exercise was conducted four weeks later.

Four panel sessions were held with lay people, combining 39 individuals altogether. Each group session involved five women and five men (except in one panel where one woman did not finish the exercise). The mean age of the 39 individuals was 40 years (with a standard deviation (SD) of 8.5), and the majority of the respondents were illiterate (61%). Two panel sessions were held with health

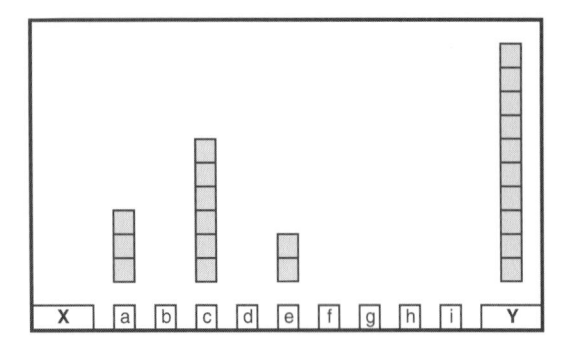

Boxes X and Y represent images of the best imaginable health state and the worst imaginable health state respectively. The handicap of the worst imaginable health state is defined by 10 units. Boxes a-i represent locally designed picture cards of 9 health states. The respondent must rate the severity of health states a-i by placing the number of units in question to the corresponding image of the health state. For example, health states represented by images a,c, and e are given disability weigts of 0.3,0.6, and 0.2, respectively.

Figure 1. Culturally adopted visual analogue scale

professionals with a total of 17 individuals, including 13 nurses and four medical doctors. Mean age was 34 years (SD = 5.8). The average number of years of practical experience was 10 (SD = 5.4). Sessions with lay people spent, on average, 74 min on the description of the hypothetical health states and the explanation of the instrument. The respondents spent, on average, 52 min to arrive at their individual valuations. The group discussions took 47 min, on average, after which individuals made their final assessments in an average of 12 min. For health professionals, these activities lasted, on average, 30, 50, 55, and 10 min, respectively.

The individual assessments from the panel sessions were converted to weights V using the following formula: $V(Q) = \text{score}(Q)/10$, where Q refers to the health states. The average disability weights were calculated from the individual weights assigned by all individuals in the panel sessions.

Results

Inter-panel reliability was assessed after the second step of elaboration in two ways: by the extent of agreement between the panels on the average weights (ANOVA) and by the extent of agreement between the panels on the ranking of the weights (Spearman rank correlation coefficient). The average weights of the four panels of lay people do not appear to diverge strongly (Table 2). Univariate testing revealed that, nevertheless, six weights differed significantly between the panels. However, these differences were never larger than 0.23. The ranking of the weights assigned by the four panels of lay people did not vary much, indicated by an average Spearman rank correlation coefficient of 0.90. The average weights elicited by the three panels of health professionals differed significantly for four health states (Table 3) but were never larger than 0.27. The average Spearman rank correlation coefficient was 0.72. Because of the small sample sizes, no further panel subgroup analyses were carried out.

Table 2. Interpanel comparison of disability weights as elicited by lay people[a]

Health state	I ($n=10$)			II ($n=10$)			III ($n=9$)			IV ($n=10$)			ANOVA	
	Mean	SD	Rank	Mean	SD	Rank	Mean	SD	Rank	Mean	SD	Rank	F	p
Severe mental disorder	0.89	0.03	1	0.88	0.06	1	0.90	0.00	1	0.89	0.09	1	0.19	0.900
Major depression	0.70	0.11	2	0.72	0.08	2	0.76	0.07	2	0.79	0.09	2	2.06	0.124
Heart problems	0.62	0.09	3	0.49	0.09	4	0.54	0.07	4	0.50	0.13	6	3.53	0.025[b]
Low back pain	0.59	0.11	4	0.41	0.10	5	0.50	0.00	6	0.53	0.11	5	6.58	0.001[b]
Asthma	0.53	0.12	5	0.60	0.14	3	0.70	0.05	3	0.63	0.11	3	3.91	0.016[b]
Diabetes	0.51	0.09	6	0.37	0.07	7	0.51	0.14	5	0.59	0.15	4	6.26	0.002[b]
Blindness	0.46	0.16	7	0.29	0.07	8	0.23	0.07	8	0.41	0.13	8	7.97	0.000[b]
Paraplegia	0.41	0.13	8	0.41	0.10	5	0.37	0.10	7	0.48	0.11	7	1.71	0.184
Deafness	0.15	0.05	9	0.17	0.05	9	0.10	0.00	9	0.23	0.08	9	9.02	0.000[b]

[a] Disability weights as measured after the second step of elaboration.
[b] Significant difference, equal variances not assumed.

Table 3. Interpanel comparison of disability weights as elicited by health professionals

Health state	Panel									ANOVA	
	I ($n=7$)			II ($n=6$)			III ($n=4$)			F	p
	Mean	SD	Rank	Mean	SD	Rank	Mean	SD	Rank		
Severe mental disorder	0.70	0.20	1	0.88	0.04	1	0.88	0.05	1	3.65	0.053
Paraplegia	0.57	0.10	2	0.43	0.23	5	0.70	0.00	3	2.98	0.043[a]
Major depression	0.57	0.19	2	0.68	0.13	2	0.80	0.00	2	3.15	0.074
Asthma	0.53	0.10	4	0.38	0.10	6	0.33	0.10	6	6.73	0.009[a]
Heart problems	0.53	0.14	4	0.58	0.10	3	0.33	0.17	6	4.75	0.027[a]
Low back pain	0.43	0.11	6	0.50	0.11	4	0.25	0.06	8	7.44	0.006[a]
Diabetes	0.36	0.11	7	0.28	0.08	8	0.38	0.05	5	1.60	0.236
Blindness	0.34	0.10	8	0.32	0.08	7	0.45	0.06	4	3.35	0.065
Deafness	0.10	0.00	9	0.10	0.00	9	0.13	0.05	9	1.78	0.204

[a] Significant difference, equal variances not assumed.

Table 4. Disability weights for the health states for lay people and health professionals

Health state	Lay people			Health professionals			Student's t	
	Mean	SD	Rank	Mean	SD	Rank	t-value	P
Severe mental disorder	0.89	0.06	1	0.81	0.16	1	2.16	0.045[a]
Major depression	0.74	0.09	2	0.66	0.17	2	1.79	0.089
Asthma	0.61	0.12	3	0.43	0.13	5	5.05	0.000[a]
Heart problems	0.54	0.11	4	0.50	0.16	4	0.89	0.381
Low back pain	0.51	0.11	5	0.41	0.14	6	2.55	0.017[a]
Diabetes	0.49	0.14	6	0.34	0.09	8	5.06	0.000[a]
Paraplegia	0.42	0.11	7	0.55	0.17	3	−2.94	0.008[a]
Blindness	0.35	0.14	8	0.36	0.09	7	−0.23	0.816
Deafness	0.16	0.07	9	0.11	0.02	9	4.57	0.000[a]

[a] Significant difference, equal variances not assumed.

Test–retest reliability, indicating the stability of respondents' valuations over time, appeared to be high. The average individual test–retest Pearson correlation was 0.90 and 0.89 for lay people and health professionals, respectively. Average test and retest disability weights for the nine health states differed only slightly.

Construct (convergent) validity of the weights was studied by a comparison with the results of the implicit rank order following from the final evaluation with an explicit rank order exercise, carried out after the final evaluation. The Spearman rank correlation coefficient equaled 0.86 and 0.94 for lay people and health professionals, respectively, indicating that both panels were consistent in their evaluations, and thus understood the valuation procedure. Based on these results, it can be concluded that the scale values derived at the panel level are sufficiently valid and reliable.

The impact of elaboration was assessed by comparison of mean disability weights between the weights of the individual valuation (step 1) and of the group discussion (step 2). For the panels of lay people, mean values of two out of nine health states (blindness and paraplegia) changed significantly, with a maximum of 0.06. Group discussion halved the variance of the responses from 0.024 to 0.012. The Spearman rank order correlation coefficient of 0.85 indicates that the ranking was not substantially affected by the elaboration. For the health professionals' panels, only the mean value for deafness changed significantly (0.05). The variance of responses decreased from 0.032 to 0.018, and the Spearman rank order correlation coefficient equaled 0.82.

Mean disability weights for the nine health states as elicited by lay people and health professionals are reported in Table 4. In comparison to that of the lay people, health professionals rated seven out of nine health states as slightly to moderately less severe. A Student's *t*-test of the difference was significant for six out of nine health states: diabetes, low back pain, severe mental disorder, asthma, paraplegia, and deafness. The differences in mean disability weights ranged from 0.05 to 0.18 and can, therefore, be regarded as small to moderate. The average Spearman rank correlation coefficient for the disability weights equaled 0.78.

Discussion

This study has shown the feasibility of eliciting disability weights in a rural African setting using a culturally adapted VAS instrument. Even if there are some concerns on the theoretical validity of the use of VAS-scores in economic evaluation, since they are not choice-based methods and they do not have a basis in economic theory, evidence shows that instruments that are more deeply rooted in economic theory do not produce reasonable results when applied in a population with a low level of formal education [25]. Earlier studies in the same context showed that respondents had problems understanding the underlying concepts of trading off time, trading off persons, and gambling in alternative, choice-based instruments such as TTO, PTO, SG [6]. Our approach, exhibiting meaningful health state and disability scenarios and feasible scaling procedures seems more appropriate in the socio-cultural conditions under study. Furthermore, regarding the high response rate and consistent results, the instrument appears to be more practical than the above-mentioned cognitively demanding techniques. The instrument scores well on inter-panel and test–retest reliability and appears to possess interval properties.

Health professionals' views matched those of lay people to a considerable extent. The rankings of the disabling effect of health states were relatively stable between the two groups, although the rankings of the intermediate states showed more variability than that of the states at both ends of the range. In comparison to that of the lay people, health professionals rated the majority of the presented health states as less severe. These findings are less convincing than those of the Dutch Study on Disability Weights [26] and that of a literature review [25] which concluded that it makes little difference whether panels to elicit disability weights are composed of health professionals or lay people.

This leads to the question of which preferences should then be used to obtain disability weights for the calculation of DALYs. Our study has shown that the evaluation of nine (frequently occurring) health states by lay people required lengthy in-depth and cognitively demanding descriptions. Measuring health state valuations of the population for every possible health state therefore seems impracticale [5]. Our study results suggest that the application of health professionals' preferences seems an acceptable alternative to elicit disability weights on a wide range of health states, at the expense of small deviations from (and most likely under-ratings of) lay people's valuation of disability weights. However, because of our small sample size, these conclusions are only tentative and more research is needed before more general conclusions can be drawn. Another alternative, in the long run, is to develop predictive models (multi-attribute utility schemes) that allow an analyst to impute health state valuations from information about the levels on various domains of health status associated with a particular state [5]. This would certainly decrease the workload as – after the initial collection of utility weights for the various domains of health states – health states only need to be described in terms of scores on domains in order to arrive at valuations. There is little experience with health profiles in developing countries [27], and more conceptual, methodological and empirical work is needed to develop robust models for this purpose. The present research can act as a first step towards this approach to obtain culturally adapted, practical, valid and reliable utility instruments.

The process of elaboration did not considerably change the aggregate mean values but affected the responses at the individual level and decreased its variation. The question arises as to whether health state valuation instruments like the culturally adapted VAS can then be used to rapidly collect lay people's preferences on disability weights of their own health state or hypothetical health states in household surveys. Our research has shown that respondents needed considerable time to understand and carry out the basic (individual) exercise, and that group discussion did alter their valuations, indicating the need for careful procedures. Furthermore, health states should preferably be valued in comparison to other health states: earlier research has shown that it is easier for people to give a value to an object if it can be compared to other objects [24]. This means that, even when measuring preferences about an individual's own health state, one should include other hypothetical health states. Rapid procedures seem, therefore, to result in less appropriate results.

There is no agreement on the role of health profiles in the context of describing health states. The GBD-study only applied bio-medically defined diagnostic labels, whereas the Dutch Study on Disability Weights has shown the importance of adding (EuroQol 5D+) functional descriptions to ease the valuation task of respondents [25]. We found that the provision of locally meaningful disability scenarios including locally designed illustrations was a necessity in the case of lay respondents. However, health professionals in our study found the descriptions somewhat approximate, which may explain the relatively large variation in their valuations compared to that of the panels of lay people.

The culturally adapted VAS instrument has been developed for the context of rural Burkina Faso to produce locally meaningful BOD estimates to foster local health policy. However, because of its explicit explorative nature, this study has only paid minor attention to the representativeness of its results to the overall population in Burkina Faso. Future research should include larger sample sizes and should assess as to what extent the study sample represents the overall population. Moreover, it should include a comprehensive list of health states in order to produce results that are useful for policy making. A further step should be to carry out more empirical studies to test whether the proposed methodology is feasible and applicable in other cultural contexts. If so, it would represent a critical advancement in acquiring BOD estimates that would be locally meaningful.

Acknowledgements

The authors are grateful to the staff from the Centre de Recherche en Santé de Nouna (CRSN) who provided many helpful comments throughout the study process. They would also like to thank Siaka Toé and Lassina Dao for their support during the interviews, Brian Anisoulard Fairman for his help in editing the paper, and two anonymous reviewers for their comments on earlier versions of this paper.

Copyright © 2002 John Wiley & Sons, Ltd.

References

1. Murray CJL, Lopez AD (eds). Global burden of disease and injury series. In *The Global Burden of Disease*, Vol 1. Harvard University Press: Boston, 1996.
2. James KC, Foster SD. Weighing up disability. *Lancet* 1999; **354**: 87.
3. Ustun TB, Rehm J, Chatterji S, Trotter R, Room R, Bickenbach J. Are disability valuations universal? Multiple-informant ranking of the disabling effects of different health conditions in 14 countries. *Lancet* 1999; **354**: 111–15.
4. Power M, Bullinger M, Harper A, WHOQOL Group. The World Health Organization WHO-QOL-100: Tests of the universality of quality of life in 15 different cultural groups worldwide. *Health Psychol* 1999; **18**: 495–505.
5. Murray CJL, Lopez AD. Progress and directions in refining the Global Burden of Disease approach: a response to Williams. *Health Econ* 2000; **9**: 69–82.
6. Sommerfeld J, Baltussen R, Metz L, Sanon M, Sauerborn R. Determinants of variance in health state valuations. Paper for WHO conference on Summary Measures on Population Health, Morocco, 2001.
7. Fox-Rushby J, Mwenesi H, Parker M, *et al.* Questioning premises: health-related quality of life in Kenya. *Qual Life Res* 1995; **4**: 428–429.
8. Amuyunzu M, Allen T, Mwenesi H, *et al.* The resonance of language: health terms in Kenya. *Qual Life Res* 1995; **4**: 388.
9. Kirigia JM. Economic evaluation in schistomiasis: valuation of health states preferences. *Health Econ* 1998; **7**: 551–556.
10. Sadana, R. A Closer Look at the WHO/World Bank Global Burden of Disease Study's Methodologies: how do poor women's values in a developing country compare with international experts? Invited paper at *Workshop on Reproductive Health & the Global Burden of Disease*, WHO Geneva, April 1998.
11. Brazier J, Deverill M. A checklist for judging preference-based measures of health related quality of life: learning from psychometrics. *Health Econ* 1999; **8**: 41–51.
12. Williams A. Calculating the global burden of disease: time for a strategic reappraisal? *Health Econ* 1999; **8**: 1–8.
13. Gold M, Siegel JE, Russell L, Weinstein M (eds). *Cost-effectiveness in health and medicine*. Oxford Publications: Oxford, 1996.
14. Torrance GW. Measurement of health utilities for economic appraisal: a review. *J Health Econ* 1986; **5**: 1–30.

15. Adam B. Values in the cultural timescapes of science. *Cultural Values* 1998; **2**: 385–402.
16. Bulmer M. Introduction: the problem of exporting social survey research. *Am Behavioral Sci* 1988; **42**: 153–167.
17. Stone L, Campbell JG. The use and misuse of surveys in international development: an experiment from Nepal. *Human Organ* 1984; **43**: 27–37.
18. Yu JH, Keown CF, Laurence W. Attitude scale methodology: cross-cultural applications. *J Int Consumer Market* 1993; **6**: 45–63.
19. Adelsward V, Sachs L. The meaning of 6.8: numeracy and normality in health information talks. *Soc Sci Med* 1996; **43**: 1179–1187.
20. Herdman M, Fox-Rushby J, Badia X. 'Equivalence' and the translation and adaptation of health-related quality of life questionnaires. *Qual Life Res* 1997; **6**: 237–247.
21. World Bank. *African Development Indicators 2000* World Bank: Washington, DC, 2000.
22. Institut National de la Statistique et de la Demographie. *Enquête Démographique et de Santé Burkina Faso 1998–1999, Rapport préliminaire*. Ministère de l'Economie et des Finances: Ouagadougou, 1999.
23. Würthwein R, Gbangou A, Sauerborn RS, Schmidt C. Measuring the local burden of disease. A study of years of life lost in Sub Saharan Africa. *Int J Epidemiol* 2001; **30**: 501–508.
24. Murray CJL. Rethinking DALYs. In *The Global Burden of Disease: A Comprehensive Assessment of Mortality and Disability from Disease, Injuries and Risk Factors in 1990 and Projected to 2020*, Murray CJL, Lopez AD (eds). Harvard University Press: Cambridge, 1996; 1–98.
25. Froberg DG, Kane RL, Methodology for measuring health-state preferences I–IV. *J Clin Epidemiol* 1989; **42**: 345–354, 459–471, 585–592, 675–685.
26. Stouthard MEA, Essink-Bot ML, Bonsel GJ, *et al*. *Disability Weights for Diseases in The Netherlands*. Department of Public Health, Erasmus University: Rotterdam, The Netherlands, 1997.
27. Shumaker SA, Berzon R (eds). *The International Assessment of Health-related Quality of Life: Theory Translation, Measurement and Analysis*. Rapid Communications: Oxford, 1995.

4.7 Gender's effect on willingness-to-pay for community-based insurance in Burkina Faso

Dong H, Kouyate B, Snow R, Mugisha F, sAuerborn R.

Health Policy 2003 May; 64(2): 153-62

Reprinted with permission from Elsevier Ireland Ltd.

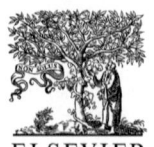

Gender's effect on willingness-to-pay for community-based insurance in Burkina Faso

Hengjin Dong [a,*], Bocar Kouyate [b], Rachel Snow [a], Frederick Mugisha [a], Rainer Sauerborn [a]

[a] *Department of Tropical Hygiene and Public Health, University of Heidelberg, Im Neuenheimer Feld 324, D-69120 Heidelberg, Germany*
[b] *Nouna Health Research Centre, Nouna, Burkina Faso*

Received 26 February 2002; accepted 30 July 2002

Abstract

The purpose was to study gender's effect on willingness-to-pay (WTP) for community-based insurance (CBI) in order to provide information for deciding enrolment unit and setting premium in Burkina Faso. A two-stage cluster sampling was used in the household survey, with each household having the same probability of being selected. One thousand one hundred and seventy-eight men and 1236 women in the 800 households were interviewed. The bidding game approach was used to elicit WTP. We found that compared to male, female had less education, lower income and expenditure, less episodes of diseases and lower ratio of becoming household head, but higher marriage rate. These characteristics influenced the WTP difference between men and women. Men were willing to pay 3666 CFA ($4.89) to join CBI, 928 CFA higher than women were. Education and economic status positively influenced WTP, implying higher years of schooling and economic status and higher WTP. Age and distance to health facility negatively influenced WTP, thus higher age and longer distance and less WTP. Based on the results from this study, we suggest that CBI should be enrolled on the basis of households or villages in order to protect vulnerable persons, such as the aged, women and the poor. In setting premium a policy-maker needs to take into account costs of the CBI benefits package, possible subsidies from government and other agencies and WTP information. WTP should never be taken as a premium because it only provides some information for the respondents' financial acceptability for a certain benefits package.
© 2002 Elsevier Science Ireland Ltd. All rights reserved.

Keywords: Willingness-to-pay; Contingent valuation method; Community-based insurance; Gender; Burkina Faso

1. Introduction

'Gender refers to women's and men's roles and responsibilities that are socially determined. Gender is related to how we are perceived and expected to think and act as women and men because of the way society is organised, not because of our biological differences' [1]. In the social and economic aspects, women are usually located primary responsibility for household and domestic labour—for the care of children, the elderly and the sick. Conversely, men are much more closely

* Corresponding author. Tel.: +49-6221-564689; fax: +49-6221-565948
E-mail address: donghengjin@yahoo.com (H. Dong).

identified with public world—with the activities of waged work and the rights and duties of citizenship [2]. Gender has been found to influence health, access to health care, quality of care, risks to get tropical infectious diseases, HIV/AIDS and other sexually transmitted diseases, violence and injuries [1]. Males are more exposed to malaria infection for occupational reasons [3]. At young ages, the prevalence of tuberculosis infection in boys and girls is similar, but a higher prevalence has been found in men of older ages [4]. More men than women are diagnosed with tuberculosis, however, women have longer delays in tuberculosis diagnosis [5,6]. Women vulnerability to HIV/AIDS has been recognised as being due to lack of knowledge and access to information, economic dependence and in many cases, forced sex [1].

Willingness-to-pay (WTP) is used to estimate utility in monetary terms. Economic theory argues that the maximum amount of money an individual is willing to pay for a commodity is an indicator of the utility or satisfaction to her of that commodity. WTP is one of the economic techniques for eliciting consumer preference. Recently WTP studies have been carried out in the various fields of health, including disease treatment, disease management, new medical technology, outcome evaluation of health care and health program, and the common used methods were the bidding game, the payment card and the take-it-or-leave-it [7,8].

Although there are many studies about gender and WTP in various areas of health and health care, there are no studies to combine gender and WTP together to identify the effect of gender on WTP in these areas. Even in the area of rural health insurance only two WTP studies have been carried out. In Ghana, a study used the bidding game method to interview five-member household heads and to assess the willingness of households (164 urban households and 142 rural households) in the informal sector to join and pay premiums for a proposed National Health Insurance scheme [9]. The study used sex as one independent variable in the multivariate analysis. But it did not describe the social and economic characteristics between sexes and did not analyse the WTP difference between sexes either. Thus the study could not provide information about the effect of gender.

Another study was done in India. The heads of 1000 households in rural area were asked directly which type of health insurance scheme they preferred and how much they were willing to pay for the chosen scheme [10]. This study did not consider the effect of sex in the multivariate analysis, so the same as the former study, it could not provide information about effect of gender on WTP.

Compared to other studies, the present study merged gender and WTP, focused on gender's effect on WTP for community-based insurance (CBI). Each household member aged 20 and more was asked WTP for him/herself. This study was carried out in rural Burkina Faso and described the characteristics of gender and quantitatively analysed the effect of gender on WTP by the indicator of WTP difference between male and female.

Our hypothesis was that WTP was related to individual preferences (utility) under certain specifications (theory of utility maximisation). An individual stating WTP of a certain amount or not is based on expected utility. If the expected utility to be derived from participating in the scheme at the stated premium is greater than the amount of the premium, an individual will opt to pay. In this context, it was assumed WTP would be affected by age, years of schooling, occupation and marital status. It would also be affected by relationship to household head, location of residency, economic and health status, and distance to health facility. The aged was expected to be willing to pay less; household head, higher income, higher education, urban people and people with poor health could be expected to be willing to pay more for the health insurance premium. Longer distance to health facility can reduce WTP.

This paper based on a WTP study for CBI in Nouna, Burkina Faso, which was a part of a larger project on the control of tropical infectious diseases. Burkina Faso has an estimated population of approximately 10.7 millions [11]. This small West African country is divided into 11 administrative health regions, which comprise 53 health districts overall, each covering a population of 200 000–300 000 individuals. Each health district has at least one hospital with surgical facilities [12].

The districts themselves are again sub-divided into smaller areas of responsibility that are organised around either a hospital or a so-called Centre de Santé et de Promotion Sociale (CSPS), the first-line health care facility in the health system. The Nouna health district, located in the Northwest of Burkina Faso, has a population of roughly 230 thousand inhabitants who are served by one district hospital and 16 CSPS.

2. Methods

2.1. Sampling procedure and sample size

The household survey, which was conducted by the project of control of tropical infectious diseases, was based on a two-stage cluster sampling procedure, with each household having the same probability of being selected. In the first stage, clusters of households were selected and in the second stage, respondent households were selected in each cluster. Overall, 800 households were selected, 480 in the rural area and 320 in the town of Nouna [13]. We used this sample and merged WTP questions into the regular household survey questionnaire. The data were collected in February 2001.

Out of the 800 households randomly selected, 776 were considered in the analysis (22 emigrated and 2 missed). In the 776 households, there were 2670 persons aged between 20 and 70. Two thousand four hundred and fourteen of them answered the WTP questions (4 refusal and 252 absentees). The response rate was 88.9% for women and 91.9% for men. There were no significant differences between the responders and non-responders in the location of residency, religion, occupation and years of schooling [14].

2.2. Household interview

The household interview and the process of eliciting WTP are described in detail in the paper of WTP study [14]. Each household member aged between 20 and 70 was randomly assigned one of 13 starting prices drawn from a range from 2000 to 8000 Franc CFA determined by pre-testing ($1 = 750 CFA). Interviewers first explained the CBI scenario to all eligible members of the household together. Then each eligible member of the household was asked for his or her own WTP by the approach of bidding game.

If the answer to the first price offered to the respondent was 'yes', the interviewer increased the bid by increments of 500 CFA until the respondent said 'no'. If the initial answer was 'no', the interviewer reduced the amount of money by 500 CFA and continued this process until the respondent said 'yes'. The last sum of money receiving a 'yes' response was used as the WTP resulting from the bidding game approach (bidding result).

2.3. Indicators and data analysis methods

We use male WTP to describe the value that a man is willing to pay for himself for CBI, and female WTP to describe the value that a woman is willing to pay for herself for the insurance. WTP difference equals male WTP minus female WTP.

Mean WTP was estimated directly from the data provided. Linear multiple regression was used to study the influence of independent variables on WTP. In the regression, WTP (bidding result) was taken as the dependent variable, individual demographic, socio-economic and other characteristics were taken as the explanatory variables. The empirical model is as follows:

$$WTP = \alpha + \beta_1 X_1 + \beta_2 X_2 + \ldots + \beta_{n-1} X_{n-1} + \beta_n X_n$$

where WTP, willingness-to-pay; α, intercept; β, coefficients of explanatory variables; X, explanatory variables.

The explanatory variables were selected based on the study hypotheses. We first considered the individual characteristics, such as age, education, religion, occupation, relation to household head, location of residency and health status. We then considered income and expenditure and last the convenience of getting health care by the variable of distance to a health facility. Episodes of diseases for the individual over three rounds of the survey were taken as the health status variable. In the project 'control of tropical infectious diseases', we have already done three waves of household surveys on the same households over 9 months.

This allowed us to add the episodes of diseases together and obtain a better health status indicator than can be obtained from only one survey. Table 1 lists the explanatory variables used in the linear regression models.

Normality of variables was tested. Income and expenditure were skewed and therefore transformed using logarithmic transformation ($x = \log(X+1)$). Outliers were considered. Outliers were excluded from the model if the studentized residuals greater than |3| [15].

3. Results

3.1. Gender characteristics

Compared to male, female had significantly lower education, farmer occupation, income, expenditure, episodes of diseases and lower ratio of becoming household head, but higher marriage rate. There were no significant differences between sexes in the aspects of age, location of residency, religion, distance to health facility and the first bid (Table 1). All significant differences between men and women came from social factors; thus implying that gender would be responsible for the gap between men and women in the WTP for CBI. Gender is the social construction of roles of men and women as mentioned before.

3.2. Willingness-to-pay by gender

We found that men were willing to pay 3666 CFA for CBI, 928 CFA more than women. Age is one of the factors that influence WTP, the aged were willing to pay less than the young. But the WTP difference between men and women was not a result of age because there was no age difference between sexes and in each age group men were willing to pay more than women (Table 2). The WTP difference between men and women varied as the cumulative ratio of bidding results changed from 0 to 100% (Fig. 1). The WTP difference is 0

Table 1
Description of explanatory variables for linear regression model and individual and other characteristics by sex

Variable name	Description	Mean			P^a
		Total ($n = 2414$)	Male ($n = 1178$)	Female ($n = 1236$)	
Individual characteristics					
Age	Age in years	39	39.41	38.61	>0.05
Single	Marital status: single = 1, else = 0	0.117	0.199	0.039	<0.001
Famihead	Household head = 1, other = 0	0.290	0.538	0.053	<0.001
Ani	Religion: traditional religion = 1, else = 0	0.085	0.094	0.076	>0.05
Occuagr	farmer = 1, other = 0	0.746	0.853	0.644	<0.001
Nouna	Location of residency, Nouna town = 1, else = 0	0.332	0.327	0.337	>0.05
Readwrit	Can read or write = 1, other = 0	0.221	0.343	0.104	<0.001
Educatio	Years of schooling	0.80	1.10	0.51	<0.001
Diseasei	Episodes of diseases of individual in 3 surveys	0.36	0.40	0.33	<0.05
Logicsh6	Individual cash income from 6 month, log 10	2.906	3.512	2.328	<0.001
Logianim	Individual animal value, log 10	2.412	3.217	1.647	<0.001
Logiexp6	Individual expenditure for 6 month, log 10	3.257	3.805	2.734	<0.001
Other characteristics					
Distance	Distance to health facility (km)	4.19	4.27	4.11	>0.05
Prixdepart	The first bid	4968	5002	4935	>0.05

[a] t-Test for age, educatio, diseasei, logicsh6, logianim, logiexp6, distance and prixdepart. χ^2-Test for single, famihead, ani, occuagr, nouna and readwrit.

Table 2
Individual WTP (CFA[a]) by sex

Variables	WTP (n)			WTP difference[b]	P[c]
	Total	Male	Female		
Total	3191 (2414)	3666 (1178)	2738 (1236)	928	<0.001
Age					
20–34	3463 (1106)	3829 (543)	3109 (563)	720	=0.01
35–49	3357 (692)	3863 (328)	2900 (364)	963	<0.001
50–64	2680 (444)	3447 (207)	2009 (237)	1438	<0.001
65+	2099 (172)	2587 (100)	1420 (72)	1167	<0.001
Marital status					
Married	3186 (2131)	3840 (943)	2666 (1188)	1174	<0.001
Single	3232 (283)	2970 (235)	4515 (48)	−1545	<0.05
Household head					
Yes	3570 (700)	3668 (634)	2626 (66)	1042	<0.05
No	3036 (1714)	3664 (544)	2745 (1170)	919	<0.001
Religion					
Traditional	4191 (205)	4715 (111)	3571 (94)	1144	<0.05
Others	3098 (2209)	3557 (1067)	2670 (1142)	887	<0.001
Occupation					
Farmer	3301 (1801)	3733 (1005)	2756 (796)	977	<0.001
Others	2867 (613)	3277 (173)	2706 (440)	571	<0.05
Location of residency					
Nouna town	2976 (802)	3232 (385)	2740 (417)	492	=0.004
Rural area	3298 (1612)	3877 (793)	2737 (819)	1140	<0.001
Read or write					
Yes	3995 (533)	4069 (404)	3764 (129)	305	>0.05
No	2963 (1881)	3456 (774)	2619 (1107)	837	<0.001

[a] US$1 = 750 CFA.
[b] WTP difference = male WTP−female WTP.
[c] t-test for WTP difference.

at 100% of the cumulative ration, about 600 CFA at 65%, about 1000 CFA at 50%, etc. Cumulative ratio of bidding results can reflect the relationship between premium and enrolment level of insurance.

Married men were willing to pay more than married women were, but unmarried women were willing to pay more than unmarried men (Table 2). This contrary result cannot change the general WTP result (men were willing to pay more than women were) because of the high marriage rate. Marriage rate for men was 80.1% and for women 96.1% (Table 1). If the men's marriage rate reached the level of women's, man in general would be willing to pay even more than woman would because married man was willing to pay more than unmarried one, implying marital status composition influences the WTP difference between men and women.

Table 2 shows us that male heads of household were willing to pay 1042 CFA more than female heads. Other males were willing to pay more than other females also, but with 919 CFA WTP difference, less than the difference between male heads and female heads.

Religion may be another factor to influence WTP. Compared to these who have no specific religions (traditional), others (such as Muslim, Christian) had relatively lower WTP for themselves (Table 2). This situation is same in male

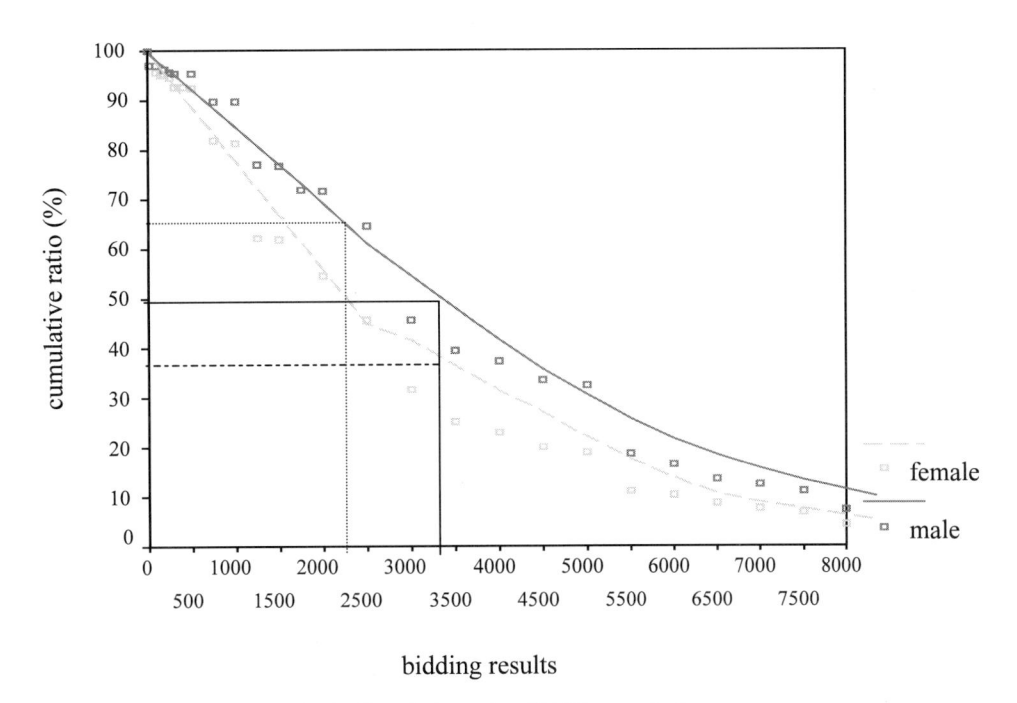

Fig. 1. Cumulative ratio of bidding results by sex.

group and female group. But men were willing to pay more than women regardless of religion. However, there was not significant difference in the composition of religions between men and women (Table 1), religion may not be the cause of WTP difference between males and females. The result of location of residency was similar to result of religious status, so the location of residency is also not the factor to influence WTP difference (Table 2).

Occupation is also an important factor to influence WTP because occupation is related to income level in most societies. We found that there were differences in WTP between occupation groups and also between male and female (Table 2). Considering the different composition of occupations between men and women (Table 1), the WTP difference in general between male and female may be affected by the occupation factor.

It is interesting to know that there was no significant difference in WTP between men and women if they could write or read, but there was significant difference if they could not (Table 2). This means that education is one factor that influences WTP and also one factor that influences WTP difference between male and female because we found that males got more years of schooling education than females in this study (Table 1).

3.3. Multivariate analysis

Many factors can influence the WTP difference between male and female. We have already described the effects of age, marital status, relationship to household head, religion, occupation, location of residency and education on WTP and WTP difference factor by factor. But the danger of single factor analysis is that when analysing the effect of one factor we cannot control the effects of other factors. Multivariate analysis can show the effect of each factor by controlling other factors. Table 3 shows the results of the multiple linear regression analysis.

There were some differences in the factors that statistically significantly influenced male and female WTP. Being single marital state significantly influenced male WTP but not female. It had unexpected negative signs, and the result was opposite to the result from single factor analysis for female WTP. Unmarried women had higher

Table 3
Coefficients of multiple linear regression for individual WTP by sex

Variables	Male WTP			Female WTP		
	B	S.E.	β	B	S.E.	β
(Constant)	1970.500*	487.041		2392.953*	309.925	
Age	−24.677*	6.772	−0.144	−27.578*	4.663	−0.177
Single	−551.831**	228.733	−0.083	−55.493	347.701	−0.005
Famihead	157.806	207.935	0.030	−225.152	294.666	−0.023
Ani	1031.892*	257.547	0.113	651.024*	233.649	0.077
Occuagr	75.681	232.675	0.010	−306.754**	144.181	−0.066
Nouna	−530.493*	204.069	−0.094	−140.629	172.720	−0.030
Educatio	75.511**	30.747	0.076	68.225	38.551	0.054
Diseasei	−5.336	103.779	−0.001	−63.555	93.039	−0.019
Logicsh6	100.470**	43.312	0.076	92.867*	33.955	0.086
Logianim	61.094	37.133	0.053	108.788*	30.710	0.101
Logiexp6	196.358*	58.417	0.117	135.939*	39.227	0.112
Distance	−54.127*	16.790	−0.109	−55.853*	13.640	−0.136
First bid	0.267*	0.039	0.187	0.172*	0.032	0.145
n	1171			1222		
F value	14.015*			13.042*		
R^2	0.136			0.123		
Std. Residual mean (S.D.)	0.000 (0.994)			0.000 (0.995)		

* $P < 0.01$.
** $P < 0.05$.

WTP than married. Education significantly influenced male WTP but not female. It, however, had the expected positive signs, higher education and higher WTP. Being a farmer did not significantly influence male WTP but it did female. Furthermore, the coefficient signs were opposite each other, positive to male and negative to female. Staying in Nouna town had an unexpected negative sign and significantly influenced male WTP but not female. Although potential value of animals had the expected positive signs for both male and female, it significantly influenced female WTP but not male one.

Both age and distance to health facility had the expected negative signs and significantly influenced both male and female WTP. However, from both values of the standardised coefficients (β) we found that female was higher than male, thus both of the factors influencing female WTP relatively stronger than male. Income and expenditure are economic indicators. They had the expected positive signs and significantly influenced both male and female WTP. Income influenced female WTP relatively stronger than male. On the contrary, expenditure influenced male WTP little stronger. Traditional religion positively influenced male and female WTP. But it influenced male WTP stronger than female WTP.

The first bid positively influenced male and female WTP, thus the starting point bias existing in both WTP estimations. Male WTP had more starting point bias than female WTP by the indication of β value.

4. Discussion

It is clear that gender is a central factor in understanding the WTP difference between male and female because we found that women had less education, lower income and higher marriage rate which were the main factors to influence WTP in this study. Other factors can also influence WTP, such as age, location of residency, distance to health facility and the first bid, but we found that there were no significant differences between men and women in this study.

Traditional African societies, there was and there still is division of labour where by women take care of household activities, subsistence agriculture, reproduction and mothering. Men are the breadwinners, tend to grow cash crops which are harvested at specific times during the year and bring in relatively large sums of money, and have greater access than women to off-farm employment. By contrast, women mainly depend on the sale of food crops that bring in small amounts of income through the year. The man's role as provider gives him control over family income and many of the major decisions [16,17]. Owing to the fact that education is associated with expectation of high incomes, a family with limited resources will take a son to school first because the daughter will get married and her roles do not necessarily require one to go to school—thus the low education observed for women.

In the study, women were found to have high marriage rates than their male counterparts. This still has to do with both the fact that women are less likely to have higher education and the fact their roles seem not to require them to stay longer as singles to acquire the skills. As such, women tend to marry when the are young and in effect, the difference is a result of different ages at marriage—women young than for men. The tend to marry young also because of the fact that their marriage is usually associated with bride price that is usually a source of income for the girl's family.

These social roles between sexes make the differences in occupation and also in income between men and women. Income and expenditure are related to ability-to-pay. Many studies have reported that WTP is positive correlation with ability-to-pay [9,18–22]. Occupation is related to income and further related to WTP. We found men earned more than women, thus resulting in the difference of WTP between them did. In this study we also found that farmer occupation negatively significantly influenced female WTP, but positively influenced male WTP although not significant. This implies that men and women may grow different crops or different acreage, resulting in different levels of income; or implies that women can obtain more income if they do not work as farmers.

Illiteracy rate is high in Burkina Faso. The female illiteracy rate is higher than male. We found that the rate of ability to read or write was 34.3% for men and 10.4% for women. Average years of schooling were 1.10 for men and 0.51 for women. Educated people may have higher income or may understand the importance of insurance more thoroughly, and put more utilities to insurance. Thus the different composition of educational levels between men and women can result in their difference in WTP.

Unmarried women were willing to pay more than unmarried men did. It is difficult to explain the reasons because we found that there were no significant differences in age and in income between them. Unmarried women maybe put more utilities for health than unmarried men do, or unmarried men were willing to pay more for other activities than for health.

The value of standardised coefficient (β) shows that the first bid has strong positive correlation with female and male WTP, thus implying that start point bias exists in the results. The danger of starting point bias is the main problem with the bidding game technique. Many studies showed that this bias existed because WTP differed markedly between different sub-samples [21–27]. For instance, Kartman et al. found that individuals were willing to pay double for the highest starting-bid group than for the lowest [22].

The purpose of WTP for CBI study is to provide information to the decision-makers about people's financial acceptability for the insurance scheme. When introducing CBI the decision-makers need to take into account the cost of the scheme, and WTP in general and also in different subgroups, such as male or female, high or middle or low income levels, young or middle age or the aged. These kinds of information can help decision-makers to set insurance premium and deciding enrolment unit.

Our study suggests that men are willing to pay more then women, the old pays less than the young, and the poor pays less than the rich. If enrolment in CBI were on the basis of individuals, young men with high income would have higher enrolment rate. For example, if the premium was set at the male 50% cumulative ratio level, the enrolment rate for men would be 50%, but for women only about 36%. If it was set at the level of female 50% cumulative ratio, the enrolment rate for women would be 50%; however for men it would be 65% (Fig. 1). In order to protect the poor, the old and women we suggest CBI should be enrolled on the basis of household or village.

WTP can provide information for setting insurance premium but its value should not be as the premium. Usually a CBI premium is based on the costs of the benefits package and shaped by subsidies from government or other agencies. If the WTP is higher than this premium, the CBI can be operated smoothly. But if the WTP is lower than this premium, the CBI cannot be operated smoothly and needs more subsidies. Otherwise the benefits package has to be changed.

While setting premium the WTP difference between a real market and a theoretical one should been taken into account also. WTP is the value elicited in the hypothetical market. It reflects people's stated preference for a hypothetical commodity or service, but not revealed preference. Revealed preference can be obtained in the real market if the commodity or service exists in the market, but for a hypothetical commodity or service the revealed preference is usually absent.

5. Conclusion

The gender characteristics in Burkina Faso are that female, compared to male, has less education, farmer occupation, lower income, expenditure, less episodes of diseases and lower ratio of becoming household head, but higher marriage rate. These characteristics influence the WTP for CBI between men and women. A decision-maker needs to take into account the gender difference in WTP in deciding the enrolment unit and in setting premium of CBI. Based on the results from this study, we suggest that CBI should be enrolled on the basis of households or villages in order to protect vulnerable persons, such as the aged, women and the poor. In setting premium a policy-maker needs to take into account costs of the CBI benefits package, possible subsidies from government and other agencies and WTP information. WTP should never be taken as a premium because it only provides some information for the respondents' financial acceptability for a certain benefits package.

Acknowledgements

This paper is one of the results of 'control of tropical infectious diseases' project in Burkina Faso financially supported by Germany Research Foundation (Deutsche Forschungsgemeinschaft) (SFB 544). It is acknowledged that in the data collection we obtained valuable help from Sanou Aboubakary, Adjima Gbangou, Yazoumé Yé and Mamadou Sanon from Nouna Health Research Centre. We are also grateful to Vinod Diwan in IHCAR, Karolinska Institute for valuable comments and suggestions.

References

[1] WHO. Gender and Health: technical paper. Geneva: World Health Organization; 1998.
[2] Doyal L. Sex, gender and health: a preliminary conceptual framework. In: Diwan VK, Thorson A, Winkvist A, editors. Gender and health. Goteborg: The Nordic School of Public Health, 1998:17–27.
[3] Sims J. Women, health and environment: an anthology. Geneva: World Health Organization, 1994.
[4] Holmes CB, Hausler H, Nunn P. A review of sex differences in the epidemiology of tuberculosis. The International Journal of Tuberculosis and Lung Disease 1998;2:96–104.
[5] Diwan VK, Thorson A. Sex, gender, and tuberculosis. Lancet 1999;353:1000–1.
[6] Long NH, et al. Longer delays in tuberculosis diagnosis among women in Vietnam. The International Journal of Tuberculosis and Lung Disease 1999;3:388–93.
[7] Diener A, O'Brien B, Gafni A. Health care contingent valuation studies: a review and classification of the literature. Health Economics 1998;7:313–26.
[8] Klose T. The contingent valuation method in health care. Health Policy 1999;47:97–123.
[9] Asenso-Okyere WK, Osei-Akoto I, Anum A, Appiah EN. Willingness to pay for health insurance in a developing economy. A pilot study of the informal sector of Ghana using contingent valuation. Health Policy 1997;42:223–37.

[10] Mathiyazhagan K. Willingness to pay for rural health insurance through community participation in India. The International Journal of Health Planning and Management 1998;13:47–67.
[11] World Bank. African Development Indicators 2000. Washington, DC: World Bank, 2000.
[12] Burkina Faso Ministry of health. Statistiques Sanitaires 1996. Ouagadougou: Burkina Faso Ministry of health, 1996.
[13] Wuertwein R, et al. The Nouna health district household survey: design and implementation. SFB Discussion Series 2001;3:1–51. Available from http://www.hyg.uni-heidelberg.de/sfb544/neues.htm.
[14] Dong H, Kouyate B, Sauerborn R. Willingness to pay for community-based insurance in Burkina Faso. SFB Discussion Series 2001;4:1–26. Available from http://www.hyg.uni-heidelberg.de/sfb544/neues.htm.
[15] Scott M. Applied logistic regression analysis. California: Sage Publications Inc, 1995.
[16] David S. Health expenditure and household budgets in rural Liberia. Health Transition Review 1993;3:57–76.
[17] Gysels M, Pool R, Nnalusiba B. Women who sell sex in a Ugandan trading town: life histories, survival strategies and risk. Social Science and Medicine 2002;54:179–92.
[18] Chiu L, Tang KY, Liu YH, Shyu WC, Chang TP. Willingness of families caring for victims of dementia to pay for nursing home care: results of a pilot study in Taiwan. Journal of Management in Medicine 1998;12(321):349–60.
[19] Chiu L, Tang KY, Shyu WC, Chang TP. The willingness of families caring for victims of stroke to pay for in-home respite care—results of a pilot study in Taiwan. Health Policy 1999;46:239–54.
[20] Cho MN, Lertmaharit S, Kamol-Ratanakul P, Saul AJ. Ex post and ex ante willingness to pay (WTP) for the ICT Malaria Pf/Pv test kit in Myanmar. Southeast Asian Journal of Tropical Medicine and Public Health 2000;31:104–11.
[21] Chestnut LG, Keller LR, Lambert WE, Rowe RD. Measuring heart patients' willingness to pay for changes in angina symptoms. Medical Decision Making 1996;16:65–77.
[22] Kartman B, Andersson F, Johannesson M. Willingness to pay for reductions in angina pectoris attacks. Medical Decision Making 1996;16:248–53.
[23] Bala MV, et al. Valuing outcomes in health care: a comparison of willingness to pay and quality-adjusted life-years. Journal of Clinical Epidemiology 1998;51:667–76.
[24] Barner JC, Mason HL, Murray MD. Assessment of asthma patients' willingness to pay for and give time to an asthma self-management program. Clinical Therapy 1999;21:878–94.
[25] Liu JT, Hammitt JK, Wang JD, Liu JL. Mother's willingness to pay for her own and her child's health: a contingent valuation study in Taiwan. Health Economics 2000;9:319–26.
[26] Phillips KA, et al. Willingness to pay for poison control centers. Journal of Health Economics 1997;16:343–57.
[27] Stalhammar NO. An empirical note on willingness to pay and starting-point bias. Medical Decision Making 1996;16:242–7.

4.8 A comparison of the reliability of the take-it-or-leave-it and the bidding game approaches to estimating willingness-to-pay in a rural population in West Africa

Dong H, Kouyate B, Cairns J, Sauerborn R.

Soc Sci Med. 2003 May;56(10):2181-9

Reprinted with permission from Elsevier.

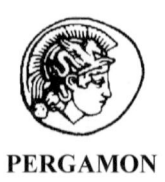

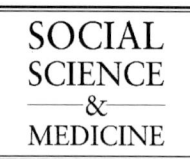

# A comparison of the reliability of the take-it-or-leave-it and the bidding game approaches to estimating willingness-to-pay in a rural population in West Africa

Hengjin Dong[a,]*, Bocar Kouyate[b], John Cairns[c], Rainer Sauerborn[a]

[a] *Department of Tropical Hygiene and Public Health, University of Heidelberg, Im Neuenheimer Feld 324, D-69120 Heidelberg, Germany*
[b] *Nouna Health Research Center, Nouna, Burkina Faso*
[c] *Health Economics Research Unit, University of Aberdeen, Aberdeen AB25 2ZD, Scotland, UK*

Abstract

The test–retest reliability of the bidding game and the take-it-or-leave-it (TIOLI) approaches to eliciting willingness-to-pay (WTP) are compared. A random sample of households in the Nouna area of Burkina Faso were interviewed twice with an interval of around 4–5 weeks. One thousand one hundred and eight individuals were asked their individual WTP for community-based health insurance. Three hundred and forty eight of these individuals were household heads who were in addition asked about their WTP for health insurance for the whole household. Median and the mean WTP were higher in the test than in the retest. Despite these differences both methods displayed moderate to good reliability (kappa values ranged from 0.467 to 0.621, Spearman correlations ranged from 0.653 to 0.701 and Pearson correlations ranged from 0.593 to 0.675). There was some evidence that the bidding game was more reliable than the TIOLI method. This study is based on larger sample size than previous studies and also is one of the first studies of the reliability of WTP in a developing country.
© 2002 Elsevier Science Ltd. All rights reserved.

Keywords: Willingness-to-pay; Contingent valuation method; Reliability; Community-based insurance; Burkina Faso

Introduction

Willingness-to-pay (WTP) studies are being increasingly undertaken in the field of health care (Diener, O'Brien, & Gafni, 1998; Klose, 1999). Most of these studies have been carried out in Western countries, but a number have been undertaken in developing countries. For example, a study in Ghana estimated the WTP to join a proposed national health insurance scheme (Asenso-Okyere, Osei-Akoto, Anum, & Appiah, 1997). There have been studies of WTP for district hospital services in rural Tanzania (Walraven, 1996), for injectable contraceptives in Egypt (Hassan, el Nahal, & el Hussein, 1994), for annual retreatment of mosquito nets with insecticide in Nigeria (Onwujekwe, Shu, Chima, Onyido, & Okonkwo, 2000), for quality improvements at government health facilities in the Central African Republic (Weaver et al., 1996), and for a rural health insurance scheme in India (Mathiyazhagan, 1998).

If contingent valuation is to inform decision making, valid and reliable methods of eliciting WTP are required. The reliability of an instrument can be assessed by asking a group of individuals the same questions at two points in time and by comparing their responses. After searching literature from Medline by the key word of 'reliability' and literature published in relevant health economics meetings we found since 1979 only eight test–retest reliability studies have been published in the health care or health related area. Most of them have investigated the reliability of the bidding game and open-ended question approaches by the correlation between test and retest responses. Only one study tested

*Corresponding author. Fax: +49-6221-565948.
E-mail address: donghengjin@yahoo.com (H. Dong).

Table 1
Summary of the results from the past test–retest reliability studies

Authors	Publication year	Country of study	Study area	Elicitation methods	Sample size for retest	Interval between test and retest	Statistical methods for reliability test	Value of statistic
Loehman et al.	1979	USA	Avoiding respiratory diseases	Open-ended question	47	3 weeks	Correlation	0.82–0.95*
Thompson et al.	1984	USA	Chronic arthritis	Open-ended question	49	Entry and exit	Correlation	0.25
Jones-Lee et al.	1985	UK	Safety	Open-ended question	210	1 month	Wilcoxon matched-pairs, signed-ranks test	No value provided**
Whittington et al.	1992	Nigeria	Drinking water (public taps)	Bidding game	166	1–2 days	% of agreement	84%
			Drinking water (private connection)	Bidding game	162	1–2 days	% of agreement	80%
O'Brien et al.	1994	Canada	Chronic lung disease	Bidding game	20	4 weeks	Correlation	0.66*
Flower et al.	1997	USA	Buying insurance for treating moderate Gaucher disease	Bidding game	52	2 weeks	Correlation	0.796*
Cho et al.	2000	Myanmar	Malaria test kit (ex post)	Bidding game	30	3 weeks	Correlation	0.78–0.9*
			Malaria test kit (ex ante)	Bidding game	30	3 weeks	Correlation	0.7–0.86*
Onwujekwe et al.	2001	Nigeria	Insecticide-treated nets	Bidding game	146	1 month	Correlation	0.34–0.51*
				TIOLI + FU***	161	1 month	Correlation	0.41–0.52*
				Haggling	139	1 month	Correlation	0.33–0.56*

*$p < 0.01$.

**$p > 0.05$ in the Wilcoxon matched-pairs, signed-ranks test means that there is no statistically significant difference in the ranks between test and retest, thus meaning the results (ranks) between test and retest are same.

***Take-it-or-leave-it with open-ended follow-up method.

the reliability of take-it-or-leave-it (TIOLI) with open-ended follow-up method. Like the bidding game and open-ended question methods, this method results in continuous data (Table 1). Five of the eight studies were carried out in high-income countries (three in USA, one in UK and one in Canada); three studies were in low-income countries (two in Nigeria and one in Myanmar). For the reliability of the bidding game, the correlation ranged 0.66–0.796 in high-income countries, 0.34–0.9 in low-income countries. It seems that the reliability of the bidding game in high-income countries is more stable than in low-income countries although there have not been enough studies undertaken to make a conclusion. There has been no information to show the reliability of TIOLI method in these previous studies. Nearly all correlation tests were statistically significant at the level of 0.01 and the correlation was positive, thus meaning that the higher the WTP in the test (the first interview) was and the higher the WTP in the retest (the second interview) would be. But the correlation was not statistically significant in the study reported by Thompson, Read, and Liang (1984). All of these studies have been conducted with relatively small numbers of respondents.

Compared with the above studies, the present study used a large sample size to test the reliability of WTP elicitation methods in the field of community-based health insurance (CBI). This is unique not only in low-income countries but also in high-income countries. The aim of this study is to assess the reliability of the bidding game and the TIOLI methods of eliciting WTP by a test–retest experiment. In addition, we compare the reliabilities of the two methods in order to know which one is more reliable. This study forms part of a project to measure WTP for community-based health insurance in the Nouna area of Burkina Faso.

The aims of the overall WTP study are to examine the willingness to pay for CBI and identify the likelihood of individuals and households opting out of the insurance scheme based on the two elicitation methods. One month before the survey was implemented a pre-test was carried out at study site. The TIOLI, the bidding game, and the payment card methods were tested. During the process, we found it was inappropriate to use the payment card because of the high illiteracy rate. We therefore decided to use the bidding game and the TIOLI. One week before the survey, a three-day workshop and a pilot study were organised. Questionnaire was used in the household interviews. The interviewers came from local areas and spoke local language as the interviewees, had middle school education, and obtained interview experiences in the former household surveys (Dong, Kouyate, & Sauerborn, 2001).

Methodology

Study site

Burkina Faso has an estimated population of approximately 10.7 millions (World Bank, 2000), is divided into 11 administrative health regions, which comprise 53 health districts overall, each covering a population of 200,000–300,000 individuals. Each health district has at least one hospital with surgical facilities (Burkina Faso Ministry of Health, 1996). The districts themselves are again sub-divided into smaller areas of responsibility that are organised around either a hospital or a so-called Centre de Santé et de Promotion Sociale (CSPS), the first-line health care facility in the health system.

Our study population, the Nouna health district, has roughly 230,000 inhabitants who are served by one district hospital and 16 CSPS. This district is located in the Northwest of Burkina Faso, about 300 km from the capital Ouagadougou. The Nouna area is a dry orchard Savannah, populated almost exclusively by subsistence farmers of different ethnic groups. The capital of province Kossi, Nouna town, is not a well-developed city, but it is a provincial economic and political centre. There is better transportation and health facilities are more conveniently located than in the rural areas. The people living in Nouna town have relatively higher education, higher income and shorter distance to health facilities compared to those living in rural areas.

Sampling and sample size

In the household survey of the wider project, a two-stage cluster sampling procedure was used, with each household having the same probability of being selected. In the first stage, clusters of households were selected and in the second stage, respondent households were selected in each cluster. Eight hundred households were selected in total, 480 in the rural area and 320 in the town of Nouna (Wuertwein et al., 2001). Four hundred households were randomly selected for the WTP test–retest reliability study. The data were collected during January and March 2001.

Household interview

The WTP questionnaire included a detailed description of the CBI, questions eliciting the respondents' WTP for the CBI, and questions about respondents' characteristics. The questionnaire was translated into the local language. Identification of household members was obtained from demographic surveillance system (DSS) and was pre-printed on the questionnaire. The DSS is a census of the entire Nouna area, which is carried out every 2 years, with vital events registrations carried out every 3 months since 1992 (Sankoh, Ye, Sauerborn, Muller, & Becher, 2001).

Each household member (including household head) aged 20–70 was randomly assigned one of the 13 starting prices for her/him. The starting prices were drawn from a range from 2000 to 8000 Franc CFA determined by pre-testing. Each household head was randomly assigned another set of 13 starting prices for the whole household from 8000 to 32,000 Franc CFA ($1 = 750 CFA). Interviewers first explained the community-based health insurance scenario to the head and all members of the household aged 20–70 together. Then the head of household was asked his/her WTP for him/her and for the whole household. Lastly, other members of the household were asked for their own WTP. In this paper, individual WTP describes the value that an individual is willing to pay for himself or herself for community-based health insurance, and household WTP describes the value that the head of household is willing to pay for health insurance for his or her whole household.

The yes/no answer to the first price offered to the respondent provided the data for the TIOLI. If the answer was 'yes', the interviewer increased the bid by increments of 500 CFA until the respondent said 'no'. If the initial answer was 'no', the interviewer reduced the amount of money by 500 CFA and continued this process until the respondent said 'yes'. The last sum of money receiving a 'yes' response was used as the WTP resulting from the bidding game approach.

The interval between the first interview (test) and the second interview (retest) was between 4 and 5 weeks. The starting prices at the second interview were exactly the same as at the first interview for each individual and each household was interviewed on both occasions by the same interviewer.

Mean and median calculation

The TIOLI results in discrete (yes/no) data and the bidding game results in continuous data. For the continuous data, based on the principles of statistics, the mean WTP was estimated directly from the data provided and the mean difference between the first and second interviews was evaluated using a t-test for paired-samples. Independent-samples t-test or one-way ANOVA were used for testing the mean difference in sub-groups, e.g., sex, location of residency, household size, etc. For the discrete (yes/no) data a non-parametric method was used to estimate the median WTP. In the reliability study, the main interest is the agreement between the first interview and the second interview in the average level and individual level. Mean and median are the common statistics to reflect the average level.

Measure of agreement between test and retest

Kappa and the proportion of responses that agreed between test and retest are the common statistics to measure the agreement for the yes/no data. Pearson and Spearman correlation coefficients are the common statistics to measure the agreement for continuous data (Altman, 1996). In this study, we used kappa and the proportion of responses to measure the agreement for the yes/no data generated by the TIOLI. We used Pearson and Spearman correlation coefficients to measure the agreement between test and retest for the continuous data generated by the bidding game. There is not a specific value of correlation coefficient above which a study is considered reliable. However, the nearer to 1 the value and the more reliable a study. In order to facilitate a comparison of the reliability of the TIOLI and the bidding game methods, the bidding responses were transformed into yes/no responses by randomly assigning a TIOLI price to each respondent (using the vector of TIOLI prices). The agreement for this artificial yes/no data between test and retest was measured by kappa in order to compare the reliability of the two methods. Kappa ranges from –1.00 to 1.00. A value of 1.00 indicates perfect agreement, a value of zero indicates no agreement better than chance, and negative values show worse than chance agreement. The strength of agreement has been defined as poor (kappa value <0.21), fair (0.21–0.40), moderate (0.41–0.60), good (0.61–0.80) and very good (0.81–1.00) (Altman, 1996).

Results

General characteristics of individuals and households

Of the 400 households randomly selected for retest, 18 were found to have emigrated. In the remaining 382 households, there were 1284 persons aged between 20 and 70 years. The WTP of each individual was elicited using both the TIOLI and the bidding game. In the first stage 1181 persons answered the questions. One hundred and three persons did not answer the questions, of these two refused to answer the questions and 101 were not present on any of the three visits. In the second stage, 1143 persons answered the questions and 141 were not present at any of the three visits. Test–retest data are available for 1108 persons because 73 answered the WTP questions in the test but were not present at the retest and 35 persons were not present at the test but answered the questions in the retest. The response rate for test and retest was 86.3%. The individual characteristics are described in Table 2.

Heads of households were in addition asked about their WTP for health insurance for their whole households. In the 382 households, 356 household heads answered the household WTP questions in the first stage, one person refused to answer the questions and 25 were not present after three visits. Three hundred and fifty eight household heads answered the questions in the second stage and 24 were not present after three visits. Test–retest data are available for 348 household heads since eight answered the WTP questions in the test but were not present in the retest and 10 were not present at the test but answered the questions at the retest. This represents a response rate of 91.1%. The household characteristics are described in Table 2.

Differences in median and mean WTP between test and retest

The median WTP (elicited by the TIOLI method) and mean WTP (elicited by the bidding game approach) are both higher in the test than in the retest (Table 3). For individual WTP, the difference in the median was 650 CFA and in the mean was 814 CFA. For household WTP, the difference in the median was 3500 CFA and in the mean was 2463 CFA. The difference is larger for males, those living in a rural area, other household members (not household heads) and the longer was the interval between test and retest. The differences in the mean (for individual and household WTP) between test and retest are statistically significant. The differences in the medians cannot be tested statistically because of the

Table 2
Individual and household characteristics

Characteristics	Individual (%)	Household (%)
Total cases	1108	348
Sex		
Male	540 (48.7)	
Female	568 (51.3)	
Age (years)	39.2	
Religion		
Traditional religion	156 (14.1)	58 (16.7)
Muslim	496 (44.8)	149 (42.8)
Other	456 (41.2)	141 (40.5)
Marriage		
Monogamy	679 (61.3)	
Polygamy	204 (18.4)	
Single	112 (10.1)	
Other	113 (10.2)	
Location of residency		
Nouna town	403 (36.4)	137 (39.4)
Rural area	705 (63.6)	211 (60.6)
Occupation		
Farmer	845 (76.3)	
Others	263 (23.7)	
Years of schooling		
0	956 (13.7)	
>0	152 (86.3)	
Household size		7.9
0–5 years old ratio (%)		18.1
65+ years old ratio (%)		6.2

non-parametric method by which these medians were estimated. The difference between urban and rural areas in the mean difference in individual WTP between test and retest was statistically significant. Also the test-retest difference in individual and household WTP was significantly lower for the shorter interview interval compared with the longer interval.

Measure of agreement between test and retest

The simplest approach to assessing agreement between test and retest is to calculate the percentage, which exactly agree. The agreement for individual WTP elicited by the TIOLI method was 79.6% ((638+244)/1108), and for household WTP was 81.3% ((238+45)/348) (Table 4). Kappa is a more satisfactory measure of agreement since it indicates agreement in excess of that expected by chance. The kappa value is 0.539 for individual WTP and 0.467 for household WTP (Table 4).

The Pearson correlation between test and retest can be used to measure reliability for the more or less continuous data generated by the bidding game method. The Pearson correlation was 0.593 for individual WTP and 0.675 for household WTP, and the Spearman correlation coefficients were 0.653 and 0.701, respectively. All of them are statistically significant at the level of 0.01.

In order to compare the reliability of the TIOLI and the bidding game the bidding results were transformed into artificial yes/no results by randomly assigning starting prices to each respondent. The simple agreement was 82.9% ((733+186)/1108) for individual WTP and 90.5% ((281+34)/348) for household WTP, kappa was 0.554 and 0.621, respectively (Table 5). Thus both the simple agreement and the kappa value of the bidding game are higher than those of the TIOLI. The difference for individual WTP is small but for household WTP it is more pronounced.

Discussion

While there are many WTP studies in the area of health economics, studies of the reliability of elicitation methods are rare. In particular, to our knowledge, only three other studies of test–retest reliability have been undertaken in a developing country. Onwujekwe, Fox-Rushby, and Hanson (2001) assess the test–retest reliability of WTP for insecticide-treated nets in southeast Nigeria. They reinterviewed household heads 1 month after the first survey and compared the reliability of a bidding game ($n = 146$), binary choice with open-ended follow-up ($n = 161$) and structured haggling ($n = 139$) using Pearson's coefficient of correlation. WTP was first assessed with respect to own personal use and then for use by other household members. The correlation was higher with respect to own use for bidding (0.51 vs. 0.34) and for haggling (0.56 vs. 0.33) but was higher for others' use in the case of binary choice with open-ended follow-up (0.52 vs. 0.41). Cho, Lertmaharit, Kamol-Ratanakul, and Saul (2000) assess the test–retest reliability of WTP for malaria test kit in Myanmar. They reinterviewed patients immediately following diagnosis of malaria (ex post, $n = 30$) and people with a prior history of malaria (ex ante, $n = 30$) 3 weeks after the first survey. They compared the reliability of a bidding game using coefficient of correlation. The correlation was 0.78–0.9 (ex post) and 0.7–0.86 (ex ante). Whittington et al. (1992) assess the test–retest reliability of WTP for drinking water in Nigeria. They reinterviewed heads of households 1–2 days after the first survey and compared the reliability of a bidding game in eliciting WTP for public taps ($n = 166$) and for private connection ($n = 162$) using percentage of agreement. The percentage of agreement was higher with respect to public taps (84%) than to private connection (80%). The interval between test and retest is very small, having a higher probability of 'memory bias'. Respondents can remember the amount they are willing to pay and easily give the same amount as before.

Table 3
Individual and household mean and median willingness-to-pay (CFA)

Variables	Median (TIOLI)			Mean (bidding game)			p^*
	Test	Retest	Difference	Test	Retest	Difference	
Individual							
Total	3000	2350	650	3569	2755	814	<0.001
Sex							>0.05
Male	3750	3250	500	4083	3223	860	<0.001
Female	2100	1750	350	3079	2310	769	<0.001
Age (years old)							>0.05
20–34	2900	2700	200	4072	3176	896	<0.001
35–49	3100	2700	400	3676	2801	875	<0.001
50–64	2550	1500	1050	2701	2025	676	<0.001
65+	1100	500	600	2178	1797	381	>0.05
Household head							>0.05
Yes	3800	2800	1000	3702	2967	735	<0.001
No	2650	2200	450	3508	2660	848	<0.001
Location of residency							<0.01
Nouna town	2750	2300	450	2886	2454	432	<0.001
Rural area	3100	2400	700	3959	2928	1031	<0.001
Interval between test and retest							<0.05
3–4 weeks	3050	2700	350	3393	2763	630	<0.001
5–6 weeks	2600	1750	850	3986	2736	1250	<0.001
Household							
Total	8500	5000	3500	10303	7840	2463	<0.001
Location of residency							>0.05
Nouna town	11500	10000	1500	9793	7653	2140	<0.001
Rural area	5000	2000	3000	10634	7962	2672	<0.001
Interval between test and retest							<0.05
3–4 weeks	8000	3500	4500	9773	7875	1898	<0.001
5–6 weeks	12000	8000	4000	11420	7768	3652	<0.001
Household size							>0.05
1–5	6000	2000	4000	8447	5818	2629	<0.001
6–10	5000	7000	−2000	10028	8031	1997	<0.001
11+	16000	12000	4000	13667	10554	3113	<0.001
0–5 years old ratio (%)							>0.05
0	2000	3000	−1000	8069	5756	2313	<0.001
1–25	11500	7500	4000	11304	8953	2351	<0.001
26+	8500	7000	1500	11153	8373	2780	<0.001

*Paired-samples t-test was used for testing the mean difference between test and retest. Independent-samples t-test and one-way ANOVA were used for testing the mean difference in sub-groups, e.g., sex, location of residency, household size, etc.

In the present study, WTP is about 25% lower in the retest compared with the test. A potential explanation for this is in terms of household food stocks. The first interview took place in January after the December harvest, whereas the second interview took place several weeks later when these stocks were at a lower level. This explanation is supported by the finding that the longer was the interval between test and retest the lower were people's WTP. Also, the difference between test and retest WTP was larger in the rural area (where

Table 4
Measure of agreement between test and retest for individual and household WTP elicited by take-it-or-leave-it

Test	Retest		Total	Kappa (SE)
	No	Yes		
Individual				
No	638	54	692	0.539 (0.026)
Yes	172	244	416	
Total	810	298	1108	
Household				
No	238	17	255	0.467 (0.055)
Yes	48	45	93	
Total	286	62	348	

Table 5
Measure of agreement between test and retest for individual and household WTP elicited by bidding game[a]

Test	Retest		Total	Kappa (SE)
	No	Yes		
Individual				
No	733	41	774	0.554 (0.028)
Yes	148	186	334	
Total	881	227	1108	
Household				
No	281	5	255	0.621 (0.059)
Yes	28	34	93	
Total	309	39	348	

[a] The bidding results were transformed into yes/no results by randomly assigning the starting prices (the first bids) to each respondent.

household food stocks are the main economic resource) than in the urban area (Table 3). That WTP is limited by ability-to-pay is appropriate because the method is attempting to elicit what the person would be prepared to forgo from current (and future) consumption to achieve an expected health improvement. Between the test and the retest, household food stocks were decreasing, and so was the ability-to-pay.

The contingent valuation method as a whole appears to be a reliable technique for eliciting WTP. The kappa values of the two WTP elicitation methods were between 0.467 and 0.621, Spearman correlations ranged from 0.653 to 0.701 and Pearson correlations ranged from 0.593 to 0.675, thus the reliability of the methods is moderate or good. Compared with the literature, the coefficients of correlation (reliability of bidding game) are higher than the study in Nigeria (Onwujekwe et al., 2001), similar to the study in Canada (O'Brien & Viramontes, 1994), but lower than the study in Myanmar (Cho et al., 2000) and in USA (Flowers, Garber, Bergen, & Lenert, 1997). It is difficult to explain the differences. The main reason may be related to the characteristics of study subjects and WTP scenarios because the bidding processes are similar and the intervals between test and retest are similar too. Our scenario is CBI, more subjective than malaria test kit and buying insurance for treating moderate Gaucher disease in other studies. The greater the extent of zero responses in the test and retest the easier it can be to demonstrate reliability. However, in the present study only 15 (1.35%) respondents stated a zero individual WTP at both interviews; and seven (2.01%) stated a zero household WTP in both interviews.

An issue in establishing test–retest reliability is the choice of interval between the first and second interview. If the interval is too long, external events might influence responses at the second interview; if too short, the respondents may remember and simply repeat their answers from the first interview (Fink, 1993). There is no general rule for selecting the interval between test and retest. Most of the studies have used an interval of 3–4 weeks (Loehman et al., 1979; O'Brien & Viramontes, 1994; Jones-Lee, Hammerton, & Philips, 1985). The interval in this study was 4–5 weeks because it was estimated that it would take the interviewers 1 month to finish the initial survey of 800 households.

A novel feature of this study is the attempt to compare directly the reliability of the bidding game and the TIOLI. The bidding results were transformed into yes/no responses by randomly assigning starting prices to each respondent because the two elicitation methods result in different types of data, which makes the direct comparison difficult or impossible. We cannot directly compare the value of kappa with the coefficients of correlation. In this study the agreement of these artificial data between test and retest suggests that the bidding game is more reliable than the TIOLI method. But we have not got literature to support this yet because to our knowledge there have been no similar studies reported in the literature. The difference in terms of reliability between the two approaches is possibly related to the culture of the society. In Burkina Faso people are used to bargaining which is more closely related to the bidding game method. It is possible that some of the respondents who answered 'yes' for the TIOLI questions in the first survey thought that they had not got a good bargain. Indeed 15.5% of the respondents changed from 'yes' to 'no' whereas only 4.9% changed from 'no' to 'yes'.

The TIOLI and the bidding game are the most commonly used elicitation methods in the contingent valuation studies (Mitchell & Carson, 1989). The TIOLI method is simpler than the bidding game since the respondent has only to make a judgment about a given price. In this respect, the TIOLI method is especially suitable for postal questionnaires or telephone interviews (Zeckhauser, 1973; Hoehn & Randall, 1987).

However, in many developing countries, and in the Nouna area in particular, face-to-face interviews are required because the people have limited education, poor reading and writing ability, and very poor telephone access. Given face-to-face interviews a bidding game becomes feasible. The bidding process will capture the highest price consumers are willing to pay (Cummings, Brookshire, & Schulze, 1986), and the process of iteration will enable the respondent to more fully consider the value of a good (Mitchell & Carson, 1989). Moreover, the bidding game is an attractive method to elicit WTP in a country, such as Burkina Faso, where people are used to bargaining and fixed-price markets are not common.

Conclusion

The test–retest reliability of the bidding game and the TIOLI method was assessed using data on the WTP for community-based health insurance in the Nouna area of Burkina Faso. An advantage of this study compared to earlier studies of the test–retest reliability of methods to elicit WTP is the larger sample used. It is also one of the first studies of test–retest reliability conducted using data from a developing country. Both methods were found to have moderate or good reliability although there were clear differences in the median and mean WTP between the two surveys. There was some evidence that the bidding game is more reliable than the TIOLI method.

Acknowledgements

This paper is one of the results of "control of tropical infectious diseases" project in Burkina Faso financially supported by Germany Research Foundation (Deutsche Forschungsgemeinschaft) (SFB 544). The Chief Scientist Office of the Scottish Executive Health Department (SEHD) funds HERU. The views expressed are those of the authors and not SEHD. It is acknowledged that in the data collection we obtained valuable help from Sanou Aboubakary, Adjima Gbangou, Yazoumé Yé and Mamadou Sanon from Nouna Health Research Centre.

References

Altman, D. G. (1996). *Practical statistics for medical research*. London: Chapman & Hall.

Asenso-Okyere, W. K., Osei-Akoto, I., Anum, A., & Appiah, E. N. (1997). Willingness to pay for health insurance in a developing economy. A pilot study of the informal sector of Ghana using contingent valuation. *Health Policy*, *42*, 223–237.

Burkina Faso Ministry of Health. (1996). *Statistiques Sanitaires 1996*. Ouagadougou: Burkina Faso Ministry of health.

Cho, M. N., Lertmaharit, S., Kamol-Ratanakul, P., & Saul, A. J. (2000). Ex post and ex ante willingness to pay (WTP) for the ICT Malaria Pf/Pv test kit in Myanmar. *Southeast Asian Journal of Tropical Medicine and Public Health*, *31*, 104–111.

Cummings, R. G., Brookshire, D. S., & Schulze, W. D. (1986). *Valuing environmental goods: A state of the arts assessment of the contingent method*. Totowa, NJ: Rowman and Allanheld.

Diener, A., O'Brien, B., & Gafni, A. (1998). Health care contingent valuation studies: A review and classification of the literature. *Health Economics*, *7*, 313–326.

Dong, H., Kouyate, B., Sauerborn, R. (2001). Willingness to pay for community-based insurance in Burkina Faso. *SFB Discussion Series* 4, University of Heidelberg, Department of Tropical Hygiene and Public Health, pp. 1–26.

Fink, A. (1993). *Evaluation fundamentals: Guiding health programs, research and policy*. London: Sage Publications.

Flowers, C. R., Garber, A. M., Bergen, M. R., & Lenert, L. A. (1997). Willingness-to-pay utility assessment: Feasibility of use in normative patient decision support systems. *Proceedings of the AMIA annual fall symposium*. Nashville, TN, 25–29 October 1997 (pp. 223–227).

Hassan, E. O., el Nahal, N., & el Hussein, M. (1994). Acceptability of the once-a-month injectable contraceptives Cyclofem and Mesigyna in Egypt. *Contraception*, *49*, 469–488.

Hoehn, J. P., & Randall, A. (1987). A satisfactory benefit cost indicator from contingent valuation. *Journal of Environmental Economics and Management*, *14*, 226–247.

Jones-Lee, M. W., Hammerton, M., & Philips, P. R. (1985). The value of safety: Results of a national sample survey. *Economic Journal*, *95*, 49–72.

Klose, T. (1999). The contingent valuation method in health care. *Health Policy*, *47*, 97–123.

Loehman, E. T., et al. (1979). Distributional analysis of regional benefits and cost of air quality control. *Journal of Environmental Economics and Management*, *6*, 222–243.

Mathiyazhagan, K. (1998). Willingness to pay for rural health insurance through community participation in India. *International Journal of Health Planning and Management*, *13*, 47–67.

Mitchell, R. C., & Carson, R. T. (1989). *Using surveys to value public goods: The contingent valuation method*. Washington, DC: Resources for the Future.

O'Brien, B., & Viramontes, J. L. (1994). Willingness to pay: A valid and reliable measure of health state preference? *Medical Decision Making*, *14*, 289–297.

Onwujekwe, O., Fox-Rushby, J., & Hanson, K. (2001). Willingness to pay for insecticide treated nets and net re-treatment: An evaluation of inter-rater and test–retest reliability. Paper presented at the *Health Economists' Study Group meeting*, City University, London, September 2001.

Onwujekwe, O., Shu, E., Chima, R., Onyido, A., & Okonkwo, P. (2000). Willingness to pay for the retreatment of mosquito nets with insecticide in four communities of south-eastern Nigeria. *Tropical Medicine & International Health*, *5*, 370–376.

Sankoh, O. A., Ye, Y., Sauerborn, R., Muller, O., & Becher, H. (2001). Clustering of childhood mortality in rural Burkina Faso. *International Journal of Epidemiology, 30*, 485–492.

Thompson, M. S., Read, J. L., & Liang, M. (1984). Feasibility of willingness-to-pay measurement in chronic arthritis. *Medical Decision Making, 4*, 195–215.

Walraven, G. (1996). Willingness to pay for district hospital services in rural Tanzania. *Health Policy Planning, 11*, 428–437.

Weaver, M., Ndamobissi, R., Kornfield, R., Blewane, C., Suthe, A., & Chopko, M., et al. (1996). Willingness to pay for child survival: Results of a national survey in Central African Republic. *Social Science & Medicine, 43*, 985–998.

Whittington, D., Smith, V. K., Okorafor, A., Okore, A., Liu, J. L., & McPhail, A. (1992). Giving respondents time to think in contingent valuation studies: A developing country application. *Journal of Environmental Economics & Management, 22*, 205–225.

World Bank. (2000). *African Development Indicators 2000*. Washington, DC: World Bank.

Wuertwein, R., Gbangou, A., Kouyate, B., Mugisha, F., Ye, Y., & Becher, H., et al. (2001). The Nouna health district household survey: Design and implementation. *SFB Discussion Series No 3*. University of Heidelberg, Department of Tropical Hygiene and Public Health (pp. 1–51).

Zeckhauser, R. (1973). Voting systems, honest preferences, and Pareto optimality. *American Political Science Review, 67*, 934–946.

4.9 Willingness-to-pay for community-based health insurance in Burkina Faso

Dong HJ, Kouyate B, Cairns J, Mugisha F, Sauerborn R.

Health Economics 2003 Oct;12(10):849-62.

Reprinted with permission from John Wiley & Sons Ltd.

HEALTH ECONOMICS
Health Econ. **12**: 849–862 (2003)
Published online 23 December 2002 in Wiley InterScience (www.interscience.wiley.com). **DOI**:10.1002/hec.771

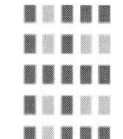

CONTINGENT VALUATION

Willingness-to-pay for community-based insurance in Burkina Faso

Hengjin Dong[a,]*, Bocar Kouyate[b], John Cairns[c], Frederick Mugisha[d] and Rainer Sauerborn[a]

[a] *Department of Tropical Hygiene and Public Health, University of Heidelberg, Germany*
[b] *Nouna Health Research Centre, Nouna, Burkina Faso*
[c] *Health Economics Research Unit, University of Aberdeen, UK*
[d] *African Population and Health Research Center, Nairobi, Kenya*

Summary

Purpose: To study the willingness-to-pay (WTP) for a proposed community-based health insurance (CBI) scheme in order to provide information about the relationship between the premium that is required to cover the costs of the scheme and expected insurance enrolment levels. In addition, factors that influence WTP were to be identified.

Methods: Data were collected from a household survey using a two-stage cluster sampling approach, with each household having the same probability of being selected. Interviews were conducted with 2414 individuals and 705 household heads. The take-it-or-leave-it (TIOLI) and the bidding game were used to elicit WTP.

Results: The average individual was willing to pay 2384 (elicited by the TIOLI) or 3191 (elicited by the bidding game) CFA (US$ 3.17 or US$ 4.25) to join CBI for him/herself. The head of household agreed to pay from 6448 (elicited by the TIOLI) or 9769 (elicited by the bidding game) CFA (US$ 8.6 or US$ 13.03) to join the health insurance scheme for his/her household. These results were influenced by household and individual ability-to-pay, household and individual characteristics, such as age, sex and education. The two methods yielded similar patterns of estimated WTP, in that higher WTP was obtained for higher income level, higher previous medical expenditure, higher education, younger people and males. A starting point bias was found in the case of the bidding game.

Conclusions: Both TIOLI and bidding game methods can elicit a value of WTP for CBI. The value elicited by the bidding game is higher than by the TIOLI, but the two approaches yielded similar patterns of estimated WTP. WTP information can be used for setting insurance premium. When setting the premiums, it is important to consider differences between the real market and the theoretical one, and between the WTP and the cost of benefits package. The beneficiaries of CBI should be enrolled at the level of households or villages in order to protect vulnerable groups such as women, elders and the poor. Copyright © 2002 John Wiley & Sons, Ltd.

Keywords willingness-to-pay; contingent valuation method; community-based health insurance; Burkina Faso; health care financing

Introduction

Health services in rural Burkina Faso, as in many Sub-Saharan countries, are characterised by low and inequitable utilisation and poor quality [1–5]. These problems prevent health care interventions from having a notable impact on health, in particular among rural poor in Burkina Faso. Low utilisation of health services is directly related to the high price relative to the household income.

*Correspondence to: Department of Tropical Hygiene and Public Health, University of Heidelberg, Im Neuenheimer Feld 324, D-69120 Heidelberg, Germany. E-mail: donghengjin@yahoo.com

Copyright © 2002 John Wiley & Sons, Ltd.

Received 26 October 2001
Accepted 28 August 2002

Health care in Burkina Faso has always imposed considerable financial costs on the users [6].

User fees were introduced in Burkina Faso in 1993 as a supplement to tax-based financing of government health services. The user fees policy combined modest fees for services and cost-recovery fees for drugs. However, utilisation of health services declined following the introduction of these fees [7,8].

One of the ways to improve the utilisation of health services is through insurance. However, formal health insurance in Burkina Faso has been limited to certain sections of the population largely excluding the rural population. For example, in Burkina Faso, social insurance is offered to salaried and state employees through the Caisse National de Securite Sociale (CNSS) and the Caisse des Retraits de Fonctionnaires (CARFO). So the only rural residents likely to have health insurance are government employees.

Secondly, community risk-sharing schemes, which are prevalent in rural Africa, can be viewed as another way to improve health care utilisation. These schemes cover a wide variety of non-health-related risks but a few cover health care expenditure [9].

Community-based insurance (CBI) is therefore being seen as a promising new tool of health system improvement for rural populations in low-income countries, particularly in Sub-Saharan Africa [10,11]. Community members pool their resources to share the financial risks of health care, own the scheme and control its management, including the collection of premiums, the payment of health care providers, and the negotiation of benefits package. Unlike private insurance, premiums are paid by households and not based on individual risk assessments. CBI has the advantage of dissociating the time of payment from the time of use of services, which is clearly better adapted than user fees to the seasonal fluctuations of revenue and expenditure flows of rural households [12]. The Government of Burkina Faso, in its recently published health plan, has also advocated community-based financing mechanisms to alleviate the health care financing crisis [13].

To ensure acceptability by the community and possibly sustainability a series of studies were conducted in Burkina Faso, including preference for benefits package of CBI [14], costing of health care intervention and premium estimation [15]. This paper reports individual and household valuations of the benefits package using contingent valuation methods. Specifically, the paper aims to examine the willingness-to-pay for CBI and to identify the likelihood of individuals and households opting out of the insurance scheme based on the take-it-or-leave-it (TIOLI) and the bidding game methods. If the expected utility to be derived from participating in the scheme at the stated premium is greater than the amount of the premium, an individual will opt to pay. It is assumed that WTP for health insurance will be affected by sex, age, years of schooling, income, residence, and health status. Female and older people are expected to be willing to pay less. Individuals with higher income, higher education, living in urban areas and people with poor health are expected to be willing to pay more for the health insurance premium. Household size and demographic composition could also influence the WTP. Larger household size and higher proportions of old or young members could increase a head of household's WTP.

There have been many WTP studies for health services in industrialised countries. The most commonly used methods have been the bidding game, the payment card and the TIOLI [16,17]. The studies have included WTP for disease treatment and management, new technology, and outcome evaluation of health care and health programmes [18–31]. However, there have been relatively few WTP studies in developing countries. Health financing has been the focus of the studies published. These studies include WTP for district hospital services [32], contraceptives [33] and the re-treatment of mosquito nets with insecticide [34]. Only two WTP studies, however, have been carried out for rural health insurance in Ghana [11] and India [35].

The bidding game method was used to assess the willingness of households (164 urban households and 142 rural households) to join and pay premiums for a proposed National Health Insurance scheme in Ghana. About 64% of the respondents were willing to pay a premium of ¢ 5000 (US$ 1 = ¢ 1650) a month for a household of five persons [11]. The study only asked the heads of the households with five members using the bidding game method, so there was no information about other household members' WTP and the relationship between household size and WTP. In India, the heads of 1000 households in rural areas were asked directly how much they were willing to pay for a rural health insurance scheme. WTP for different types of medical benefits was estimated. Most households selected a comprehensive medical care benefit and were willing to pay Rs.163.48 per year (US$ 1 = Rs. 47.43). Socioeconomic factors and physical accessibility to quality health services were found to be significant determinants of WTP [35].

The current study used two methods to elicit individual WTP and household head's WTP for his/her household. Two approaches can provide more information than one method. Moreover, instead of relying on the household head, individual WTP was also elicited in order to understand which individual characteristics may be associated with opting out of the scheme if insurance premiums are set on an individual basis.

Methodology

Study site

Burkina Faso has an estimated population of approximately 10.7 millions [36]. It is divided into 11 administrative health regions, which comprise 53 health districts overall, each covering a population of 200 000 to 300 000 individuals. Each health district has at least one hospital with surgical facilities [37]. The districts themselves are again sub-divided into smaller areas of responsibility that are organised around either a hospital or a so-called Centre de Santé et de Promotion Sociale (CSPS), the first-line health care facility in the health system.

The study population, the Nouna health district, has roughly 230 000 inhabitants who are served by one district hospital and 16 CSPS. This district is located in the Northwest of Burkina Faso, about 300 Km from the capital Ouagadougou. The Nouna area is a dry orchard Savannah, populated almost exclusively by subsistence farmers of different ethnic groups.

Sampling procedure and sample size

This study was a part of a larger project on the control of tropical infectious diseases in Burkina Faso. The household survey conducted by the project was based on a two-stage cluster sampling procedure, with each household having the same probability of being selected. In the first stage, clusters of households were selected and in the second stage, respondent households were selected in each cluster. Overall, 800 households were selected, 480 in the rural area and 320 in the town of Nouna [38]. This sample was a true indication of the overall population. The subjects in this study were household members aged 20 to 70. The average number of adults per household in Nouna is about 2.5. Thus, 800 households should yield approximately 2000 data points, which would be enough for a WTP study suggested by Mitchell and Carson [39]. The WTP questions were merged into the regular household survey questionnaire. The data were collected during January and March 2001.

Household interview

A pilot study of the TIOLI, the bidding game, and the payment card methods was undertaken at the study site one month before the main survey. The payment card was found to be inappropriate because of the high illiteracy rate and was dropped from the main survey.

A three-day workshop for training interviewers was organised one week before the survey. The interviewers came from the locality, spoke the local language, had middle school education, and had obtained interview experience in previous household surveys. Questions about respondents' characteristics were merged into the household survey questionnaire. A detailed description of the CBI scenario and the WTP questions were included as a separate module in the household survey questionnaire. The questionnaire was translated into the local language.

Household members were identified from the demographic surveillance system, a census of the entire Nouna area, which is carried out every two years, with vital events registrations carried out every three months since 1992 [40]. The names of household members aged 20 to 70 were pre-printed on the WTP module. Each member was randomly assigned one starting price, which was also pre-printed. The 13 starting prices for individuals (ranging from 2000 to 8000 Franc CFA) and the 13 starting prices for the whole household (ranging from 8000 to 32 000 Franc CFA) (US$ 1 = 750 CFA) were based on the CBI scenario and the results of the pilot.

The interviewers first explained the CBI scenario to the head and all members of the household together. Then the head of household was asked his/her WTP for him/herself and for the whole household. Lastly, other members of the household were asked for their own WTP. In this paper 'individual WTP' describes the value that an individual is willing to pay for him/herself, and 'household WTP' describes the value that the head of household is willing to pay for his/her whole household.

The yes/no answer to the first price offered to the respondent provided the data for the TIOLI. If the answer was 'yes', the interviewer increased the bid by increments of 500 CFA until the respondent said 'no'. If the initial answer was 'no', the interviewer reduced the amount of money by 500 CFA and continued this process until the respondent said 'yes'. The last sum of money receiving a 'yes' response was used as the WTP resulting from the bidding game approach.

Regression analysis

Selecting regression models: The nature of the data determined the available choices for the regression models. For the bidding game, mean WTP was estimated directly from the data provided. Linear multiple regression was used to study the influence of individual and household variables on WTP. The empirical model is as follows:

$$\text{WTP} = \alpha + \beta_1 X_1 + \beta_2 X_2 + \cdots + \beta_{n-1} X_{n-1} + \beta_n X_n$$

where WTP is the willingness-to-pay, α the intercept, β the coefficients of explanatory variables and X the explanatory variables.

Logistic regression was used to estimate the median WTP and to study the influence of independent variables using the TIOLI data. The dependent variable was the yes/no answer to the first bid. The probability of a yes answer was modelled as a Logit function as follows:

$$\log \frac{\text{Prob(yes)}}{1 - \text{Prob(yes)}} = \alpha + \beta_1 X_1 + \beta_2 X_2 + \cdots + \beta_n X_n$$

where Prob(yes) is the probability of answer 'yes', α the intercept, β the coefficients of explanatory variables and X the explanatory variables.

Cameron proposed a simple and more direct way of estimating the median WTP from Logit (and probit) models estimated from the TIOLI data [41]. The formula is $\log(p/(1-p)) = \alpha + \beta x$ bid. The probability $p(=\text{Prob(yes)})$ is set at 0.5, yielding the median WTP $= -\alpha/\beta$.

Explanatory variables: The explanatory variables were selected based on the study hypotheses and relevant knowledge. The amount people are willing to pay for CBI is affected by many factors. For example, knowledge about the importance of insurance, ability-to-pay, and individual characteristics may influence their WTP. The multivariate analysis included household and individual characteristics, including economic characteristics. Accessibility of health care was measured by the distance to the nearest health facility. Two health status variables were used, episodes of disease for the individual, and the household over the previous three rounds of the household survey.

Regression model diagnostics: The correlation matrix of variables was used to assess collinearity. There was no evidence of collinearity ($r^2 > |0.9|$) [42] between any pairs of variables. Following tests of normality the income and expenditure variables were transformed using a logarithmic transformation ($x = \log(X + 1)$). Outliers were excluded from the model if the studentised residuals were greater than $|3|$ [43].

Results

General characteristics of individuals and households

Out of the 800 households randomly selected, 776 were included in the analysis (22 had emigrated and two were missed). These households contained 2670 eligible subjects of whom 2414 (90.4%) responded to the questions about WTP for themselves (four refusals and 252 absentees). There were no significant differences in key variables such as religion, location of residence, occupation and years of schooling between the responders and the non-responders. There were significant differences, however, in sex, age, and marital status. Women had a higher response rate than men, older people had a higher response rate than young people, and married persons had a higher response rate than single persons (Table 1).

In the 776 households, 705 (90.0%) heads of the households answered the household WTP questions (one refusal and 70 absentees). There were no significant differences between the responders and

Table 1. The individual characteristics and response rate (%)

Characteristics	Total	Response[a] (%)	No response (%)	$P=$[b]
Total cases	2670	2414 (90.4)	256 (09.6)	
Sex:				0.009
Male	1325	1178 (88.9)	147 (11.1)	
Female	1345	1236 (91.9)	109 (08.1)	
Age (years)	38.7	39.0	35.8	0.001
Religion:				0.111
Traditional religion	218	205 (94.0)	13 (06.0)	
Muslin	1654	1484 (89.7)	170 (10.3)	
Other	798	725 (90.0)	73 (09.1)	
Marriage:				0.0003
Monogamy	1509	1375 (91.1)	134 (08.9)	
Polygamy	549	504 (91.8)	45 (08.2)	
Single	337	283 (84.0)	54 (16.0)	
Other	275	252 (91.6)	23 (08.4)	
Location of residency:				0.317
Nouna town	895	802 (89.6)	93 (10.4)	
Rural area	1775	1612 (90.8)	163 (09.2)	
Occupation:				0.135
Farmer	1981	1801 (90.9)	180 (09.1)	
Others	689	613 (89.0)	76 (11.0)	
Years of schooling:				0.071
0	2309	2097 (90.8)	212 (09.2)	
>0	361	317 (87.8)	44 (12.2)	

[a] Response means that the number of individuals who have answered the willingness to pay questions.
[b] t-test for age, χ^2 test for other variables.

the non-responders in the location of residence, religion, household size, proportion of children 0–5 years old, proportion of adults 65+ years old, household economic and medical expenditure variables (Table 2).

Median and mean WTP

Median individual WTP elicited by the TIOLI was 2384 CFA. Individuals living in Nouna town were willing to pay more than those living in rural areas (3008 vs 1947 CFA). The probability of accepting the bids decreased as the amount of the bids increased (Figure 1). The probability of accepting the lowest bid (2000 CFA) was 0.64 and only 0.19 for the highest bid (8000 CFA).

Mean individual WTP elicited by the bidding game was 3191 CFA with a standard deviation of 3923, one third higher than the median elicited by the TIOLI. But, individuals living in Nouna town were willing to pay average 2976 CFA (standard deviation 2442), less than those living in rural areas (mean 3298 and standard deviation 4478). About 3.5% were zero bids for individual WTP and 1.1% of bids were higher than 10 000 CFA (Figure 2). As expected, these outlier responses are strongly related to income. 59% of persons with zero bids had no income in the past six months, compared to 33% for the sample as a whole. Individuals bidding zero also had a lower income than the average level (21 043 vs 48 571 CFA). The income of high-bid persons was higher than the average level (54 920 vs 48 571 CFA). The cumulative percentage of bidding results for individual WTP showed that 15% of the respondents gave bidding results higher than 5000 CFA, and another 15% gave bidding results lower than 1000 CFA. 70% of the respondents gave bidding results between 1000 to 5000 CFA (Figure 2).

Median household WTP elicited by the TIOLI was 6448 CFA, about three times as much as the individual WTP. Figure 3 shows the relationship between the probability of accepting the bid and the amount of the bid for household WTP. As expected, the probability of accepting the bid decreases as the amount of the bid increases. The probability of accepting the bid ranges from 0.49 for the lowest bid (8000 CFA) to only 0.09 for the highest bid (32 000 CFA).

Table 2. The household characteristics and response rate (%)

Characteristics	Total	Response[a] (%)	No response (%)	$P=$[b]
Total cases	776	705 (90.9)	71 (09.1)	
Location of residency:				0.315
Nouna town	296	265 (89.5)	31 (10.5)	
Rural area	480	440 (91.7)	40 (08.3)	
Religion:				0.117
Traditional religion	77	74 (96.1)	3 (03.9)	
Muslin	461	419 (90.0)	42 (09.1)	
Other	238	212 (89.1)	26 (10.9)	
Household size	8.0	8.1	7.3	0.280
0–5 years old percentage	17.2	16.9	19.9	0.102
65+ years old percentage	6.0	6.1	4.8	0.526
Household agricultural value (CFA)[c]	197080	203927	129100	0.152
Household animal value (CFA)[c]	332007	348877	164496	0.114
Household total medical expenditure in past month (CFA)[c]	923	949	667	0.117
Household expenditure on Western medicine in past month (CFA)[c]	698	702	646	0.724

[a] Response means that the number of household who have answered the willingness to pay questions.
[b] χ^2 for location of residency and religion, t-test for other variables.
[c] log 10 transformed data for t-test. 1 USD = 750 CFA.

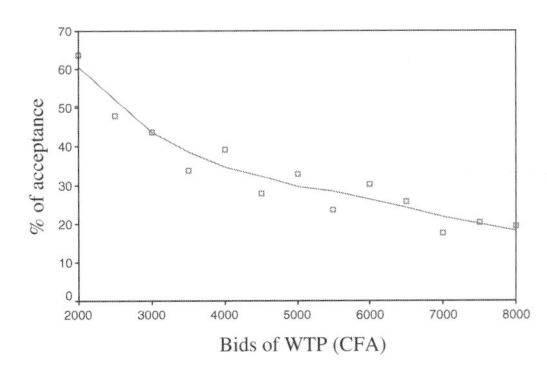

Figure 1. Individual acceptance rate (%) and bids (CFA) (by TIOLI method)

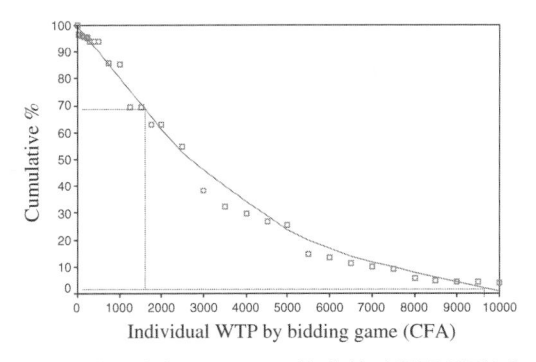

Figure 2. Cumulative percentage of individual WTP (CFA) (by bidding game method)

Mean household WTP elicited by the bidding game was 9769 CFA with a standard deviation of 8249, 51.5% higher than the median elicited by the TIOLI, and three times as much as the mean individual WTP. About 3.8% were zero bids for household WTP and 1.0% of bids were higher than 35 000 CFA (Figure 4). The cumulative percentage of bidding results for household WTP showed that 15% of the respondents had bidding results higher than 17 500 CFA, and another 15% had bidding results lower than 2500 CFA. 70% of the respondents had bidding results between 2500 to 17 500 CFA (Figure 4).

The impact of factors on individual WTP in TIOLI

Logistic regression analysis showed that age, distance to health facility and the starting bid had negative effects, reducing the probability of accepting the bids. The coefficients showed that distance to health facility had a stronger negative relationship with the probability of accepting and the starting bid's negative influence was not strong. Traditional religion, sex, family head, individual expenditure and household expenditure on Western medicine had a stronger positive

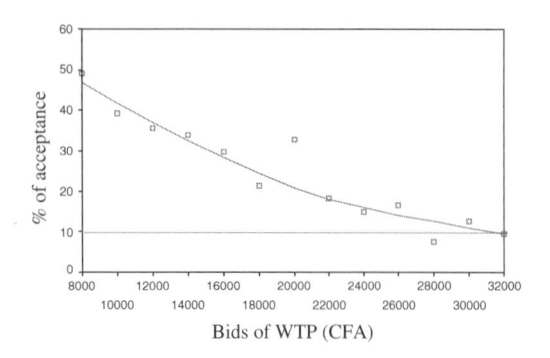

Figure 3. Household acceptance rate (%) and bids (CFA) (by TIOLI method)

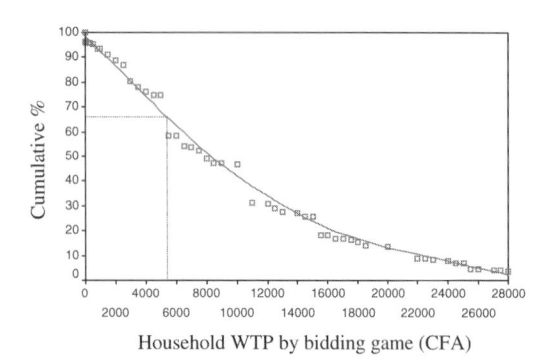

Figure 4. Cumulative percentage of household WTP (CFA) (by bidding game method)

influence on the probability of accepting the bids. All variables had the hypothesised signs (Table 3).

The impact of factors on household WTP in TIOLI

Logistic regression analysis showed that only three factors significantly influenced the probability of accepting the bids for the household WTP. Higher household expenditure on Western medicine and more years of schooling for the household head were associated with a higher probability of accepting the bids. The starting bid had a negative effect on the probability of accepting (Table 4).

The impact of factors on individual WTP in bidding game

Linear regression analysis showed that age, living in Nouna town, and distance to health facility had negative effects on bidding results, reducing the value of WTP. However, individual cash income, expenditure, household medical expenditure, age, sex, education, monogamy, traditional religion, and the starting bid had positive effects on the bidding results, increasing the value of WTP. Almost all variables had the hypothesised signs, except the living in Nouna town. The standardised coefficients of variables (Beta) show the strength between the dependent variable (bidding result) and the independent variables. The value of the starting bid had the strongest positive influence on the bidding result (Beta = 0.17). Conversely, age had the strongest negative influence on the bidding result (Table 3).

The impact of factors on household WTP in bidding game

Linear regression analysis showed that household expenditure in the past six months, household expenditure on Western medicine in the past month, years of schooling of the household head and the starting bid had statistically significant effects on the bidding results. All effects were positive, as hypothesised, increasing the bidding value. Education had the strongest positive influence on the bidding results. The next strongest influence was the starting bid. The higher the value of the starting bid the higher the bidding results, as in the case of the individual WTP (Table 4).

Discussion

The main results of this study were that individuals were on average willing to pay 2384 or 3191 CFA to join the CBI for themselves. Depending on the method chosen, individual ability-to-pay and individual characteristics influenced this average. The heads of households were on the average willing to pay 6448 or 9769 CFA to join the CBI for their households. The household head's individual characteristics and household ability-to-pay also influenced the average level. These estimates cannot be compared directly with other studies because the scenario, elicitation method and regression model were different. Mathiyazhagan used an 'open-ended' question method [35] and Asenso-Okyere used an ordered probit

Table 3. Coefficients of the logistic and linear regressions for full sample excluding outliers (individual WTP)

Variables	Logistic regression[a]			Linear regression[b]		
	B	S.E.	Exp(B)	B	S.E.	Beta
(Constant)	0.674*	0.264	1.963	1618.656**	259.364	
Individual cash income of 6 months	0.071*	0.028	1.074	93.081***	27.512	0.078
Individual expenditure for 6 months	0.139***	0.036	1.149	142.776***	33.585	0.101
Individual animal value	0.076***	0.024	1.079	97.334***	24.174	0.089
Individual episodes of diseases in 3 surveys	−0.017	0.071	0.983	−67.527	70.575	−0.019
Household expenditure on Western medicine in the past month	0.120***	0.038	1.128	169.299***	40.156	0.081
Age	−0.022***	0.004	0.978	−24.638***	4.037	−0.145
Sex	0.287**	0.131	1.333	327.496*	133.249	0.065
Education (years of schooling)	0.065***	0.022	1.067	75.411**	22.626	0.068
Monogamy	0.195	0.116	1.215	250.807*	113.078	0.049
Single	−0.270	0.205	0.764	−264.328	204.434	−0.034
Traditional religion	0.651***	0.169	1.918	916.790***	175.839	0.101
Household head	0.351*	0.154	1.420	255.663	157.261	0.046
Living in Nouna town	−0.071	0.130	0.931	−285.284*	130.024	−0.053
Distance to health facility	−0.049***	0.012	0.952	−54.740***	10.823	−0.116
Starting price	−0.00036**	0.00003	1.000	0.231**	0.026	0.170
n	2401			2397		
R^2	0.226			0.162		

*$P \leq 0.05$. **$P \leq 0.01$.
[a] Model test: χ^2 value = 424.571, $p < 0.01$, correct % = 72.1.
[b] Model test: F value = 30.684, $p < 0.01$, Standard residual mean = 0.000 and standard deviation = 0.997.

Table 4. Coefficients of the logistic and linear regressions for full sample excluding outliers (household WTP)

Variables	Logistic regression[a]			Linear regression[b]		
	B	S.E.	Exp(B)	B	S.E.	Beta
(Constant)	0.014	1.121	1.014	−915.935	2800.682	
Household agricultural value	−0.128	0.075	0.880	−60.638	201.135	−0.014
Household cash income of 6 months	0.018	0.111	1.018	389.248	267.079	0.060
Household animal value	0.023	0.072	1.023	91.208	178.681	0.023
Household expenditure for 6 months	0.222	0.202	1.248	1048.683*	518.338	0.094
Household episodes of diseases in 3 surveys	−0.030	0.048	0.970	−170.103	127.190	−0.052
Household expenditure on Western medicine in the past month	0.323**	0.093	1.381	805.791**	270.269	0.112
Household size	0.010	0.022	1.010	77.012	59.590	0.060
0–5 years percentage (number of 0–5 years old/household size)	0.404	0.811	1.498	2928.537	2079.212	0.057
Old percentage (number of 65+ years old/household size)	−1.013	0.981	0.363	−1037.241	2059.609	−0.022
Age	−0.008	0.010	0.992	−34.421	24.260	−0.066
Sex	0.894	0.459	2.444	1330.388	1076.127	0.052
Education (years of schooling)	0.153**	0.040	1.166	564.222**	114.505	0.196
Monogamy	−0.100	0.243	0.904	453.492	633.798	0.029
Single	0.128	0.621	1.136	−783.139	1720.080	−0.018
Traditional religion	0.471	0.335	1.602	1226.972	906.787	0.050
Living in Nouna town	−0.298	0.304	0.742	−325.843	784.294	−0.021
Distance to health facility	−0.046	0.028	0.955	−110.957	64.637	−0.075
Starting price	−0.00013**	0.00002	1.000	0.131**	0.036	0.130
n	694			699		
R^2	0.273			0.167		

*$P \leq 0.05$. **$P \leq 0.01$.
[a] Model test: χ^2 value = 138.529, $p < 0.01$, correct % = 78.4.
[b] Model test: F value = 7.583, $p < 0.01$, Standard residual mean = 0.000 and standard deviation = 0.987.

model [11]. But WTP was found to be positively correlated with income, a proxy ability-to-pay, a result found in several other studies [11,26,27,44–46]. Asenso-Okyere reported that the premium level households were willing to pay was significantly influenced by dependency ratio, income, sex, health care expenditures and education [11]. In the present study, age, traditional religion, marital status and distance to health facility were also found to significantly influence people's WTP.

Almost all-explanatory variables had the hypothesised signs in both the linear and logistic models, except the location of residence. The effect of location of residence on individual WTP elicited by the bidding game method was negative. This result is unexpected, because urban people are usually wealthier and better educated and would be expected to have higher WTP. The larger standard deviation in rural areas might be one reason to explain it.

In this study, the response rates ((eligible interviewees – refusals – absentees)/eligible interviewees) for individual WTP and household WTP were high, more than 90%. Excluding absentees, the response rates were even higher, 99.8% (2414/2418) for individual WTP and 99.9% (705/706) for household WTP. There were no significant differences in household characteristics between the households that answered the WTP questions and the ones that did not (including absentees). But there were significant differences in some individual characteristics (sex, age, and marital status) between the responding persons and the non-responding persons. These differences may have had some influence on the results, because in both linear and logistic regression models for individual WTP, the variable sex and age were significant. Men were willing to pay more and older people were willing to pay less. Any bias created by the non-responders would not be, however, large enough to change the sign of the results.

The bidding game process is simple and the respondent can easily make a choice. This process will capture the highest price consumers are willing to pay [47], and the process of iteration will enable the respondent to more fully consider the value of the amenity [39]. The main disadvantage is the starting point bias. The TIOLI is also simpler and the respondent has only to make a judgement about a given price [48,49]. But this method needs large sample and an appropriate price range. The bidding result was found to be higher than the result from the TIOLI method. Both methods yielded similar results regarding factors associated with WTP, in that higher WTP values were obtained for higher income levels, higher medical expenditure, higher education, younger people and males. It is not clear which method is superior, however, because there is no 'gold standard' method in the contingent valuation studies.

The first bid was included in the linear regression analysis in order to access the extent of any starting point bias. There was clear evidence of starting point bias for both individual and household WTP. Many studies have found this bias by demonstrating that WTP differs markedly between different sub-samples [20,26,27,29,50–52]. For instance, Kartman et al. found that those facing the highest starting-bid group had a WTP twice that of those facing the lowest starting-bid [24]. Whether it is possible to develop techniques to correct for starting point bias is an issue for future research.

Although there were outliers, zero bids and exceptionally high bids, in the WTP bidding results, the strategic bias was small in this study, because zero bids and high bids were related to income level. Thus, WTP is positively associated with ability-to-pay, which has theoretical validity.

The test-retest (with an interval of around four to five weeks) reliability of the bidding game and the TIOLI were also compared in this study. Both methods displayed moderate to good reliability [Dong HJ, Kouyate B, Cairns J, Sauerborn R. A comparison of the reliability of the take-it-or-leave-it and the bidding game approaches to estimating willingness-to-pay in a rural population in West Africa. *Soc Sci Med* 2002, accepted].

From the policy point of view, the WTP value can be used to estimate the premium of insurance. In this aspect, the median and mean values of WTP are very important information. But the median value is estimated on the basis of 50% of accepting the bid. It doesn't mean that in real life 50% of people are willing to join the insurance at the price of that bid. There are always some differences in the real market and the theoretical one. The relationship between people's behaviour in a hypothesised market and their behaviour in the real market needs further study.

The relationship between the bids and the acceptance rates (shown in Figures 1 and 3) could potentially provide valuable information for setting the premium. However, the data have some shortcomings, in that the lowest bid (8000 CFA) for household WTP was too high (the probability of accepting the bid was less than 50%). Decision-makers might want to know what uptake would be at lower annual premiums. With hindsight it would have been better has the lowest starting bid been 4000 CFA.

Household WTP was much less than the individual WTP multiplied by household size. The reasons may be that household heads did not give other members of household the same weight as themselves in their WTP. This information should be carefully taken into consideration when setting the premiums. If the enrolment unit for CBI were the household, the premium for a household estimated by individual WTP would be much higher than that estimated by household WTP.

From a public health point of view, since CBI aims to protect vulnerable, groups and to avoid adverse selection, that enrolment should be on the basis of the household or village. If the enrolment of CBI were based on individuals, women, the elderly, and the poor who are willing to pay less, could easily be excluded. The studies in Ghana and India did not shed light on this issue because they only interviewed the heads of the households [11,35]. The number of disease episodes had a negative relationship with WTP, although the coefficient of the variable was not significant. This implies that more episodes of diseases are related to a lower WTP, which could reflect the association between disease and poverty.

Mugisha has estimated the cost of the CBI scenario [15]. He first estimated the unit cost of relevant services, then the total cost in the study sample based on the actual utilisation of services and on health needs, finally the cost per capita to the population. However, this is likely to be an under-estimation, because the actual utilisation on which it was based did not cover all service items in the CBI scenario due to the lack of appropriately detailed data. It is estimated that the cost per capita was 1673 CFA (actual utilisation) and 9638 CFA (need-based), including 58% government subsidies. If government subsidies are maintained, then the cost per capita to the population is 703 and 4048 CFA, respectively. Thus, if the CBI premium is set on the basis of cost recovery, the premium for the average household with 8 members is 5624 and 32 384 CFA, based on actual utilisation and need, respectively. Based on the WTP elicited by the TIOLI, the coverage rate will be ∼50 and 10%, respectively (Figure 3). Based on the WTP elicited by the bidding game, the rate will be from less than 5 to 65% (Figure 4).

More research is needed in order to set an appropriate premium. For example, to what extent will utilisation be stimulated by the introduction of insurance. Also there is a need to study alternative ways to cover the financial gap between WTP and the premium based on health needs. If the household coverage is set at 50%, the gaps are 25 936 (32 384–6448, TIOLI) and 22 615 (32 384–9769, bidding game) CFA, 2.3 to 4.0 times the WTP. An analysis should be done to determine the impact of increasing government subsidies as opposed to reducing the coverage rate.

Conclusion

Both bidding game and TIOLI methods can elicit the WTP for CBI in areas with a high illiteracy rate. Depending on the method used, estimated WTP for annual health insurance in rural Burkina Faso was 2384 or 3191 CFA for individuals and 6448 or 9769 CFA for the household heads on behalf of their households. The value elicited by the bidding game is higher than that elicited by the TIOLI. But the two approaches yielded similar patterns of estimated WTP, in that higher values were obtained for higher income levels, higher medical expenditures, higher education, younger people and males. A starting point bias was present in the bidding game. When setting the premium using WTP information, differences between the real market and the theoretical one must be considered, as well as differences between the WTP and the cost of the benefits package. The results of the study also show that CBI enrolment should be on the basis of the household or village in order to protect the vulnerable persons such as woman, the elderly and the poor.

Acknowledgements

This work was supported by the collaborative research grant 'SFB 544' of the German Research Society (DFG). Health Economics Research Unit (HERU) at University of Aberdeen is funded by the Chief Scientist Office of the Scottish Executive Health Department (SEHD). The views expressed in this paper are those of the authors and not the SEHD. The authors would like to thank Sanou Aboubakary, Adjima Gbangou,

Yazoumé Yé and Mamadou Sanon from Nouna Health Research Centre for their valuable help during the data collection process. We are also grateful to Cheryl Cashin and Osman A. Sankoh for helpful comments and suggestions.

Appendix A: Community-based health insurance scenario

Introduction

Sickness needs to be treated immediately and it is not possible to wait. If you don't have the money available, then you will need to borrow it from your neighbour or sell your sheep or chickens. While you run around trying to get the money together, the sick person suffers. And many times it happens that you come back with the money only to find out that the sick person has died.

In order to solve this financial problem, an agency is planing to set one health insurance in your community. If you join the insurance and pay an annual premium, you don't need to pay for the following health services provided in Nouna health district area for a period of one year.

Benefits package

Drugs: all essential and generic drugs which you already buy in your pharmacy, either at the first line health facility level or at the Nouna hospital level. The insurance will not pay for drugs sold in private drugstores.

Impregnated bednets will be covered (1 per household).

Laboratory tests: all costs of laboratory tests that have been prescribed by the public health agent are covered if they are being carried out in public health facilities.

Inpatient stays: when you are hospitalised, the insurance will cover up to 30 days inpatient stays during a year.

Urgent transport by ambulance from your village to Nouna hospital will be covered. This will only be when sickness puts your life in danger and you need to be treated urgently at the Nouna hospital (for example: a woman who is bleeding during delivery of her child, hernia, non-obstetrical emergencies (child in a coma) ...). The decision to order the ambulance will be made by a nurse or a medical doctor.

Surgery: general surgery and delivery complications, extraction of teeth and circumcision are not included.

X-rays will be covered if the doctor thinks it is necessary.

Organisation of the insurance scheme

A committee selected from your villages will manage the scheme. Some of the premiums will be kept at village level by the committee to cover the provision of drugs. The insurance scheme proposes that some of your premium will be combined with some of the money from other villages (such as Bouraso, Koro, and Toni) and this money will cover the provision of other services. This money will be kept and managed by another committee elected from all the villages.

The premiums will be kept in a bank. The committee chair and a treasurer have a right to withdraw money from the bank and to pay health facilities. An annual audit will ensure that funds are used rationally.

The committee will give a financial report of the scheme to local government every year. In each health facility, there will be a community worker who will be paid by the insurance. His responsibilities are to facilitate the relationship between insured patients and the health facility and to make sure the patients receive the benefits, such as drugs.

Enrolment and payment

You need to pay an annual premium for joining the insurance payable in December or January. Credit is not allowed. Each insured person will be given an insurance card with a photo, name, age, sex and address. After you pay the premiums, then you can enjoy the benefits of insurance immediately. If you don't pay the premiums, you have to pay for all service 'out-of-pocket'. For example, if you are a pregnant woman, you have to pay for prenatal care and delivery. Also, if there is a delivery complication, you have to pay for the surgery.

Reimbursement procedure

Insured patients don't need pay money to see a doctor for the services that are covered by the insurance. The money will be paid by the committee. But patients will have to pay for services not covered by the insurance. If the patients have problems seeing a doctor, they can contact the community worker at the health facility.

The insurance covers only treatments prescribed by public agents (and not by private agents). The covered treatments are limited to the Nouna health district area. The insurance will not cover any services rendered outside the Nouna health district. Also, no transport out of the district will be covered by the insurance.

References

1. Sauerborn R, Nougtara A, Sorgho G et al. Assessment of MCH services in the district of Solenzo, Burkina Faso. II. Acceptability. *J Trop Pediatr* 1989; **35**(Suppl 1): 10–13.
2. Sauerborn R, Nougtara A, Diesfeld HJ. Low utilisation of community health workers: results from a household interview survey in Burkina Faso. *Soc Sci Med* 1989; **29**: 1163–1174.
3. Sauerborn R, Berman P, Nougtara A. Age bias, but no gender bias, in the intra-household resource allocation for health care in rural Burkina Faso. *Health Transit Rev* 1996; **6**: 131–145.
4. Krause G, Schleiermacher D, Borchert M et al. Diagnostic quality in rural health centres in Burkina Faso. *Trop Med Int Health* 1998; **3**: 100–107.
5. Baltussen R, Yé Y, Haddad S, Sauerborn R. Perceived quality of care of primary health care services in Burkina Faso. *Health Policy Plan* 2002; **17**: 42–48.
6. Sauerborn R, Nougtara A, Latimer E. The elasticity of demand for health care in Burkina Faso. *Health Policy Plan* 1994; **9**: 185–192.
7. Sauerborn R, Zombre S, Some F et al. *The rationale and feasibility of community-based insurance in rural Burkina Faso*. Discussion paper, University of Heidelberg, Department of Tropical Hygiene and Public Health, 2001.
8. Mugisha F, Kouyate B, Gbangou A, Sauerborn R. Examining out-of-pocket expenditure on health care in Nouna, Burkina Faso: implication for health policy. *Tropical Med Int Health* 2002; **7**: 187–196.
9. Sommerfeld J, Sanon M, Kouyate B et al. Informal Risk-Sharing Arrangements (IRSAS) in rural Burkina Faso: lessons for the development of Community-Based Insurance (CBI) I. *Int J Health Plann Mgmt* 2002; **17**: 147–163.
10. Creese A, Bennett S. Rural risk-sharing strategies. In: *Innovations in Health Care Financing. World Bank Discussion Paper No. 365*. George J Schieber, (ed.). The World Bank: Washington, DC, 1997: 163–182.
11. Asenso-Okyere WK, Osei-Akoto I, Anum A et al. Willingness to pay for health insurance in a developing economy. A pilot study of the informal sector of Ghana using contingent valuation. *Health Pol* 1997; **42**: 223–237.
12. Sauerborn R, Nougtara A, Hien M et al. Seasonal variations of household costs of illness in Burkina Faso. *Soc Sci Med* 1996; **43**: 281–290.
13. Burkina Faso Ministry of health. Project de Document de Politique Sanitaire Nationale (PSN). 2000.
14. Kouyaté B, Sanou M, Mugisha F et al. Community preference for a benefit package under community-based insurance. *Centre de Recherche en Sante de Nouna—Discussion paper series, No 2 Nouna, Burkina Faso* 2001.
15. Mugisha F. Health care system and household response to costs associated with illness in Nouna, Burkina Faso. University of Heidelberg, dissertation, 2001.
16. Diener A, O'Brien B, Gafni A. Health care contingent valuation studies: a review and classification of the literature. *Health Econ* 1998; **7**: 313–326.
17. Klose T. The contingent valuation method in health care. *Health Pol* 1999; **47**: 97–123.
18. Anderson G, Black C, Dunn E et al. Willingness to pay to shorten waiting time for cataract surgery. *Health Aff (Millwood)* 1997; **16**: 181–190.
19. Appel LJ, Steinberg EP, Powe NR et al. Risk reduction from low osmolality contrast media. What do patients think it is worth? *Med Care* 1990; **28**: 324–337.
20. Barner JC, Mason HL, Murray MD. Assessment of asthma patients' willingness to pay for and give time to an asthma self-management program. *Clin Ther* 1999; **21**: 878–894.
21. Coley CM, Li YH, Medsger AR et al. Preferences for home vs hospital care among low-risk patients with community-acquired pneumonia. *Arch Intern Med* 1996; **156**: 1565–1571.
22. Johannesson M. Economic evaluation of lipid lowering – a feasibility test of the contingent valuation approach. *Health Policy* 1992; **20**: 309–320.
23. Johannesson M, Jonsson B, Borgquist L. Willingness to pay for antihypertensive therapy results of a Swedish pilot study. *J Health Econ* 1991; **10**: 461–473.
24. Johannesson M, O'Conor RM, Kobelt-Nguyen G et al. Willingness to pay for reduced incontinence symptoms. *Br J Urol* 1997; **80**: 557–562.
25. Zethraeus N. Willingness to pay for hormone replacement therapy. *Health Econ* 1998; **7**: 31–38.
26. Chestnut LG, Keller LR, Lambert WE et al. Measuring heart patients' willingness to pay for changes in angina symptoms. *Med Decis Making* 1996; **16**: 65–77.

27. Kartman B, Andersson F, Johannesson M. Willingness to pay for reductions in angina pectoris attacks. *Med Decis Making* 1996; **16**: 248–253.
28. Granberg M, Wikland M, Nilsson L *et al*. Couples' willingness to pay for IVF/ET. *Acta Obstet Gynecol Scand* 1995; **74**: 199–202.
29. Liu JT, Hammitt JK, Wang JD *et al*. Mother's willingness to pay for her own and her child's health: a contingent valuation study in Taiwan. *Health Econ* 2000; **9**: 319–326.
30. Gore PR, Madhavan S. Consumers' preference and willingness to pay for pharmacist counselling for non-prescription medicines. *J Clin Pharm Ther* 1994; **19**: 17–25.
31. Dixon S, Shackley P. Estimating the benefits of community water fluoridation using the willingness-to-pay technique: results of a pilot study. *Community Dent Oral Epidemiol* 1999; **27**: 124–129.
32. Walraven G. Willingness to pay for district hospital services in rural Tanzania. *Health Pol Plan* 1996; **11**: 428–437.
33. Hassan EO, el Nahal N, el Hussein M. Acceptability of the once-a-month injectable contraceptives Cyclofem and Mesigyna in Egypt. *Contraception* 1994; **49**: 469–488.
34. Onwujekwe O, Shu E, Chima R *et al*. Willingness to pay for the retreatment of mosquito nets with insecticide in four communities of southeastern Nigeria. *Trop Med Int Health* 2000; **5**: 370–376.
35. Mathiyazhagan K. Willingness to pay for rural health insurance through community participation in India. *Int J Health Plann Manage* 1998; **13**: 47–67.
36. World Bank. *African Development Indicators 2000*. World Bank: Washington DC, 2000.
37. Burkina Faso Ministry of health. *Statistiques Sanitaires 1996*. Ouagadougou: Burkina Faso Ministry of Health, 1996.
38. Wuertwein R, Gbangou A, Kouyate B *et al*. The Nouna health district household survey: design and implementation. *SFB Discussion Series No 3* 2001.
39. Mitchell RC, Carson RT. *Using Surveys to Value Public Goods: The Contingent Valuation Method*. Resources for the Future: Washington, DC, 1989.
40. Sankoh OA, Ye Y, Sauerborn R *et al*. Clustering of childhood mortality in rural Burkina Faso. *Int J Epidemiol* 2001; **30**: 485–492.
41. Cameron T. A new paradigm for valuing non-market goods using referendum data: maximum likelihood estimation by censored logistic regression. *J Environ Econ Manage* 1988; **15**: 355–379.
42. Kleinbaum D, Kupper L, Muller K. *Applied Regression Analysis and Other Multivariable Methods*. PWS-KENT Publishing Company: Boston, 1988.
43. Scott Menard. *Applied Logistic Regression Analysis*. Sage Publications Inc.: California, 1995.
44. Chiu L, Tang KY, Liu YH *et al*. Willingness of families caring for victims of dementia to pay for nursing home care: results of a pilot study in Taiwan. *J Manag Med* 1998; **12**: 349–360, 321.
45. Chiu L, Tang KY, Shyu WC *et al*. The willingness of families caring for victims of stroke to pay for in-home respite care–results of a pilot study in Taiwan. *Health Pol* 1999; **46**: 239–254.
46. Cho MN, Lertmaharit S, Kamol-Ratanakul P *et al*. Ex post and ex ante willingness to pay (WTP) for the ICT Malaria Pf/Pv test kit in Myanmar. *Southeast Asian J Trop Med Public Health* 2000; **31**: 104–111.
47. Cummings RG, Brookshire DS, Schulze WD. *Valuing Environmental Goods: A State of the Arts Assessment of the Contingent Method*. Rowman and Allanheld: Totowa, NJ, 1986.
48. Zeckhauser R. Voting systems, honest preferences, and Pareto optimality. *Amer Political Sci Rev* 1973; **67**: 934–946.
49. Hoehn JP, Randall A. A satisfactory benefit cost indicator from contingent valuation. *J Environ Econ Manage* 1987; **14**: 226–247.
50. Bala MV, Wood LL, Zarkin GA *et al*. Valuing outcomes in health care: a comparison of willingness to pay and quality-adjusted life-years. *J Clin Epidemiol* 1998; **51**: 667–676.
51. Phillips KA, Homan RK, Luft HS *et al*. Willingness to pay for poison control centers. *J Health Econ* 1997; **16**: 343–357.
52. Stalhammar NO. An empirical note on willingness to pay and starting-point bias. *Med Decis Making* 1996; **16**: 242–247.

4.10 Differential willingness of household heads to pay community-based health insurance premia for themselves and other household members

Dong H, Kouyate B, Cairns J, Sauerborn R.

Health Policy Plan. 2004 19(2): 120-6.

Reprinted with permission from Oxford University Press.

Differential willingness of household heads to pay community-based health insurance premia for themselves and other household members

HENGJIN DONG,[1] BOCAR KOUYATE,[2] JOHN CAIRNS[3] AND RAINER SAUERBORN[1]

[1]Department of Tropical Hygiene and Public Health, University of Heidelberg, Heidelberg, Germany, [2]Nouna Health Research Centre, Nouna, Burkina Faso and [3]Health Economics Research Unit, University of Aberdeen, Aberdeen, UK

Objective: This study compares household heads' willingness-to-pay (WTP) for community-based health insurance (CBI) for themselves with their WTP for other household members, in order to provide information for policy makers on setting the premium and choosing the enrolment unit.

Method: A random sample of 698 heads of households was interviewed in the northwest of Burkina Faso and a bidding game approach was used to elicit WTP. Factors associated with differences in WTP were identified, including characteristics of the household head and of the household.

Results: Mean WTP by the heads of households for insurance for themselves (3575 CFA) was twice their mean WTP per capita for the household as a whole (1759 CFA). The old have a lower WTP than the young, females have lower WTP than males, the poor have a lower WTP than the rich, and that those with less schooling have a lower WTP than those with more years of schooling.

Conclusion: The differences in household heads' WTP for insurance for themselves and their WTP to insure their households as a whole need to be considered when setting the insurance premium. WTP information can assist decision makers with the complex problem of choosing the enrolment unit and setting the premium.

Key words: willingness to pay, contingent valuation method, community-based health insurance, preference, health care financing, Burkina Faso

Introduction

Community-based health insurance (CBI) is viewed by many as a promising new tool for health system improvement for rural populations in low-income countries, particularly in sub-Saharan Africa (Creese and Bennett 1997). It is a means of providing insurance coverage for rural communities unlikely to benefit immediately from either a social or private health insurance scheme (Asenso-Okyere et al. 1997). CBI has the advantage of dissociating the time of payment from the time of use of services, which is clearly better adapted than user fees to the seasonal fluctuations of revenue and expenditure flows of rural households (Sauerborn et al. 1996).

This paper compares the willingness-to-pay (WTP) of household heads for CBI for themselves and for their entire household. WTP is used to estimate utility in monetary terms. According to economic theory the maximum amount of money an individual is willing to pay for a commodity or service is an indicator of the utility or satisfaction to her of that commodity. It is usually elicited by a contingent valuation method, which circumvents the absence of actual markets by presenting consumers with hypothetical markets in which they have the opportunity to buy the good or service.

A number of studies of WTP for health benefits to others have been undertaken. Viscusi et al. (1987) compared WTP to reduce pesticide risks to oneself and to one's children. Agee and Crocker (1996) estimated parental WTP to reduce the risk of neurological impairment in their children. Liu et al. (2000) asked a sample of 700 mothers in Taiwan how much they were willing to pay for preventive medicine to protect themselves and their children from suffering a cold. Finally, Onwujekwe et al. (2002) asked 1519 household heads in south-east Nigeria open-ended questions to elicit WTP for insecticide-treated nets for indigent members of the community.

In the present study household heads in northwest Burkina Faso are asked about their WTP for health insurance for themselves *and* for their entire household. Although two studies have previously asked household heads about their WTP for health insurance for the whole household, neither study compared the WTP of the household head for insurance for themselves with their WTP for insurance for the entire household (Asenso-Okyere et al. 1997; Mathiyazhagan 1998). Such a comparison is important because it can provide information relevant to the choice of whether the enrolment unit should be individual or household, and to setting the premium.

Methodology

Study site, sampling procedure and sample size

The household survey, which was conducted as part of a project on the control of tropical infectious diseases in Nouna, Burkina Faso, was based on a two-stage cluster sampling procedure, with each household having the same probability of being selected. In the first stage, clusters of households were selected and in the second stage, respondent households were selected in each cluster. The Nouna health district, located in the northwest of Burkina Faso, has a population of roughly 230 000 inhabitants who are served by one district hospital and 16 Centres de Santé et de Promotion Sociale, the first-line health care facility in the health system. Overall, 800 households were selected, 480 in the rural area and 320 in the town of Nouna (Wuertwein et al. 2001). The WTP questions were merged into the regular (two to three times a year) household survey questionnaire. The data were collected during January and March 2001.

Out of the 800 randomly selected households, 776 were included in the analysis (22 had moved elsewhere) and two households could not be located at the time of the survey. In the 776 households, 705 (90.0%) heads of the households answered the household WTP questions (one refused and 70 were absent from the household at the time of the survey). Out of the 705 heads, seven heads didn't answer the individual WTP questions, leaving 698 cases available for analysis. The proportion of zero values was 4.7% for individual WTP and 3.9% for WTP for the whole household. There were no significant differences between the responders and non-responders in terms of location of residence, religion, household size, proportion of children 0–5 years old, proportion of adults 65+ years old, household economic variables and previous medical expenditures (Dong et al. 2003a).

Household interview

The pilot study, household interview, CBI benefit package and the process of eliciting WTP are described in detail elsewhere (Dong et al. 2003a). The interviewer first explained the CBI scenario to the household head. The head of household was then asked his/her WTP for him/herself and for the whole household including him/herself. Each household head was randomly assigned one of 13 starting prices drawn from a range from 2000 to 8000 CFA for him/herself and another set of 13 starting prices for the whole household from 8000 to 32 000 CFA with a interval of 500 Franc CFA (US$1 = 750 CFA). The starting prices were informed by the expected cost of the CBI benefit package and the results from a pilot WTP study.

If the answer to the first price offered to the respondent was 'yes', the interviewer increased the bid by increments of 500 CFA until the respondent said 'no'. If the initial answer was 'no', the interviewer reduced the amount of money by 500 CFA and continued this process until the respondent said 'yes'. The last sum of money receiving a 'yes' response was used as the WTP resulting from the bidding game approach. This procedure results in more conservative WTP values than one using the mid-point between the last 'yes' response and the final 'no' as the WTP value.

WTP measures and data analysis methods

Individual WTP describes the value that a household head is willing to pay for him/herself for CBI, and household WTP describes the value that the head of household is willing to pay for health insurance for his/her whole household. WTP per capita is household WTP divided by the number of persons in the household.

Mean WTP is estimated directly from the data provided. Multiple linear regression is used to study the influence of individual and household variables on WTP because the WTP data are continuous and the proportion of zero WTP values is low. The empirical model is as follows:

$$WTP = \alpha + \beta_1 X_1 + \beta_2 X_2 + \ldots + \beta_{n-1} X_{n-1} + \beta_n X_n$$

WTP = willingness-to-pay

α = intercept

β = coefficients of explanatory variables

X = explanatory variables

Individual WTP and WTP per capita are likely to depend to a large extent on the expected benefits from insurance and the ability-to-pay the premium. These in turn are likely to be influenced by a number of characteristics of the household head and of the household. Cash income and expenditure in the previous 6 months and the value of agricultural produce and animals will influence the ability to pay. Household size and its composition in terms of age and gender, and the age and gender of the household head, may influence both expected benefit from health insurance and the ability to pay.

The level of recent medical expenditure by the household may also influence the expected benefit. Household heads with poorer health or in households with poorer health are expected to be willing to pay more for the health insurance premium because of their greater capacity to benefit. The number of episodes of disease for the head of household and total disease episodes in the household (recorded over three rounds of the household survey) are used to measure health status. The expected benefit may also depend on the distance to the nearest health facility. Those with more years of schooling would be expected to have a higher WTP because they may perceive the benefits to be greater.

Table 1 lists the explanatory variables used in the linear regression models.

Table 1. Household and household head characteristics

Variable name	Description	Mean (s.d.)
Household variables		
Logagrih	Household agricultural value, log10	4.41 (1.76)
Loghcsh6	Household cash income from 6 month, log 10	4.59 (1.16)
Loghanim	Household animal value, log 10	4.31 (1.84)
Loghexp6	Household expenditure for 6 month, log 10	4.72 (0.68)
Diseaseh	Episodes of diseases of household in 3 surveys	2.13 (2.31)
Logmcsth	Household total medical expenditure for past month, log 10	0.65 (1.29)
Loghwmex	Household western medical expenditure for past month, log 10	0.34 (1.03)
Household size		8.02 (5.74)
0–5 years old percentage	0–5 year old/household size	0.17 (0.15)
65+ years old percentage	65+ year olds/household size	0.06 (0.15)
Male percentage	Number of males/household size	0.52 (0.20)
Household head individual variables		
Age	Age in years	49.25 (14.19)
Sex	Male = 1, female = 0	0.91
Education	Years of schooling	0.97 (2.62)
Monogamy	Monogamy = 1, else = 0	0.63
Single	Single = 1, else = 0	0.03
Traditional religion	Traditional religion = 1, else = 0	0.11
Residing in Nouna town	Location of residency, Nouna town = 1, else = 0	0.38
Diseasei	Episodes of disease of individuals in 3 surveys	0.60 (0.90)
Health facility variables		
Distance	Distance to health facility (km)	3.74 (5.01)

P-P Normal Probability Plots were applied to check whether variables were normally distributed. Income and expenditure were skewed and therefore transformed using a logarithmic transformation ($x = \log(X+1)$). Outliers were excluded from the model if the studentized residuals were greater than |3| (Scott 1995). Analysis of residuals was used to assess the appropriateness of the model. The results showed that the model was appropriate (residual mean 0, variance 0.984 to 0.985) (Table 2). If all assumptions were met, the residual mean would be 0 and the variance would be 1. A Ramsey reset test and a test for heteroscedasticity (Donaldson et al. 1998) were used to further test the models (Table 2). The test results were not statistically significant. Thus there are not evident problems with the specification of the model or violations of the assumption of constant variance.

Results

Household and household head characteristics

Respondents had a mean age of 49 years and on average 1 year of schooling. Ninety-one per cent of them were male and 38% lived in Nouna town. Households had on average eight members and a cash income in the previous 6 months of 145 865 CFA (mean) or 63 000 CFA (median) and agricultural produce valued at 203 995 CFA (mean) or 104 000 CFA (median). Of the 698 respondents, 33 were not willing to pay anything for health insurance for themselves and 27 of these were not willing to pay for the household as a whole.

Mean WTP and WTP per capita by sub-group

Table 3 shows the mean premium household heads are willing to pay for themselves and the mean WTP per capita grouped by various individual and household characteristics. Household heads' WTP for themselves was double their WTP per capita. This difference between individual WTP and WTP per capita and all the other WTP differences reported in the table (except with respect to marital status) are statistically significant.

There are differences between sub-groups in individual WTP and in WTP per capita. Unmarried household heads were willing to pay more for themselves and others than married household heads, but this was not statistically significant. Household heads residing in Nouna town were willing to pay relatively less for themselves and more for other household members than those in rural areas. As the household size increases the WTP difference increases. The presence of children in a household is associated with a higher WTP for own insurance and a lower WTP per capita.

Factors influencing individual WTP and WTP per capita

Table 2 shows the results of the multivariate analysis with individual WTP and WTP per capita as dependent variables.

Age of household head had a negative coefficient and significantly influenced individual WTP and WTP per capita. Male gender and years of schooling had the expected positive associations. Male gender significantly influenced WTP per capita, and education significantly influenced both individual WTP and WTP per capita. Single marital state had a positive association and significantly influenced WTP per capita. Residing in Nouna town, religion and episodes of disease did not have a statistically significant impact.

Household income and expenditure in the past 6 months

Table 2. Individual and per capita WTP

Variables	Individual WTP		WTP per capita	
	B (S.E.)	Beta	B (S.E.)	Beta
(Constant)	78.714 (963.199)		2215.877 (608.193) **	
Household head's individual variables				
Age	–16.903 (8.408) *	–0.094	–11.936 (5.344) *	–0.100
Sex	735.162 (397.842)	0.082	699.459 (252.989) **	0.119
Education	115.259 (38.706) **	0.117	125.626 (24.588) **	0.194
Monogamy	90.777 (215.650)	0.017	–159.213 (136.582)	–0.046
Single	71.436 (603.186)	0.005	734.702 (372.855) *	0.076
Traditional religion	538.670 (310.887)	0.063	–41.711 (194.934)	–0.008
Residing in Nouna town	–457.422 (269.328)	–0.086	–219.535 (170.301)	–0.063
Diseasei	4.036 (116.883)	0.001	76.393 (74.013)	0.041
Household variables				
Logagrih	13.020 (69.777)	0.009	–42.080 (44.138)	–0.044
Loghcsh6	183.452 (91.495) *	0.081	21.083 (58.221)	0.014
Loghanim	27.293 (61.812)	0.020	–16.201 (39.117)	–0.018
Loghexp6	404.000 (171.454) *	0.105	62.144 (108.954)	0.025
Diseaseh	–42.308 (49.870)	–0.038	–55.893 (31.465)	–0.077
Logmcsth	369.510 (108.334) **	0.185	229.642 (68.591) **	0.177
Loghwmex	–50.257 (129.327)	–0.020	–131.149 (80.975)	–0.080
Household size	–51.038 (21.074) *	–0.114	–99.703 (13.311) **	–0.339
0–5 years old percentage	286.579 (709.337)	0.016	–364.544 (451.357)	–0.031
65+ years old percentage	–1732.663 (721.045) *	–0.104	–357.854 (457.705)	–0.033
Male percentage	–10.313 (5.093) *	–0.081	–3.404 (3.228)	–0.041
Health facility and other variables				
Distance	–37.467 (22.111)	–0.073	–29.465 (13.992) *	–0.088
First bid (individual WTP)	0.304 (0.049) **	0.220		
First bid (household WTP)			0.019 (0.008) *	0.086
n	692		692	
F value	8.164**		11.092**	
R^2	0.204		0.258	
Std. Residual mean (s.d.)	0.000 (0.985)		0.000 (0.985)	
Ramsey reset test	F (3673) = 1.36		F (3677) = 2.22	
	p = 0.253		p = 0.085	
Heteroscedasticity test	Chi^2 (1) = 0.81		Chi^2 (1) = 3.45	
	p = 0.367		p = 0.063	

* $p < 0.05$; ** $p < 0.01$.

both had a positive impact on WTP, but it was only statistically significant in the case of individual WTP. The size of the household had a significantly negative impact on both individual WTP and WTP per capita. Greater distance to the health facility had the expected negative association, reducing individual WTP and WTP per capita, although it was only statistically significant in the latter case. The starting bid had the expected positive impact on individual WTP and WTP per capita. The impact was particularly marked in the case of individual WTP.

Discussion

Mean WTP is usually advocated for use in cost-benefit analysis and median WTP is advocated for pricing, although both of them can provide valuable information for price setting. However, if the WTP data were normally distributed the mean WTP would equal the median WTP. This article focuses on the household head's WTP for CBI for him/herself and for the household. Median WTP in this sample has been analyzed in detail elsewhere (Dong et al. 2003a). This study has emphasized characteristics of the household and of the head of household. From a provider perspective, expected quality of health services, availability of essential drugs and distance to a health facility are policy relevant influences on WTP for CBI. Only distance to a health facility varied in a measurable manner across households in this study. The impact of quality of care and drug availability will need further studies.

This study suggests that the individual WTP of household heads for health insurance is on average twice their WTP per capita, that the old have a lower WTP than the young, that females have lower WTP than males, that the poor have a lower WTP than the rich, and that those with less schooling have a lower WTP than those with more years of schooling. The results in Table 3 suggest that there might be interesting differences between men and women with respect to WTP for themselves and WTP per capita, and it is not difficult to identify reasons for such differences (Liu et al. 2000). However, the standard errors for male and female WTP are large and there are 10 men for every woman in the sample, so it is not appropriate to make much of this finding. A key relationship is that between WTP and household size. This

Table 3. Household heads' individual mean WTP (CFA[a]) and WTP per capita

Variables	Sample size	Individual WTP (s.d.)	WTP per capita (s.d.)	WTP difference (s.d.)	p[b]
Total	698	3575 (3255)	1759 (2683)	1816 (2495)	<0.001
Sex					=0.001
Male	634	3668 (3271)	1748 (2674)	1919 (2533)	
Female	64	2653 (2962)	1859 (2797)	794 (1798)	
Religion					<0.05
Traditional	73	4122 (3547)	1714 (2148)	2408 (3005)	
Others	625	3511 (3217)	1764 (2740)	1747 (2422)	
Marriage					>0.05
Married	676	3535 (3236)	1700 (2660)	1835 (2509)	
Single	22	4818 (3663)	3545 (2825)	1273 (1983)	
Location of residency					=0.001
Nouna town	263	3460 (2670)	2053 (2340)	1407 (2418)	
Rural area	435	3645 (3564)	1581 (2859)	2064 (2511)	
Household size					<0.001
1–5	250	3617 (4102)	2890 (4047)	727 (2341)	
6–10	282	3612 (2645)	1338 (1105)	2274 (2300)	
11+	166	3449 (2729)	768 (625)	2681 (2472)	
0–5 years old percentage					<0.001
0	222	3386 (4230)	2595 (4220)	791 (2368)	
1–25	292	3573 (2698)	1212 (1143)	2361 (2379)	
26+	184	3806 (2661)	1616 (1579)	2190 (2459)	
65+ years old percentage					<0.001
0	520	3800 (3404)	1915 (2936)	1885 (2482)	
1–10	59	3928 (3054)	898 (761)	3030 (2819)	
11–20	61	2611 (1913)	1103 (1347)	1508 (1758)	
21+	58	2210 (2697)	1917 (2362)	293 (2154)	
Male percentage					<0.001
0	25	2962 (3663)	2670 (3853)	292 (1584)	
1–25	32	3062 (2242)	1557 (1318)	1505 (1725)	
26–50	336	3705 (2731)	1779 (2064)	1926 (2726)	
51–75	243	3529 (2761)	1362 (1408)	2167 (2399)	
76+	62	3562 (6455)	2940 (6471)	623 (1414)	

[a] US$1 = 750 CFA.
[b] t-test or one-way ANOVA test for WTP difference.

inverse relationship suggests that, even when controlling for household income and expenditure, number of household members reflects ability to pay rather than capacity to benefit.

Also suggested is that medical expenditure (logmcsth) is significantly associated with both higher individual WTP and higher WTP per capita, and age is significantly associated with both lower individual WTP and lower WTP per capita. Medical expenditure can be taken as an indicator of economic status like income and total expenditure. These findings imply that the poor and the aged are vulnerable groups that need to be taken into consideration when determining the arrangements for CBI.

Before discussing the implications of these results, it is important to consider possible limitations of the analysis. One potential limitation lies in the unfamiliarity of the respondents with CBI and with the questions used to elicit their WTP. However, care was taken to explain the principle of CBI. Also a separate study of the reliability of the WTP estimates suggested that reliability was moderate to good (Dong et al. 2003b). Another potential limitation relates to the strong evidence of starting point bias. The value of the standardized coefficient (Beta) shows that the first bid has a strong positive correlation particularly with individual WTP but also with WTP per capita. Starting point bias is the main problem with the bidding game technique. Many studies have shown this bias with WTP differing markedly among different sub-samples (Chestnut et al. 1996; Kartman et al. 1996; Stalhammar 1996; Phillips et al. 1997; Bala et al. 1998; Barner et al. 1999; Liu et al. 2000). For instance, Kartman and colleagues (1996) found that individuals in the highest starting-bid group were willing to pay double that of those in the lowest. Thirteen different starting points were used in this study, in part so that the results would be less vulnerable to starting point bias.

Finally, it is possible that household heads did not give as careful consideration to their responses when reporting WTP for the entire household. But similar models explained individual WTP and WTP per capita (the only differences in association were for insignificant coefficients) and a higher proportion of variation in WTP is explained by the WTP per capita model. This does not support the suggestion that household heads were less careful in providing WTPs for the entire household.

What are the implications for premium setting and whether enrolment should be on an individual or household basis? In considering this it is necessary to specify the objective of CBI. For example, suppose it was to maximize numbers enrolled subject to a breakeven constraint. The solution will depend on the expected cost of the benefits provided when enrolment is restricted to household heads and when it is extended to all household members, and on the likely demand for insurance at different premia. The insurance premium could differ according to household size; for example, households might be categorized into those with less than 6, 6 to 10 and more than 10 members, and each group would then pay a different premium. WTP per capita for different household sizes multiplied by household size can provide useful information for those setting the insurance premium.

Clearly choice of enrolment unit and the setting of premia are complex problems but ones which in principle WTP data can help address. Demand for health insurance can be predicted for different enrolment units and for different insurance premia. Of course these choices cannot be solely resolved by using WTP data to maximize the number enrolled. It is also necessary to consider broader issues, in particular, financial sustainability. However, the analysis of WTP for CBI can help to identify the likely consequences of different policies.

Conclusion

Household heads' valuation of the benefits of health insurance to themselves differs from their valuation of the benefits to other members of the household. This difference may be related to economic status, gender and other social and economic characteristics of the households. These differing valuations can provide information for policy-makers for setting the premium for CBI and for deciding whether the enrolment unit should be the individual or the household. The results imply that the premium for CBI needs to be adjusted for economic status and household size or the poor need to be given exemptions or subsidies; otherwise, the poor will have less access to CBI than the rich. The results also imply that the household might be a better unit of enrolment in terms of protecting other household members (not household head) such as women, elders and children.

References

Agee DM, Crocker TD. 1996. Parental altruism and child lead exposure: inferences from the demand for chelation therapy. *Journal of Human Resources* **31**: 677–91.

Asenso-Okyere WK, Osei-Akoto I, Anum A, Appiah EN. 1997. Willingness to pay for health insurance in a developing economy: a pilot study of the informal sector of Ghana using contingent valuation. *Health Policy* **42**: 223–37.

Bala MV, Wood LL, Zarkin GA et al. 1998. Valuing outcomes in health care: a comparison of willingness to pay and quality-adjusted life-years. *Journal of Clinical Epidemiology* **51**: 667–76.

Barner JC, Mason HL, Murray MD. 1999. Assessment of asthma patients' willingness to pay for and give time to an asthma self-management program. *Clinical Therapeutics* **21**: 878–94.

Chestnut LG, Keller LR, Lambert WE, Rowe RD. 1996. Measuring heart patients' willingness to pay for changes in angina symptoms. *Medical Decision Making* **16**: 65–77.

Creese A, Bennett S. 1997. Rural risk-sharing strategies. In: Schieber JG (ed) *Innovations in Health Care Financing*. World Bank Discussion Paper No. 365. Washington DC: World Bank, p. 163–82.

Donaldson C, Jones AM, Mapp TJ, Olson JA. 1998. Limited dependent variables in willingness to pay studies: applications in health care. *Applied Economics* **30**: 667–77.

Dong H, Kouyate B, Cairns J, Mugisha F, Sauerborn R. 2003a. Willingness to pay for community-based insurance in Burkina Faso. *Health Economics* **12**: 849–62.

Dong H, Kouyate B, Cairns J, Sauerborn R. 2003b. A comparison of the reliability of the take-it-or-leave-it and the bidding game approaches to estimating willingness-to-pay in a rural population in West Africa. *Social Science and Medicine* **56**: 2182–9.

Kartman B, Andersson F, Johannesson M. 1996. Willingness to pay for reductions in angina pectoris attacks. *Medical Decision Making* **16**: 248–53.

Liu JT, Hammitt JK, Wang JD, Liu JL. 2000. Mother's willingness to pay for her own and her child's health: a contingent valuation study in Taiwan. *Health Economics* **9**: 319–26.

Mathiyazhagan K. 1998. Willingness to pay for rural health insurance through community participation in India. *International Journal of Health Planning and Management* **13**: 47–67.

Onwujekwe O, Chima R, Shu E et al. 2002. Altruistic willingness to pay in community-based sales of insecticide-treated nets exists in Nigeria. *Social Science and Medicine* **54**: 519–27.

Phillips KA, Homan RK, Luft HS et al. 1997. Willingness to pay for poison control centers. *Journal of Health Economics* **16**: 343–57.

Sauerborn R, Nougtara A, Hien M, Diesfeld HJ. 1996. Seasonal variations of household costs of illness in Burkina Faso. *Social Science and Medicine* **43**: 281–90.

Scott M. 1995. *Applied logistic regression analysis*. Thousand Oaks, CA: Sage Publications Inc.

Stalhammar NO. 1996. An empirical note on willingness to pay and starting-point bias. *Medical Decision Making* **16**: 242–7.

Viscusi WK, Magat WA, Huber J. 1987. An investigation of the rationality of consumer valuations of multiple health risks. *Rand Journal of Economics* **18**: 465–79.

Wuertwein R, Gbangou A, Kouyate B et al. 2001. The Nouna health district household survey: design and implementation. *SFB Discussion Series* **3**: 1–51.

Acknowledgements

This paper arises from the 'control of tropical infectious diseases' project in Burkina Faso financially supported by the German Research Foundation (Deutsche Forschungsgemeinschaft) (SFB 544). The Health Economics Research Unit (HERU) at the University of Aberdeen is funded by the Chief Scientist Office of the Scottish Executive Health Department (SEHD). The views expressed in this paper are those of the authors and not the SEHD. Sanou Aboubakary, Adjima Gbangou, Yazoumé Yé and Mamadou Sanon from Nouna Health Research Centre provided invaluable help with data collection. We are also grateful to Frederick Mugisha for valuable comments and suggestions.

Biographies

Hengjin Dong, Ph.D., is a Research Fellow in the Department of Tropical Hygiene and Public Health at the University of Heidelberg in Germany.

Bocar Kouyate works at the Nouna Health Research Centre at Nouna, Burkina Faso.

John Cairns, MPhil., is Professor in Health Economics at the Health Economics Research Unit, University of Aberdeen, Scotland, UK.

Rainer Sauerborn, Ph.D., is a Professor in the Department of Tropical Hygiene and Public Health at the University of Heidelberg in Germany.

Correspondence: Hengjin Dong, PhD, Department of Tropical Hygiene and Public Health, University of Heidelberg, Im Neuenheimer Feld 324, D-69120 Heidelberg, Germany. E-mail: donghengjin@yahoo.com or hengjin.dong@urz.uni-heidelberg.de

4.11 The two faces of enhancing utilization of health-care services: determinants of patient initiation and retention in rural Burkina Faso

MUGISHA F, KOUYATE B, DONG H, CHEPNG'ENO G, SAUERBORN R.

BULL WHO 82 (8), AUGUST 2004, 572-579

Reprinted with permission from World Health Organization.

The two faces of enhancing utilization of health-care services: determinants of patient initiation and retention in rural Burkina Faso

Frederick Mugisha[1], Kouyate Bocar[2], Hengjin Dong[3], Gloria Chepng'eno[4], & Rainer Sauerborn[5]

Objective To explore the factors that determine whether a patient will initiate treatment within a system of health-care services, and the factors that determine whether the patient will be retained in the chosen system, in Nouna, rural Burkina Faso.

Methods The data used were pooled from four rounds of a household survey conducted in Nouna, rural Burkina Faso. The ongoing demographic surveillance system provided a sampling framework for this survey in which 800 households were sampled using a two-stage cluster sampling procedure. More than one treatment episode was observed for a single episode of illness per patient. The multinomial logit model was used to explore the determinants of patient initiation to systems of modern, traditional and home treatment, and a binary logit model was used to explore the determinants of patient retention within the chosen health-care provider system.

Findings The results suggest that the determinants of patient initiation and their subsequent retention are different. Household income, education, urban residence and expected competency of the provider are positive predictors of initiation, but not of retention, for modern health-care services. Only perceived quality of care positively predicted retention in modern health-care services.

Conclusion Interventions focusing on patient initiation and patient retention are likely to be different. Policies directed at enhancing initiation for modern health-care services would primarily focus on reducing financial barriers, while those directed at increasing retention would primarily focus on attributes that improve the perceived quality of care.

Keywords Delivery of health care/statistics; Health services accessibility; Patient acceptance of health-care/psychology/statistics; Patient satisfaction/economics; Patient compliance; Fees and charges; Health services/standards; Home nursing/utilization; Choice behavior; Medicine, Traditional; Quality of health care; Health services, Indigenous/utilization; Socioeconomic factors; Rural health services; Policy making; Sampling studies; Burkina Faso (*source: MeSH, NLM*).

Mots clés Délivrance soins/statistique; Accessibilité service santé; Acceptation des soins/psychologie/statistique; Satisfaction malade/économie; Observance prescription; Tarifs et honoraires; Services santé/normes; Soins infirmiers domicile/utilisation; Comportement choix; Médecine traditionnelle; Qualité soins; Service santé indigène/utilisation; Facteur socio-économique; Service santé milieu rural; Choix d'une politique; Etude échantillon; Burkina Faso (*source : MeSH, INSERM*).

Palabras clave Prestación de atención de salud/estadística; Accesibilidad a los servicios de salud; Aceptación de la atención de salud/psicología/estadística; Satisfacción del paciente/economía; Cooperación del paciente; Tarifas y honorarios; Servicios de salud/normas; Cuidados domiciliarios de salud/utilización; Conducta de elección; Medicina tradicional; Calidad de la atención de salud; Servicios de salud autóctonos/utilización; Factores socioeconómicos; Servicios rurales de salud; Formulación de políticas; Muestreo; Burkina Faso (*fuente: DeCS, BIREME*).

Arabic

Bulletin of the World Health Organization 2004;82:572-579.

Voir page 578 le résumé en français. En la página 578 figura un resumen en español.

Introduction

Enhancing the utilization of health-care services has two faces: one, increasing initiation of patients to appropriate treatment and two, ensuring their subsequent retention. Initiation refers to the choice of health-care services made by the patient seeking treatment for the first time, while retention refers to a follow-up visit to the same health-care services in order to seek treatment for the same episode of illness. The former deals primarily with reducing barriers that prevent access to appropriate treatment, including financial constraints, reducing distances to health-care

---

[1] Associate Research Scientist, African Population and Health Research Center, Shelter-Afrique Centre, PO Box 10787, 00100 GPO, Nairobi, Kenya (email: fmugisha@aphrc.org). Correspondence should be sent to this author.
[2] Director, Nouna Health Research Center (CRSN), Nouna, Burkina Faso.
[3] Research Fellow, Department of Tropical Hygiene and Public Health, Heidelberg University, Heidelberg, Germany.
[4] Research Trainee, African Population and Health Research Center (APHRC), Nairobi, Kenya.
[5] Director, Department of Tropical Hygiene and Public Health, Heidelberg University, Heidelberg, Germany.
Ref. No. **03-003335**
(*Submitted: 19 March 2003 – Final revised version received: 15 October 2003 – Accepted: 18 February 2004*)

facilities, and improving education. The latter, retention, deals with maintaining appropriate treatment and ensuring proper monitoring in the case of patients who have a chronic disease or who have not been cured by the first treatment. Although initiation has been the subject of extensive research (*1–7*), retention has received less attention. Of the few studies on retention that have been conducted, one concerns health-care switching behaviour of patients with malaria in a Kenyan rural community (*8*), and one relates to gynaecological care (*9*). Other studies that have looked at switching have mainly been concerned with insurance providers (e.g. *10, 11*) and drug regimes (e.g. *12*).

The reason for the concentration of research efforts on initiation may be the assumption that the factors that determine initiation into a health-care system are the same as those that determine retention, and the fact that the number of patients to be retained is a small proportion of the number required to initiate treatment. However, if the determinants of initiation and retention are different, then there may be a need to look more closely at existing policies and strategies in order to ensure that both types of determinant are taken into account. Moreover, if the determinants of retention are likely to have a multiplier effect on the determinants for initiation, then the effect on overall utilization may be much greater. For example, if people were to choose a health-care provider on the basis of advice from a neighbour (the "neighbourhood effect"), a person who is dissatisfied with their own experience of treatment received will be less likely to advise a neighbour to initiate treatment.

In the dataset from rural Burkina Faso used in this paper, we observed multiple episodes of treatment, in chronological order, for a single episode of illness, per person. We explored the determinants of patient initiation to treatment and their subsequent retention, if a second treatment episode was sought.

Methods

Sampling procedure and data collection

The data used to explore the determinants of initiation into a health-care system and of retention in that system were pooled from four rounds of a household survey conducted in Nouna, rural Burkina Faso. The survey was carried out within the framework of the ongoing demographic surveillance system (DSS), which involves the quarterly collection of demographic and health data from the same household members. A two-stage cluster sampling procedure was used in urban and rural areas of Nouna. During the first stage of cluster sampling, clusters were selected at random from rural areas (twenty clusters) and from urban areas (seven clusters). In the second stage, respondent households were selected at random from each of these 27 clusters. In total, 800 households were selected into the sample; 480 of these were in rural areas and 320 were in urban areas, representing 62% and 38% of all the households in these areas, respectively. All observations for the four rounds of the survey were pooled to obtain a sample that was of sufficient size to allow both patient initiation and retention to be analysed.

Individuals were asked whether or not they had been ill in the preceding one month. Each individual reporting an episode of illness was asked whether he/she had sought treatment from a health-care worker, a traditional healer or a relative/friend/self. For each episode of illness, individuals who had had more than one episode of treatment were asked to report the chronological order in which they had sought treatment from health-care providers. For example, a person who decided to go to the modern health-care provider and later change to the traditional healer would report "modern" for the first episode of treatment and "traditional" for the second. For each episode of treatment, we collected additional information on the perceived quality of the care received and expenditure necessary. This chronology of events allowed us to examine whether a patient had sought more than one episode of treatment and, if so, whether the patient had changed health-care provider (i.e. had switched) or not (i.e. had been retained).

Definition of variables

Commonly used variables are listed in Table 1, while others are described in the text.

Treatment choice was divided into three distinct systems of health care; "home", including treatment by self, friend, or relative; "modern", including treatment by health-care personnel including a nurse, midwife, doctor, pharmacist or dentist; and "traditional", including treatment with herbs and other African traditional medicines administered by the traditional healer.

Retention was coded as 0 when a patient was retained in a health-care system (home, modern or traditional) for at least two episodes of treatment and 1 if the patient had switched from one system to another during the same episode of illness. Thus if a patient had sought treatment from a health-care worker in a health clinic and then went to a hospital, the patient was considered to be retained in the modern system of health care. Likewise, if a person had sought treatment from a hospital during the first episode of treatment and went to the traditional healer during the second episode of treatment for the same illness, the person was considered to have changed system and had therefore not been retained by the modern system.

For *type of illness*, malaria and fever were coded as 1, and other illnesses (e.g. diarrhoea, snake-bite, influenza, stroke, mumps) as 0. The literature suggests that people are less likely to seek treatment if they perceive the illness to be malaria (*5*). *Total health care expenditure* during the first episode of treatment comprised expenditure on transport, medication and consultation. *Reasons for treatment choice* included lack of money for an alternative, trust in the perceived competency of the system, and nearest choice. This was coded as 1 for competency and 0 otherwise. *Perceived quality of care* is considered to be a summary of the different attributes of the health-care provider in the opinion of the patient. It was defined on a five-likert scale, for which 1, 2, 3, 4 and 5 represented "very poor", "poor", "fair", "good" and "very good" perceived quality, respectively, although for the analysis these were regrouped to "poor", "fair" and "good". *Education* of the head of the household was considered and classified as primary, secondary or alphabetization (a form of adult education in which people are taught to read and write, and also involves limited skills training).

Statistical analysis

To explore the determinants of patient retention we used a binomial logit model, in which we concurrently compared patients who did not switch health-care providers with those who did, and with patients who did not seek a second episode of treatment. A multinomial model was used to concurrently compare different treatment choices for the first episode of treatment. The multinomial logit model can be thought of as an extension of the binary logit model (*13*). The multinomial logit model allows the effects of the independent variables to differ for each system of health-care provision. It can be thought of as simultaneously estimating binary logits for all possible comparisons

Results

The results suggest that the factors determining whether a patient is initiated into a system of health care and factors determining whether a patient is retained by that system are different. While household income, education, and type of illness determine the initial choice of provider (i.e. initiation), they do not determine whether patients switch health-care providers for subsequent treatment, if the illness requires more than one episode of treatment.

Table 2 shows the distribution of patients who sought treatment from the three health-care provider systems for the first episode of treatment. The results show that a greater proportion of rural residents seek health care from home and traditional systems. Patients who sought treatment from the modern system had had a higher level of education than those who sought treatment from the traditional system. Most patients (and a similar proportion of patients in each case) who chose the modern or the traditional systems did so because of perceived confidence in the provider. The head of the household was more likely to seek treatment from the traditional or modern systems than were other members of the same household. Malaria was more likely to be treated at home.

Table 3 shows the distribution of patients who were retained, chose to switch to another system or never sought a second episode of treatment. The results show that men, the employed, those who had confidence in the provider system at the time of initiating treatment and household heads were more likely to change provider. Patients with malaria, rather than any other illness, and patients with a lower level of education were less likely to seek a second episode of treatment, and patients in urban areas were more likely to be retained than patients in rural areas.

Determinants of choice at initiation of treatment
Modern versus home treatment

The multinomial logit model was used to compare the factors influencing choice of health-care provider for modern versus home, traditional versus home, and traditional versus modern systems (Table 4). When modern treatment was compared to

Table 1. **Definition and coding of commonly-used variables**

Variable	Definition	Mean	Coding
Sex	Sex of the individual	0.50	1 = male, 0 = female
Cma	Household head	0.24	1 = household head, 0 = other
Mala	Type of illness	0.36	1 = malaria, 0 = other illnesses
Residence	Residence type	0.37	1 = urban, 0 = rural
Hcome	Annual household income	696 203	Numerical values
Employ	Paid employment	0.19	1 = yes, 0 = no
Cost	The total expenditure on health care for the first episode of treatment	1 546	Numerical value in CFA francs (currency of Burkina Faso)

Table 2. **Distribution (%) of patients at initiation of treatment, Nouna, Burkina Faso**

Variable	Category	Treatment system		
		Home (n = 966)	Modern (n = 323)	Traditional (n = 113)
Sex	Male	51.8	46.8	48.7
	Female	48.2	53.2	51.3
Residence	Rural	64.8	54.8	69.0
	Urban	35.2	45.2	31.0
Paid employment	Yes	15.7	27.2	27.4
	No	84.3	72.8	72.6
Education	None	67.8	56.5	71.7
	Primary	15.2	17.4	12.4
	Secondary	15.3	25.1	8.0
	Alphabetization	1.7	1.0	7.9
Reason for choice	Confidence in provider	41.6	61.9	64.6
	Others	58.4	38.1	35.4
Household head	Yes	22.4	27.2	28.3
	No	77.6	72.8	71.7
Illness category	Malaria	41.5	32.2	2.7
	Other illness	58.5	67.8	97.3
Total		68.9	23.0	8.1

Table 3. **Distribution (%) of patients according to whether they were retained by a provider at second episode of treatment, Nouna, Burkina Faso**

Variable	Category	Retained (n = 57)	Switched (n = 110)	No second treatment (n = 1235)
Health-care provider	Home	2.4	7.35	90.3
	Modern	8.4	7.74	83.9
	Traditional	6.2	12.39	81.4
Sex	Male	51.8	61.4	49.7
	Female	48.2	38.6	50.3
Residence	Rural	73.6	57.9	62.1
	Urban	26.4	42.1	37.9
Paid employment	Yes	27.3	36.8	17.8
	No	72.7	63.2	82.2
Education	None	59.1	56.1	66.5
	Primary	22.7	22.8	14.5
	Secondary	14.6	17.5	17.2
	Alphabetization	3.6	3.6	1.8
Reason for choice	Confidence in provider	37.3	68.4	48.2
	Others	63.7	31.6	51.8
Household head	Yes	30.9	36.8	22.8
	No	69.1	63.2	77.2
Illness category	Malaria	18.2	22.8	38.5
	Other illness	81.8	77.2	61.5
Total		**7.8**	**4.1**	**88.1**

home treatment, it was found that the perceived competency of the modern system, household income, whether an individual is employed and having secondary education versus no education positively influence people seeking modern health care, and this effect is significant at the 99% confidence level. Those that perceive themselves to be suffering from malaria are less likely to seek modern treatment. Women are also more likely to seek modern treatment than their male counterparts, with a result that was significant at the 95% confidence level.

Traditional versus home treatment

We compared factors determining whether a patient sought treatment in the traditional system or at home. Patients who perceived the traditional system to be competent were more likely to use it. Perceived competency of the provider was more important for persons choosing the traditional system than for those choosing the modern system (1.02 versus 0.77), although not statistically significant. The effect of employment is significant and is greater for the traditional system than the modern system, i.e. employed people were more likely to choose the traditional system. Patients with malaria were less likely to seek treatment from the modern or traditional systems than to treat themselves at home, and those who did seek treatment outside the home were most likely seek it from the modern system, rather than the traditional system. Patients living in households with lower incomes were more likely to use the traditional system.

Traditional versus modern treatment

Comparison of the factors determining whether a patient sought treatment in the traditional or the modern system, showed that persons aged 36–46 years were more likely to seek traditional health care than younger or older people. A higher household income, alphabetization rather than having no education, and the perception of the illness to be malaria had a negative effect on the likelihood of seeking care from the traditional system. Patients from households in which at least one member had had a secondary-school education were more likely to seek health care from the traditional system.

Determinants of patient retention

When comparing patient switching and patient retention during the second episode of treatment (Table 5), three key findings emerge. First, patients that perceived the quality of care during the first episode of treatment to be poor were more likely to switch to another provider system. Second, patients that had confidence in the provider at initiation of treatment were more likely to switch to another provider at the second treatment. Third, those that sought treatment at the modern facility were more likely to switch to either traditional or self-treatment. According to these results, the competency of the health-care provider was perceived before any encounter with the provider, while the quality of care was perceived after the first episode of treatment. Therefore, while the quality of care is determined after experiencing treatment, perceived competency of the provider is determined before that experience. It was anticipated that perceived quality of care would be most highly correlated with choice of the modern health-care provider. The model was run separately to determine the correlation between perceived quality of health care and type of health-care system, but this did not improve the specification of the model nor affect results.

When persons who switched or who were retained for the second episode of treatment were compared with patients who did not seek a second episode of treatment, a similar pattern in respect of perceived quality of health care again emerged (Table 5).

Patients who perceived the quality of the first treatment to be poor sought a second episode of treatment. Other statistically significant results suggest that patients who perceived the provider to be competent at the start of the treatment process were more likely to switch than those who did not seek a second treatment, although this was not the same for those who maintained treatment with the same provider. Patients in urban areas were less likely to be retained than those in rural areas. Finally, when switching was compared with not seeking a second episode of treatment, it was found that patients who went to a modern health-care provider for the first episode of treatment were more likely to switch to another provider than to refrain from seeking further treatment.

Comparing determinants of patient initiation and retention

We set out to explore whether the determinants of initiation into and retention by a particular health-care provider differ if the patient seeks a second treatment option for the same episode of illness. The results suggest that the determinants do indeed differ. The perceived competency of the provider is an important determinant of choice and has the strongest effect for the modern health-care system. It is also significant in determining switching, that is, patients who had perceived the health-care provider to be competent chose to switch to another provider. Other than perceived provider competency, none of the factors that determine patient initiation are the same as those that determine whether a patient switches health-care providers.

Discussion

We were motivated to compare determinants of patient initiation and patient retention by the fact that, although enhancing utilization of health services encompasses two faces — initiation of patients to seek treatment in a particular system, and retention by that system should the illness require further treatment or in the case of future illnesses — only initiation has been a subject of extensive research (1–7). However, if the determinants differ, it is likely that different policy options may be required in order to increase utilization of modern health services.

Of the few studies relevant to retention, one concerns health-care switching behaviour of patients with malaria in a Kenyan rural community (8), and one relates to gynaecological care (9). In the former, based on ethnographic interviews, the author suggests that patients are more likely to start with self-treatment at home and to decide on the basis of their progress whether or not to switch to treatment from another provider. The author proposes that this allows the patient to minimize expenditure incurred as a result of the illness. It is also suggested that people are subsequently more likely to choose treatments available outside the home, including visiting a private health-care practitioner, a government health centre or a hospital, when the situation becomes serious. In the second study in women who had return appointments at an academic primary care centre for internal medicine, 23% of the 121 patients who initially had been treated by a non-primary care centre gynaecological-care provider indicated that they did not plan to return. Other studies that have looked at switching have mainly concerned insurance providers (e.g. 10, 11). The authors of one study (10) explored the effect of the adoption by the University of California of a policy of limiting its contribution to the cost of the least expensive insurance plan. The results suggest that out-of-pocket premiums increased for roughly one-third of University of California employees and individuals facing premium increases of less than US$ 10 were roughly five times more likely to switch insurance plans than those whose premiums remained constant. Another study undertook a consumer survey to gauge the importance of 41 variables in making the decision to enrol or re-enrol/switch health maintenance organization. Using logistic regression analysis, they concluded that variables associated with access to emergency care services had the greatest impact on decisions to switch. This was contrary to results of other studies, which ranked access to emergency care much lower (11).

Table 4. **Logit coefficients for a multinomial logit model of patient choice during the initiation of treatment, Nouna, Burkina Faso**

Comparison[a]		Logit coefficients for									
									Education[b]		
		reason	sex	cma	mala	urban	hcome	employ	pri	sec	alph
M/H	$\beta_{M/H}$	0.77	-0.31	0.28	-0.46	-0.28	0.12	0.53	0.11	0.69	-0.69
	$\exp(\beta_{M/H})$	2.16	0.74	1.33	0.63	0.76	1.13	1.70	1.12	2.00	0.50
	ρ	<0.01	0.04	0.11	<0.01	0.26	0.01	0.01	0.43	0.01	0.31
T/H	$\beta_{T/H}$	1.02	0.01	-0.03	-3.15	-0.43	-0.53	0.93	-0.64	1.11	-0.35
	$\exp(\beta_{T/H})$	2.77	1.02	0.97	0.04	0.65	0.59	2.53	0.53	3.03	0.70
	ρ	<0.01	0.96	0.90	<0.01	0.23	0.04	0.01	0.11	0.04	0.46
T/M	$\beta_{T/M}$	0.25	0.31	-0.31	-2.70	-0.15	-0.63	0.40	-0.75	1.80	-1.05
	$\exp(\beta_{T/M})$	1.28	1.38	0.73	0.07	0.86	0.53	1.49	0.47	6.05	0.35
	ρ	0.29	0.20	0.29	<0.01	0.71	0.01	0.28	0.08	0.02	0.03
Number of observations											1401
Likelihood ratio χ^2 ($df = 20$)											212.12
Pseudo R^2											0.10

[a] M = modern, H = home, T = traditional.
[b] Level of education: pri = primary; sec = secondary; alph = alphabetization.

Table 5. **Logit coefficients for a multinomial logit model of patient switching and retention at second treatment episode, Nouna, Burkina Faso**

Comparison[a]		Logit coefficients for												
		Perceived quality of care[b]		reason	hcome	Education[c]			employ	mala	sex	urban	Health-care system	
		Q-fair	Q-good			pri	sec	alph					Modern	Traditional
S/R	$\beta_{S/R}$	-0.61	-1.53	1.24	0.00	-0.58	0.00	-0.85	0.20	0.69	0.50	0.72	1.01	0.11
	$\exp(\beta_{S/R})$	0.54	0.22	3.47	1.00	0.56	1.00	0.43	1.22	2.00	1.65	2.06	2.73	1.12
	ρ	0.13	0.02	<0.01	0.95	0.29	1.00	0.20	0.68	0.13	0.16	0.17	0.01	0.84
S/N	$\beta_{S/N}$	-3.10	-5.62	1.38	0.00	0.31	1.11	0.22	0.81	0.67	0.61	-0.71	1.48	0.23
	$\exp(\beta_{S/N})$	0.05	0.00	3.99	1.00	1.36	3.02	1.24	2.24	1.96	1.84	0.49	4.41	1.26
	ρ	<0.01	<0.01	<0.01	0.31	0.54	0.23	0.71	0.06	0.09	0.06	0.15	<0.01	0.66
R/N	$\beta_{R/N}$	-2.48	-4.09	0.14	0.00	0.89	1.11	1.07	0.61	-0.02	0.11	-1.43	0.48	0.12
	$\exp(\beta_{R/N})$	0.08	0.02	1.15	1.00	2.42	3.03	2.91	1.84	0.98	1.11	0.24	1.61	1.13
	ρ	<0.01	<0.01	0.58	0.19	0.03	0.17	0.03	0.08	0.95	0.65	<0.01	0.10	0.75

Number of observations: 1392
Likelihood ratio χ^2 (df = 26): 375.60
Pseudo R^2: 0.30

[a] S = switched providers at second treatment episode; R = retained by provider at the second treatment episode; N = no second treatment sought.
[b] Perceived quality of health care during the first treatment episode: Q-fair, perceived to be fair, Q-good, perceived to be good.
[c] Level of education: pri = primary; sec = secondary; alph = alphabetization.

The fact that while household income, urban residence, type of illness, and education are significant determinants of patient initiation into a treatment system, they do not determine patient retention, and that only the perceived quality of care during the initial treatment does is in line with health belief models (15). One of the key descriptors of the health belief model is the perceived benefit of taking action; taking action toward the prevention of disease or toward dealing with an illness is the next step to expect after an individual has accepted that they are susceptible to a disease and recognized it as serious. During the initial episode of treatment, the patient chooses a system of health-care services because the associated benefits are perceived to be higher than those of alternative systems. However, at the second episode of treatment, the quality of care previously experienced is used as a learning opportunity and the patient will only return to the same provider if there is a perceived benefit. These results are similar to those of studies reviewed above in which switching was determined by the enrolment experience in the case of the health maintenance organization and emergency services (11), prices in the case of insurance plans (10) and the motivation to reduce costs, in the case of Nyamongo's study in rural Kenya (8).

We recognize that the variable "perceived quality of care" used in the paper is not decomposable into different attributes, such as availability of drugs, conduct of personnel, equipment and costs (16), but is taken as an index of the different attributes. We therefore suggest that further research could attempt to decompose the five-likert-scale to identify different attributes of quality, as perceived by patients. In this case, the same instrument would elicit information on different attributes of quality and an overall assessment of quality using a likert scale.

The likelihood that a patient will switch from the modern health-care facilities, i.e. will not be retained, deserves comment. This has been investigated in a number of studies and the quality of modern health-care services has repeatedly been found to be poor (15, 16). Baltussen et al. (16) used an instrument containing a 20-item scale, including four subscales related to personnel practices and conduct, adequacy of resources and services, healthcare delivery, and financial and physical accessibility, which was administered to 1081 users of 11 health-care centres, found that overall, the urban hospital was rated less highly than the average rural health-care centre. Drug availability and financial accesibility to health services were identified as the two main priorities for health policy action. Krause et al. (17) presented a quantitative estimate of community effectiveness of treatment for malaria in Nouna, Burkina Faso, on the basis of population surveys, observational studies of health services and user surveys. They estimated the overall community effectiveness to be 3%, that is, efficacy of treatment with antimalarial drugs was reduced drastically by lack of effective distribution and administration.

Household income has been shown elsewhere to predict utilization of health care services (2, 4, 18). In this study, households with higher incomes were more likely to choose modern health care. A study in the United Republic of Tanzania (4) showed that socioeconomic status of the respondent's family predicted utilization of modern health-care services. Similarly, lack of money was a significant barrier to utilization of dental services, and income also predicted use of primary curative services in South Africa (2). Financial barriers were also reported in Zambia (19) and Burkina Faso (5). On the other hand, poorer households were more likely to use the traditional system. Perceived poverty predicted utilization of traditional health care services in the United Republic of Tanzania (4). The results of this study therefore agree with those of other studies showing that the higher the household income, the greater the likelihood that the household uses modern health-care services. Therefore minimizing financial barriers is likely to have a bigger impact in improving utilization of modern health-care services than previously thought. This is because it is likely to shift patients from the traditional to modern health-care services, at least at initiation of treatment.

Employed people are more likely to seek treatment from the modern and traditional systems than at home, although the magnitude of effect is higher for the modern than for the traditional system. This is in agreement with the findings of a study in South Africa that showed that employed people were more likely to use primary curative services than unemployed people (2).

In this study, when the type of illness was perceived as malaria, the patients' preference was for home treatment, followed by modern and finally traditional treatment. In previous work (5), we showed that people chose home treatment for malaria because they perceived that they were sufficiently competent to treat the illness. Type of illness was also a significant determinant of choice of modern treatment in South Africa (2).

Policy implications and conclusion

The immediate implication of our results for health-care policy is that interventions focusing on patient initiation and patient retention are likely to be different. For example, interventions to enhance patient initiation would probably focus on reducing financial barriers, since people with low incomes are less likely to use modern health-care services. Interventions to increase patient retention would primarily focus on improving attributes of health services that are likely to ameliorate the perceived quality of care. Therefore focusing only on patient initiation does not sufficiently capture the full picture and misses an important aspect that is likely to affect overall utilization of health-care services. ∎

Conflicts of interest: none declared.

Résumé

Les deux aspects du renforcement de l'utilisation des services de santé : déterminants du premier recours à un système de soins de santé et de la fidélité du patient au système choisi dans les régions rurales du Burkina Faso

Objectif Explorer les facteurs qui déterminent le premier recours à un système de soins de santé et la fidélité du patient au système choisi, à Nouna, dans une région rurale du Burkina Faso.

Méthodes Les données utilisées ont été regroupées à partir de quatre passages d'une enquête dans les ménages réalisée à Nouna, dans une région rurale du Burkina Faso. Le système de surveillance démographique a fourni le cadre d'échantillonnage de cette enquête, au cours de laquelle 800 ménages ont été vus selon la méthode du sondage par grappes à deux degrés. On a observé plus d'un épisode de traitement par épisode de maladie par patient. On a utilisé un modèle logit multinomial pour explorer les déterminants du premier recours à un système de traitement – moderne, traditionnel ou à domicile – et un modèle logit binaire pour explorer les déterminants de la fidélité au système choisi.

Résultats D'après les résultats, les déterminants du premier recours à un système de soins de santé et de la fidélité du patient au système choisi sont différents. Pour les services de santé modernes, le revenu du ménage, le niveau d'études, la résidence en zone urbaine et la compétence attendue du prestataire de soins sont des facteurs prédictifs positifs du premier recours à un système de soins, mais non de la fidélité du patient, pour laquelle seule la qualité perçue des soins était un facteur prédictif positif.

Conclusion Les interventions axées sur le premier recours d'un patient à un système de soins de santé et sur sa fidélisation seront probablement différentes. Les politiques visant à augmenter le premier recours à un système de traitement dans des services de santé modernes seront probablement axées sur la réduction des obstacles financiers, tandis que celles qui visent à fidéliser les patients seront principalement axées sur les aspects qui améliorent la qualité perçue des soins.

Resumen

Las dos facetas del fomento de la utilización de los servicios de salud: factores determinantes del comienzo del tratamiento y de la retención de los pacientes en la Burkina Faso rural

Objetivo Estudiar en Nouna, Burkina Faso rural, los factores que determinan si un paciente iniciará el tratamiento necesario dentro de un sistema de servicios de atención de salud, así como los factores que determinan si el paciente permanecerá o no en el sistema elegido.

Métodos Los datos proceden de cuatro tandas de una encuesta de hogares realizada en Nouna, localidad rural de Burkina Faso. El sistema de vigilancia demográfica en marcha permitió incluir a 800 hogares en un procedimiento de muestreo del conglomerados en dos etapas. Se observó más de un episodio de tratamiento por episodio de la enfermedad del paciente. Se usó un modelo logit multinomial para estudiar los factores determinantes del tratamiento inicial de los pacientes en el marco de sistemas de tratamiento moderno, tradicional y domiciliario, y un modelo logit binario para analizar los factores determinantes de la retención de los pacientes en el sistema elegido de dispensadores de salud.

Resultados Los datos obtenidos parecen indicar que los factores determinantes del inicio del tratamiento por el paciente y de la retención posterior de éste son diferentes. Los ingresos familiares, la educación, el entorno urbano y la competencia esperada del dispensador son factores predictivos positivos del primer contacto, pero no de la retención, en el caso de los servicios de atención de salud modernos. El único factor predictivo positivo de la retención en tales servicios, en cambio fue la calidad de atención percibida.

Conclusión Las intervenciones tenderán a ser distintas según se centren en el comienzo del tratamiento de los pacientes o en la retención de los mismos. Las políticas dirigidas a facilitar el contacto inicial con los servicios de atención de salud modernos se centrarían principalmente en la reducción de los obstáculos financieros, mientras que las orientadas fundamentalmente a aumentar la retención se centrarían en los factores que mejoran la calidad de atención percibida.

Arabic

References

1. Darkaoui N, De Brouwere V, Zayyoun A, Filali H, Belouali R, Gouaima F, et al. [Utilization of hospital emergency services for primary care (study at the Children's Hospital of Rabat, Morocco)]. *Revue d'Epidémiologie Santé Publique* 1999;47 Suppl 2:2S53-64. In French.
2. Goldstein S, Price M. Utilisation of primary curative services in Diepkloof, Soweto. *South African Medical Journal* 1995;85:505-8.
3. Katung P. Socio-economic factors responsible for poor utilisation of the primary health care services in a rural community in Nigeria. *Niger Journal of Medicine* 2001;10:28-9.
4. Masatu M, Lugoe W, Kvale G, Klepp KI. Health services utilization among secondary school students in Arusha region, Tanzania. *East African Medical Journal* 2001;78:300-7.
5. Mugisha F, Kouyate B, Gbangou A, Sauerborn R. Examining out-of-pocket expenditure on health care in Nouna, Burkina Faso: implications for health policy. *Tropical Medicine and International Health* 2002;7:187-96.
6. Sauerborn R, Nougtara A, Diesfeld H. Low utilization of community health workers: results from a household interview survey in Burkina Faso. *Social Science and Medicine* 1989;29:1163-74.
7. Tursz A, Crost M. [An epidemiologic study of health care seeking behavior of children under 5 years of age by sex in developing countries]. *Revue d'Epidémiologie Sante Publique* 1999; 47 Suppl 2:2S133-56. In French.
8. Nyamongo I. Health care switching behaviour of malaria patients in a Kenyan rural community. *Social Science and Medicine* 2002;54:377-86.
9. Shiang E, Epstein A, Goldman L. Who provides gynecologic care? *American Journal of Preventive Medicine* 1985;1:15-21.
10. Buchmueller T, Feldstein P. The effect of price on switching among health plans. *Journal of Health Economics* 1997;16:231-47.
11. Ho F, Chen Y. Switching HMO providers. Dissatisfaction with emergency access cited as the primary reason for disenrollment. *Marketing Health Services* 1998;18:23-7.
12. Langman M, Kahler KH, Kong SX, Zhang Q, Finch E, Bentkover JD, et al. Drug switching patterns among patients taking non-steroidal anti-inflammatory drugs: a retrospective cohort study of a general practitioners database in the United Kingdom. *Pharmacoepidemiology and Drug Safety* 2001,10:517-24.
13. Scott Long J. *Regression models for categorical and limited dependent variables.* London: SAGE Publications; 1997.
14. Begg C, Gray R. Calculation of polychotomous logistic regression parameters using individualized regressions. *Biometrika* 1984;71:11-8.
15. Kloeblen A, Batish S. Understanding the intention to permanently follow a high folate diet among a sample of low-income pregnant women according to the Health Belief Model. *Health Education Research* 1999;14:327-38.
16. Baltussen R, Ye Y, Haddad S, Sauerborn R. Perceived quality of care of primary health care services in Burkina Faso. *Health Policy and Planning* 2002;17:42-8.
17. Krause G, Sauerborn R. Comprehensive community effectiveness of health care. A study of malaria treatment in children and adults in rural Burkina Faso. *Annals of Tropical Pediatrics* 2000;20:273-82.
18. Ntabaye M, Scheutz F, Poulsen S. Household survey of access to and utilisation of emergency oral health care services in rural Tanzania. *East African Medical Journal* 1998;75:649-53.
19. Kaona F, Siajunza M, Manyando C, Khondowe S, Ngoma G. Utilisation of malarial drugs at a household level: results from a KAP study in Choma, southern province and Mporokoso, northern province of Zambia. *Central African Journal of Medicine* 2000;46:268-70.

4.12 The feasibility of community-based health insurance in Burkina Faso

Dong H, Mugisha F, Gbangou A, Kouyate B, Sauerborn R

Health Policy 69 (2004): 45-53

Reprinted with permission from Elsevier.

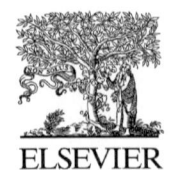

The feasibility of community-based health insurance in Burkina Faso

Hengjin Dong [a,*], Frederick Mugisha [b], Adjima Gbangou [c], Bocar Kouyate [c], Rainer Sauerborn [a]

[a] *Department of Tropical Hygiene and Public Health, University of Heidelberg, Im Neuenheimer Feld 324, D-69120 Heidelberg, Germany*
[b] *African Population and Health Research Center (APHRC), Shelter Afrique Center, Longonot Road, P.O. Box 10787-00100 GPO, Nairobi, Kenya*
[c] *Nouna Health Research Centre, Nouna, Burkina Faso*

Received 13 June 2003; accepted 1 December 2003

Abstract

To ensure the acceptability of community-based insurance (CBI) by the community and its sustainability, a feasibility study of CBI was conducted in Burkina Faso, including preference for benefit package of CBI, costing of health services, costing of the benefit package and willingness-to-pay (WTP) for the package. Qualitative methods were used to collect information about preferences for the benefit package. Cost per unit health services, health demand obtained from household survey and physician-judged health needs were used to estimate the cost of the benefit package. The bidding game method was used to elicit household head's WTP for the package. We found that there were strong preferences for inclusion of high-cost health services such as operation, essential drugs and consultation fees in the benefit package. It is estimated that the cost of the package per capita was 1673 CFA (demand-based) and 9630 CFA (need-based), including 58% government subsidies (€ 1 = 655 CFA). The average household head with eight household members agreed to pay from 7500 (median) to 9769 CFA (mean) to join the CBI for his/her household. The WTP results were influenced by household characteristics, such as location, household size and age composition. Under certain assumptions (household as the enrolment unit, median household head's WTP as premium for the average household, 50% enrolment rate), it would be feasible to run CBI in Nouna, Burkina Faso if enrolees' health demand did not increase by more than 28% or if the underwriting of the initial losses was covered by extra funds.
© 2004 Elsevier Ireland Ltd. All rights reserved.

Keywords: Community-based health insurance; Feasibility; Burkina Faso

1. Introduction

Health services in rural Burkina Faso, as in many Sub-Saharan countries, are characterised by low and inequitable utilisation and poor quality [1–5]. These problems prevent health care from having a notable

* Corresponding author. Tel.: +49-6221-564689; fax: +49-6221-565948.
E-mail address: donghengjin@yahoo.com (H. Dong).

impact on health, in particular among rural poor in Burkina Faso. Low utilisation of health services is directly related to their high price in relation to the household income. Health care in Burkina Faso has imposed considerable financial costs on the users [6].

User-fees were introduced in Burkina Faso in 1993 as a supplement to tax-based financing of government health services. The user-fee policy combined modest fees for services and cost-recovery fees for drugs. However, utilisation of health services continued to decline following the introduction of these fees [7,8].

One of the ways to improve the utilisation of health services is through insurance. However, formal health insurance in Burkina Faso has been limited to certain sections of the population largely excluding the rural population. For example, in Burkina Faso social insurance is offered to salaried and state employees through the Caisse National de Sécurité Sociale (CNSS, national social security fund) and the Caisse de Retraite des Fonctionnaires (CARFO, national social security fund for retired state employees). So the only rural residents likely to have health insurance are government employees.

In addition, community risk-sharing schemes, which are prevalent in rural Africa, can be viewed as another way to improve health care utilisation. At present, these schemes cover a wide variety of non-health-related risks but a few cover health care expenditure [9].

Community-based insurance (CBI) is therefore being seen as a promising new tool to improve health system for rural populations in low-income countries, particularly in Sub-Saharan Africa [10,11]. Community members pool their resources to share the financial risks of health care, own the scheme and control its management, including the collection of premiums, the payment of health care providers, and the negotiation of the benefit package. Unlike private insurance, premiums are paid by households and are not based on individual risk assessments. CBI has the advantage of dissociating the time of payment from the time of use of services, which is clearly better adapted than user-fees to the seasonal fluctuations of revenue and expenditure flows of rural households [12]. The Government of Burkina Faso, in its recently published health plan, has also advocated community-based financing mechanisms to alleviate the health care financing crisis [13].

It is found that there are four well-identifiable types of community-based health care financing schemes in developing countries. In community-managed user-fees, resource mobilization relies mainly on out-of-pocket payments at the point of contact with providers but the community is actively involved designing these fees and managing the collection, pooling, and allocation of the funds mobilized in this way. In community-based prepayment schemes, the community collects payments in advance of treatment and then manages these resources in paying for providers. In community provider-based health insurance, providers serving a particular community collect the prepayments themselves. In linked community health fund or revolving fund, the community acts as "agent" to reach rural and excluded populations on behalf of the formal government or social health insurance system via contracts or agreements. In our study, we plan to design a scheme similar to community-based prepayment schemes [14].

To ensure the CBI's acceptability by the community and its possible sustainability a series of studies related to the feasibility of CBI were conducted in Burkina Faso. The studies include preference for benefit package of CBI [15], costing of health services and costing of the benefit package [16,17], and household valuations of the benefit package using contingent valuation methods [18,19]. The paper aims to link the results of the relevant studies in order to understand the feasibility of running CBI in Nouna by examining community's acceptability for CBI, examining local people's preference for the CBI benefit package, and estimating the CBI premium on the basis of cost of the package and household head's WTP for the package.

2. Methods

2.1. Study site

Burkina Faso has an estimated population of approximately 10.7 millions [20]. It is divided into 11 administrative health regions, which comprise 53 health districts overall, each covering a population of 200,000–300,000 individuals. Each health district has at least one hospital with surgical facilities [21]. The districts themselves are again sub-divided into smaller areas of responsibility that are organised around either a hospital or a so-called Centre de Santé et de Promotion Sociale (CSPS), the first-line health care facility in the health system.

The Nouna health district has roughly 230,000 inhabitants who are served by one district hospital and 16 CSPS. This district is located in the Northwest region of Burkina Faso, about 300 km from the capital Ouagadougou. The Nouna area is a dry orchard Savannah, populated almost exclusively by subsistence farmers of different ethnic groups. The study site comes from the Nouna health district. It covers the catchment area of the Nouna hospital and four CSPS (Koro, Bourasso, Dara and Toni) for a total population of 60,000. The Nouna demographic surveillance system is undertaken in this area.

2.2. Benefit package preference study

Qualitative and quantitative methods were applied in the data collection for preference of benefit package [15]. In the pilot study, three key informant interviews were done by using non-structured questionnaire in order to obtain people's preferences for the benefit package of CBI. Based on the results of key informant interviews a semi-structure questionnaire about benefit package was developed. This was followed by 14 focus group discussions in order to obtain a relative comprehensive list of health services that are likely to be included in the CBI. The participants were purposively selected based on the criteria of sex, age, location (different villages and Nouna town), ethnicity and religion.

In the main study, a household survey was carried out in order to draft the services included in the benefit package according to the frequencies. One hundred and sixty households were purposively selected for interview based on the criteria of location (rural or urban), rich and poor. Eighty households (40 rich and 40 poor) were from rural areas and another 80 (40 rich and 40 poor) from Nouna town. The sample size was not calculated, but based on budget. One representative from each household was asked to tick off the health services (on a list) that are likely to be included in the package. After interviews, we found the data from 157 households to be useful.

After drafting the benefit package, in-depth interviews were done in order to ensure that the benefit package reflected the preferences of local people. Thirty-two representatives from the 157 validated households were selected for in-depth interview. The interviewers went to the homes of the selected representatives to show the list of the health services that would be likely to be included in the CBI and asked them if the services were the ones they really wanted and the reasons for their choice. We found the results were the same as the ones from the household survey, so the benefit package was finalized after the in-depth interviews. In the pilot and main studies, drawings were used to show the content of each health service in order to make respondents understand the services better.

2.3. Cost estimation

Cost estimation was done using all the four first line health facilities and one district hospital using the year 2000 as a base year [16,17]. Average costing was used in the cost estimation and the costs were estimated by the "step down" accounting procedure. Costs were annualised assuming a length of life of 3 years for equipment, 4 years for motorbikes and 20 or 30 years for the building depending on the construction materials. A real interest rate of 3% was used in annualisation of cost [17].

The first step was to identify line item expenses from annual reports to districts and the sources of finance for these items, including the government, facilities, and local communities. The government resources included all resources that were provided to the health facility by the government, no matter whether the resources were out of government coffers or donations. The facility resources included all resources generated by the health facility, such as funds generated through charges in the fee-for-service system and the sale of drugs. Community resources were those contributed by the individuals in the community collectively. For example, the community contributes bricks to build a dispensary, or makes contributions in cash.

The second step was identifying other resources within the health facilities that were not on the line item reports and their sources. These resources included in-kind donations, buildings, equipment, vaccines and salaries of government employees.

The third step involved identifying cost categories. There are three cost categories: the overhead, intermediate and final cost categories. Overhead categories produce only services that are consumed by other departments of the health facility, not directly by patients. Intermediate cost categories produce services that are used by other departments but also provide services directly to patients. Final cost categories provide services directly to patients, not to other departments. In this study the overhead category was administration; the intermediate cost category was drugs and consumables; and the final cost categories were maternity, family planning, inpatient, outpatient, training, vaccination and well child.

The fourth step was allocating the resource costs to the different cost categories. The fifth step was allocating the overhead cost to intermediate and final cost categories, and intermediate cost categories to the final cost categories. As a rule of thumb, the basis for allocating specific proportions of each cost centre's costs to other cost centres reflected consumption of the source cost category resources by the receiving cost category. And the last step was allocating the costs of the final categories to each type of health services. Thus, we can easily estimate unit cost of each health service.

2.4. Willingness-to-pay study

Household survey was used to collect household head's WTP for his/her whole household. Two-stage cluster sampling technique was used to select 800 households, 480 in the rural area of Nouna district and 320 in the town of Nouna. Detailed information about household survey and WTP study has been presented in earlier publication [18]. The subjects in this study were household heads. The data were collected during January and March 2001.

Before the survey a pilot study was done to test the commonly used three methods eliciting WTP [18]. We found the payment card was not reasonable because of high illiteracy rate, so in the main study we used the take-it-or-leave-it and the bidding game methods to elicit WTP. In this article we only used the results from the bidding game. Each household head was randomly assigned one of 13 starting prices (ranging from 8000 to 32000 Franc CFA, €1 = 655 CFA), which was pre-printed on the questionnaire. The starting prices were set based on the CBI benefit package and the results of the pilot study.

If the initial answer was 'yes', the interviewer increased the bid by increments of 500 CFA until the respondent said 'no'. If the initial answer was 'no', the interviewer reduced the amount of money by 500 CFA and continued this process until the respondent said 'yes'. The last sum of money receiving a 'yes' response was used as the WTP resulting from the bidding game approach.

2.5. Health demand and health need

Household survey provided data not only for WTP but also for health demand. All illness episodes were recorded in the survey. For each illness episode reported, the type of health care sought was also reported. The options were self-care, household care, traditional healer, community-health worker and professional modern health care. For the latter, consultations at the dispensary and hospital level, drug prescription and inpatient admission were distinguished. These were aggregated to compile the current demand for health care (utilisation) from local CSPS and Nouna hospital.

Three physicians who have had extensive clinical experience of working on the study site assigned to each illness episode the health services which they judged necessary based on their clinical judgement, personal experience and on national diagnosis and treatment guidelines of the Burkina Faso Ministry of Health. They used the following steps to judge the necessary health needs. They first identified all acute and chronic illnesses reported in the household survey, grouped the illnesses by age (0–4 years, 5–14 years and >14 years) and perceived severity (mild, moderately severe and severe). Two physicians assigned one or several of the eight health services (Table 1) that were in their view needed to treat the reported illness. They were therefore unaware of their colleague's assessment. Then they did so for three degrees of perceived illness severity and for three age groups. Lastly in case of non-agreement in the health services assigned by the two physicians, a third physician discussed and "arbitrated" the assignment with them.

3. Results

3.1. Benefit package

People preferred that the CBI covered essential drugs, laboratory tests, inpatient stays, surgery,

Table 1
Cost of the benefits package per capita based on health needs and current demand (CFA[a])

Intervention (1)	Cost per volume (2)	Based on health needs		Based on current demand	
		Volume per capita (3)	Cost per capita (4) = (2) × (3)	Volume per capita (5)	Cost per capita (6) = (2) × (5)
Major surgery	20846	0.028	584		
Minor surgery	6949	0.017	118		
Drugs (OP)[b]	3739	0.859	3212	0.224	837
Ambulance	16000	0.037	592		
X-ray	4611	0.056	258		
Laboratory	2739	0.275	753		
Inpatient admissions	10634	0.202	2148	0.030	319
Consultation (OP)	2127	0.924	1965	0.243	517
Total			9630		1673

[a] €1 = 655 CFA.
[b] OP: outpatient.

X-rays, consultation fees and urgent transportation (ambulance services) in the benefit package.

Drugs included all essential and generic drugs prescribed by doctors at local CSPS or Nouna hospital, which could be purchased in pharmacies, either at CSPS or at the Nouna hospital. The CBI would not pay for drugs sold in private drugstores. Laboratory tests included tests prescribed by doctors at local CSPS or Nouna hospital if they were carried out in the Nouna public health facilities. Inpatient stays included thirty inpatient days during a year. Surgery included general surgery and delivery complications at CSPS and Nouna hospital. X-rays would be that a doctor thought necessary and could be carried out at Nouna public health facilities. Consultation fees meant the cost for outpatient consultations.

Urgent transportation by ambulance from patient's village to Nouna hospital would be covered. This would only occur when a given condition puts a patient's life in danger and the patient needs to be treated urgently at the Nouna hospital, e.g., a woman who is bleeding during delivery (of her child), hernia, non-obstetrical emergency (child in a coma). The decision to order the ambulance would be made by a nurse, a mid-wife or a medical doctor.

3.2. Cost of the benefit package

3.2.1. Unit cost of health services
The cost per unit health service ranged from 20,846 to 2127 CFA (Table 1). For one major surgery, the cost was 20,846 CFA and for a consultation, the cost was 2127 CFA. According to the analysis carried out on finance sources, it emerged that the government currently covers 58% of the service cost, and therefore patients are exempted to this extent.

3.2.2. Cost of the benefit package per capita based on current demand
Based on the current demand and the cost per unit health service, the cost of the benefit package per capita was 1673 CFA in 2000 (Table 1), 58% of which had already been paid by the government.

3.2.3. Cost of the benefit package per capita based on health needs
Based on the judged health needs and cost per unit health service, the cost of the benefit package per capita was 9630 CFA in 2000 (Table 1). In which, the government paid 58%. The per capita cost of the benefit package based on health needs is 5.76 times as much as that based on current demand.

3.3. Household head's WTP for the benefit package

It is found that the elicited WTP was valid because the elicited WTP was positively related to the ability-to-pay [18]. It is also found that the method of the bidding game was reliable by a test-retest experiment in this study [19].

Median household head's WTP for his or her whole household for the benefit package was 7500 and mean

Table 2
Household head's willingness-to-pay for his/her household (CFA[a])

Variables	Sample size	Mean (S.D.)	Median
Total	705	9769 (8249)	7500
Location of residency			
Nouna town	265	10185 (8429)	10000
Rural area	440	9518 (8138)	7250
Household size			
1–5	251	8825 (8501)	6000
6–10	286	9847 (8021)	7500
11–15	104	11106 (8128)	10000
16+	64	10945 (8160)	10000
0–5 years old ratio (%)			
0	223	8016 (8104)	5000
1–25	296	10536 (8240)	10000
26+	186	10649 (8150)	10000

[a] €1 = 655 CFA.

Table 3
Mean WTP by initial prices

Initial prices	n	Accepting (%)	Median	Mean	S.D.
8000	51	49.0	7500	6922	4270
10000	51	39.2	6000	7070	4734
12000	59	35.6	7500	8605	7708
14000	47	34.0	10000	8479	5378
16000	64	29.7	10000	10398	8081
18000	56	21.4	5000	8455	7346
20000	55	32.7	10000	11887	8542
22000	55	18.2	7500	10564	8267
24000	47	14.9	7500	10253	9626
26000	54	16.7	10000	12861	9589
28000	65	7.7	7500	10516	8467
30000	48	12.5	6000	9552	9196
32000	53	9.4	7000	10849	11358

Note: (1) Unit of the initial prices, median, mean and standard deviation is CFA (€1 = 655 CFA). (2) Correlation $r = -0.07$ ($P > 0.05$), between initial price (starting point) and median WTP. (3) Correlation $r = -0.95$ ($P < 0.01$), between initial price and % accepting the initial price. (4) Correlation $r = 0.71$ ($P < 0.01$), between initial price and mean WTP. (5) Correlation $r = 0.88$ ($P < 0.01$), between initial price and standard deviation (S.D.).

was 9769 CFA with a standard deviation of 8249 (Table 2). Households located in Nouna town had a higher mean WTP and median WTP. The mean or median WTP increased with the increasing household size and the proportion of young children.

The initial prices may affect the amount of WTP. It is found that the initial price correlated significantly with the percentage of accepting the price ($r = -0.95$), mean WTP ($r = 0.71$) and standard deviation ($r = 0.88$). However, there was no significant correlation between the initial prices and median WTP ($r = -0.07$) (Table 3). We also found that the all percentages of accepting the initial prices were lower than 50%, only the percentage of accepting the lowest initial price reached 49% (Table 3).

3.4. Use of the results in designing CBI

3.4.1. Setting premium

In our earlier publication we found that the individual WTP (individual pays for herself or himself for the insurance) was shaped by income, age and gender [18]. Young males with high income were willing to pay more than others did. In order to protect the poor, the older and females, household as an enrolment unit would be better.

In setting the premium, we assumed that the enrolment unit would be a household, the average household size would be eight with four adults and four children (based on the results from the household survey), the enrolment rate would be 50%, and a child would pay 30% of the amount an adult would pay in order to reduce the economic burden for the households with many children. Thus, the premium for an average household would equal to the average household WTP (7500 CFA), an adult would pay 1442 ($7500/(4 + 4 \times 0.3)$) and a child would pay 433 CFA. The premium for each household varies with the household size and composition of adults and children. For example, the premium for a household with four adults and four children would be 7500 ($1442 \times 4 + 433 \times 4$), for a household with two adults and six children would be 5482 CFA.

3.4.2. Projection of CBI balance

It is important to project the CBI cost and revenue balance in order to see the feasibility. In addition to the above assumptions, we further assumed that the government would continue to pay 58% of the cost and the CBI would cover the whole study site in 3 years. The whole site has 7340 households. The CBI will be offered to 2446 households in the first year, 4892 households the second year and the all households the third year. The CBI would be profitable if enrolees would not change their health-seeking behaviour and

Table 4
Projection of CBI balance based on current demand

	1st year	2nd year	3rd year
Number of planned households	2446	4892	7340
Enrolment rate	0.5	0.5	0.5
Number of enrolled households	1223	2446	3670
Premium/household (CFA[a])	7500	7500	7500
Revenue (CFA)	9172500	18345000	27525000
Cost/household[b] (CFA)	5621	5621	5621
Total cost (CFA)	6874483	13748966	20629070
Management cost (5% of revenue)	458625	917250	1376250
Current year balance (CFA)	1839392	3678784	5519680
Cumulative balance (CFA)	1839392	5518176	11037856

[a] €1 = 655 CFA.
[b] $5621 = 1673 \times 42\% \times 8$.

Table 5
Projection of CBI balance based on health needs

	1st year	2nd year	3rd year
Number of planned households	2446	4892	7340
Enrolment rate	0.5	0.5	0.5
Number of enrolled households	1223	2446	3670
Premium/household (CFA[a])	7500	7500	7500
Revenue (CFA)	9172500	18345000	27525000
Cost/household[b] (CFA)	32357	32357	32357
Total cost (CFA)	39572611	79145222	118750190
Management cost (5% of revenue)	458625	917250	1376250
Current year balance (CFA)	−30858736	−61717472	−92601440
Cumulative balance (CFA)	−30858736	−92576208	−185177648

[a] €1 = 655 CFA.
[b] $32357 = 9630 \times 42\% \times 8$.

keep the same health demand (Table 4). The revenue and cost of CBI would reach the balance point if the enrolees' health demand would increase by 28%. After that, the CBI would have a deficit. If the health demand would become equivalent to the health services resulting from needs, the deficit would be quite large (Table 5). Thus, the underwriting of the initial losses covered by extra funds would be necessary in order to keep the CBI survival.

4. Discussion

To our knowledge, this is the first article in developing countries to study the feasibility of CBI by examining community's acceptability; examining people's preference for the benefit package; estimating professionally defined health care needs on the basis of comprehensive population-based morbidity data, rather than on hospital or health post records; and using these data with the cost of the package and household head's WTP for the package together to estimate premium level for CBI.

From the methodological point of view, the gap between expressed demand and professionally defined health needs, the difference between people's behaviour at a hypothetical market (WTP) and their behaviour in the real market need to be discussed while using the data to judge the feasibility.

CBI, like other types of insurance, has the social function to protect the socially marginalised, such as the poor, women, children and the older; and the financial function to make sure that people can obtain health services when needed without financial problems. Compared to uninsured people, insured one may have less financial barrier to access health care. This makes some of health needs to be converted to health demand, increasing the cost of health services and resulting in the cost increase of CBI. If this transfer rate were larger than 28%, the planned CBI in Nouna district would go bankrupt unless it could obtain extra external financial support.

We used median household head's WTP to set premium in this study, and the premium was about 6.3% of the median annual household expenditure (118,650 CFA). From the theoretical point of view, this is affordable. However, WTP is a product of a hypothetical market, does not equal to the amount in a real market. This is called inference bias, referring to the phenomena that the preferences have changed from the time of the study to the time the results are used for decision making. To our knowledge, only one article identified the inference bias [22]. It was found that according to the bidding results, 22–71% of respondents were willing and able to pay for the connections to new water systems and actually did in 3 years; 88–100% of them were not able to pay for the connections and actually did not in 3 years [22]. That we used median household head's WTP as premium for whole household is based on the assumption of 50% enrolment rate. If people changed their preference at the time to buy CBI, the enrolment rate could be reduced at the premium level, which will reduce the CBI financial pool and make it go bankrupt more easily. We are planning to investigate the inference bias after the implementation of CBI in Nouna district.

Other weaknesses of the WTP study such as starting point bias may affect the reasonable estimation of premium. We did find that there was starting point bias [18]. The data presented in Table 3 also show clear effects of starting point (initial price). The starting point correlates significantly with the mean WTP, but not with the median WTP. This further strengthens the use of the median WTP for setting the insurance premium. The initial prices were higher in this study because the highest percentage of accepting the initial prices was only 49%, although they were estimated based on the results from the pilot study and the cost of the benefit package. In retrospect, it would have been better to have designed the survey with fewer starting prices over a small range to make the sub-sample size of each initial price larger and the mean and median WTP of each initial price more stable.

Feasibility of CBI is not only a product of premium but also that of other factors such as its institutional framework. In the technical report, Musan summarised the lessons learned from the study of existing CBI schemes [23]. He found that 'community participation is important to the success of a CBI scheme. Such participation needs to be active to that the community has real empowerment in decision making. Failure in risk management is one of the greatest threats to the viability of the CBI schemes. Provider staffs require training to appreciate the need for the scheme so that they may handle the client/patient with the respect they deserve. Marketing to the community is very important. This is very important in the initial design of the scheme and should go on throughout the life of the scheme to ensure that membership levels are kept high. Underwriting of the initial losses by the government or a donor can help the scheme set low rates at the beginning but may also give a false sense of affordability to the community'.

Considering the lessons learned from existing CBI schemes and the results from this feasibility study, we think it is feasible to run CBI in Nouna, Burkina Faso under certain assumptions. Some of the assumptions are that the household is the enrolment unit, premium for the average household equals to median household head's WTP, enrolee's health demand increases by less than 28% or the underwriting of the initial losses will be covered by externally generated funds. However, more is needed to make the CBI successful, such as community participation in decision-making, training providers and CBI-oriented marketing to the community.

5. Conclusion

It is feasible to implement CBI in Nouna, Burkina Faso based on the results and assumptions of this study. The average household premium for the insurance based on the median household head's WTP is about 6.3% of the annual household expenditure. However, it is needed to have more support for the success of the CBI. The underwriting of the initial losses need to be covered by extra funds. Community needs to take part in more relevant process of decision-making. CBI-oriented providers' training and marketing to the community need to be enforced.

Acknowledgements

This work was supported by the collaborative research grant 'SFB 544' of the German Research Society (DFG). The authors would like to thank Sanou Aboubakary, Adjima Gbangou, Yazoumé Yé and Mamadou Sanon from Nouna Health Research Centre for their valuable help during the data collection process. The authors would like to thank Manuela De Allegri, Subhash Pokhrel and Budi Hidayat in the Department of Tropical Hygiene and Public Health, Heidelberg University for their valuable comments.

References

[1] Sauerborn R, Nougtara A, Sorgho G, et al. Assessment of MCH services in the district of Solenzo, Burkina Faso. II. Acceptability. Journal of Tropical Pediatrics 1989;35(Suppl 1):10–3.

[2] Sauerborn R, Nougtara A, Diesfeld HJ. Low utilisation of community health workers: results from a household interview survey in Burkina Faso. Social Science & Medicine 1989;29:1163–74.

[3] Sauerborn R, Berman P, Nougtara A. Age bias, but no gender bias, in the intra-household resource allocation for health care in rural Burkina Faso. Health Transit Review 1996;6:131–45.

[4] Krause G, Schleiermacher D, Borchert M, et al. Diagnostic quality in rural health centres in Burkina Faso. Tropical Medicine & International Health 1998;3:100–7.

[5] Baltussen R, Yé Y, Haddad S, Sauerborn R. Perceived quality of care of primary health care services in Burkina Faso. Health Policy and Planning 2002;17:42–8.

[6] Sauerborn R, Nougtara A, Latimer E. The elasticity of demand for health care in Burkina Faso. Health Policy and Planning 1994;9:185–92.

[7] Sauerborn R, Zombre S, Some F, et al. The rationale and feasibility of community-based insurance in rural Burkina Faso. Discussion paper, Department of Tropical Hygiene and Public Health, University of Heidelberg; 2001.

[8] Mugisha F, Kouyate B, Gbangou A, Sauerborn R. Examining out-of-pocket expenditure on health care in Nouna, Burkina Faso: implication for health policy. Tropical Medicine & International Health 2002;7:187–96.

[9] Sommerfeld J, Sanon M, Kouyate B, et al. Informal risk-sharing arrangements (IRSAS) in rural Burkina Faso: lessons for the development of Community-Based Insurance (CBI) I. International Journal of Health Planning and Management 2002;17:147–63.

[10] Creese A, Bennett S, Rural risk-sharing strategies. In: George J. Schieber, editor. Innovations in health care financing. World Bank Discussion Paper No. 365. Washington DC: The World Bank; 1997. p. 163–82.

[11] Asenso-Okyere WK, Osei-Akoto I, Anum A, et al. Willingness to pay for health insurance in a developing economy. A pilot study of the informal sector of Ghana using contingent valuation. Health Policy 1997;42:223–37.

[12] Sauerborn R, Nougtara A, Hien M, et al. Seasonal variations of household costs of illness in Burkina Faso. Social Science & Medicine 1996;43:281–90.

[13] Burkina Faso Ministry of health. Project de Document de Politique Sanitaire Nationale (PSN); 2000.

[14] Preker AS, Carrin G, Dror D, et al. Rich poor difference in health care financing. In: Health care financing for rural and low-income populations, the role of communities. Washington D.C.: The international Bank for Reconstruction and Development, The World Bank; 2002.

[15] Kouyaté B, Sanou M, Mugisha F, et al. Community preference for a benefit package under community-based insurance. Centre de Recherche en Sante de Nouna—Discussion paper series, No. 2 Nouna. Burkina Faso; 2001.

[16] Mugisha F, Health care system and household response to costs associated with illness in Nouna, Burkina Faso. University of Heidelberg (dissertation); 2001.

[17] Mugisha F, Kouyate B, Dong H, Sauerborn R. Costing health care interventions at primary health facilities in Nouna, Burkina Faso. African Journal of Health Sciences 2002;9:63–73.

[18] Dong HJ, Kouyate B, Cairns J, Mugisha F, Sauerborn R. Willingness to pay for community-based insurance in Burkina Faso. Health Economics 2003;12:849–62.

[19] Dong HJ, Kouyate B, Cairns J, Sauerborn R. A comparison of the reliability of the take-it-or-leave-it and the bidding game approaches to estimating willingness-to-pay in a rural population in West Africa. Social Science & Medicine 2003; 56:2181–9.

[20] World Bank. African Development Indicators 2000. Washington D.C.: World Bank; 2000.

[21] Burkina Faso Ministry of Health. Statistiques Sanitaires 1996. Ouagadougou: Burkina Faso Ministry of Health; 1996.

[22] Griffin CC, Briscoe J, Singh B, Ramasubban R, Bhatia R. Contingent valuation and actual behavior: predicting connections to new water systems in the State of Kerala, India. World Bank Economics Review 1995;9:373–95.

[23] Musan SN. Community-based health insurance experiences and lessons learned from East and Southern Africa. Technical Report No. 34. Bethesda, MD: Partnerships for Health Reform Project, Abt associates Inc.; 1999.

5 Biochemistry-based health care research

5.1 Introduction

BOUBACAR COULIBALY[1,2](✉), JANA K. EUBEL[1,2] STEPHAN GROMER[2,] R. HEINER SCHIRMER[2](✉)

[1] *Centre de Recherche en Santé de Nouna (CRSN), Nouna, Burkina Faso*

Tel.: +226 20 53 70 43
Email: boubacar@fasonet.bf

[2]*Biochemiezentrum Heidelberg, Im Neuenheimer Feld 504, D-69120 Heidelberg, Germany*

Tel.: +49 (6221) 544171
Email: Heiner.Schirmer@bzh.uni-heidelberg.de

BC and JKE contributed equally to this report

> The test for our progress *in medicine and science*, as well as in economy, is not what we can add to the affluence of those who have much, the test is how much we can supply for those who have too little of everything
> *(after Franklin D. Roosevelt 1937)*

From the bench at the CRSN to the field

Biochemical research at the CRSN in Nouna has laid the grounds for the clinical trials on methylene blue/chloroquine (BlueCQ) as an antimalarial drug combination. These biochemical studies encompass new methods for the determination of hemoglobin and methemoglobin, biochemical tests for vitamin B_2-deficiency in malnutrition, as well as the miniaturization of screening tests for G6PD deficiency and other enzyme variations in red blood cells. In the course of these studies we have developed a perspective which is so far neglected in industrialized countries: Biochemistry can contribute – possibly more than other biomedical disciplines – not only to more comprehensive but also to more affordable health care.

Lifestyle versus emergency genes: The genomic dilemma of affluent societies

In this context we study emergency genes and the corresponding proteins. Here we can only sketch the basis of this project. Biochemical evolution of man has been shaped for more than 100 000 generations by coping with chronic emergencies such as starvation and parasitic diseases as selecting factors. On the other hand, there are virtually no genes protecting man from affluence and a luxurious lifestyle which have prevailed as a wide-spread phenomenon in Western societies only for two generations – by far too short a time for genomic adaptations. Diseases like gout, obesity, diabetes, hypercholesteremic cardiovascular disease must also be studied under the aspect that the responsible "bad" gene ensembles have emergency obligations like rigorously saving purines, biochemical energy, and steroids for the organism. In the same vein, many so called hereditary conditions like G6PD deficiency protect in a subtle way from infectious diseases like malaria. It is obvious that the positive roles of emergency genes can be studied more appropriately in West Africa than in West Europe but these genes and their regulation are equally important in both regions: Affluence-associated diseases on the one hand and biochemical protection from privation on the other are only two sides of the same medal and must be studied in a concerted effort.

RESULTS AND DISCUSSION

Novel indications for affordable established drugs. The case of methylene blue

Biochemistry can certainly promote drug finding. Whenever a protein from a pathogen is purified it should be tested as a target of known drugs which fulfill two criteria: they must have been registered as drugs already for another medical indication and they must be affordable for those patients who will need them the most. A case in point is methylene blue (MB; Figure 1), the standard drug against methemoglobinemia in children and against ifosfamide-induced neurotoxicity in cancer patients (Schirmer et al. 2003; chapter 5.2). We study the biochemistry of MB in order to reintroduce it as an antimalarial drug (Guttmann and Ehrlich, 1898).

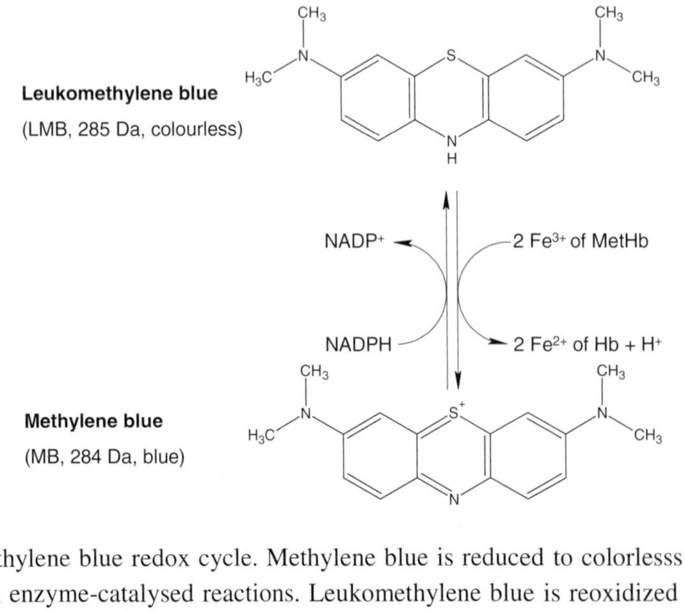

Leukomethylene blue
(LMB, 285 Da, colourless)

NADP⁺ ← — 2 Fe^{3+} of MetHb

NADPH — → 2 Fe^{2+} of Hb + H^+

Methylene blue
(MB, 284 Da, blue)

Figure 1: Methylene blue redox cycle. Methylene blue is reduced to colorlesss leukomethylene blue by NADPH in enzyme-catalysed reactions. Leukomethylene blue is reoxidized to methylene blue by numerous cellular oxidants such as methemoglobin (MetHb or Hi). Another important oxidant is O_2 which is reduced to H_2O_2 by leukomethylene blue.

MB acts as an inhibitor of hemoglobin degradation in the digestive organelles of *Plasmodium falciparum*, probably by preventing the oxidation of hemoglobin to methemoglobin. MB has at least two other target molecules in the malarial parasite, namely the enzymes glutathione reductase and thioredoxin reductase.

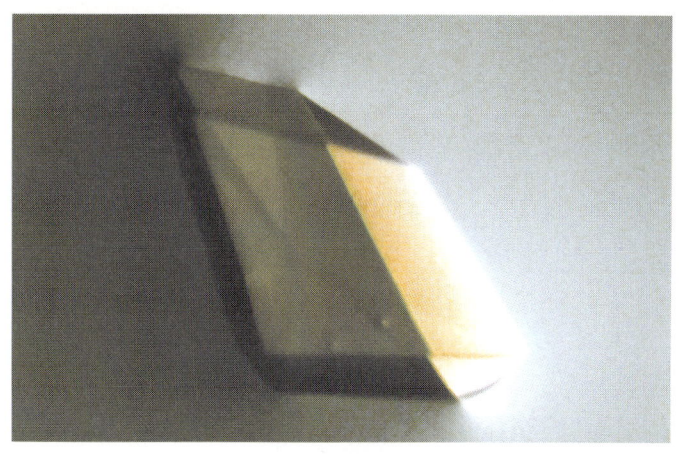

Figure 2: Crystal of *Plasmodium falciparum* glutathione reductase. The enzyme is colored yellow because it contains FAD, a vitamin B_2 derivative, as a cofactor (from Coulibaly 2004).

For these enzymes MB acts not only as a non-competitive inhibitor but also as a subversive substrate. A subversive agent is a molecule that converts an antioxidative disulfide reductase into a prooxidant enzyme. Thus MB is reduced to leuko-MB by glutathione reductase at the expense of NADPH and the resulting leukomethylene blue is reoxidized by molecular oxygen to give hydrogen peroxide or by methemoglobin (Figure 1). MB can also be reduced in spontaneous reactions by NADPH, the second order rate constant being $6.5\ M^{-1}\ s^{-1}$ at 37 °C and pH 7.3, by vitamin C and by dithiols such as thioredoxin and dihydrolipoamide (Eubel et al. 2004). Taken together, these data indicate that MB is a very active redox-cycling agent in situ.

It is important to study if the binding site of MB from where it inhibits glutathione reduction is identical with the site where MB acts as an electron-accepting substrate. This question can be addressed by subjecting crystals of glutathione reductase to X-ray diffraction analysis (Sarma et al. 2003). Figure 2 shows a glutathione reductase crystal. The enzyme is yellow because this is the colour of its prosthetic group FAD, a riboflavin derivative. When MB binds in these crystals they turn green. One binding site of MB appears to be the cavity between the two subunits of glutathione reductase. This site is shown as a blue structure at the bottom of Figure 3. The figure also shows other sites – in red and yellow - where ligands can bind to the enzyme (Sarma et al. 2003).

Methylene blue *per se* inhibits parasite growth but, in addition it may influence the activity of other antimalarial drugs. As a subversive inhibitor of glutathione reductase and thioredoxin reductase, MB decreases the concentration of glutathione in the parasite. A low glutathione level favors the antiparasitic activity of chloroquine (Becker et al. 2003, Ginsburg 2003, Ziebuhr et al. 2004). Therefore we study the possibility that the drug combination (chloroquine + methylene blue, BlueCQ) counteracts chloroquine resistance (collaboration with Professor Katja Becker, Giessen, Germany). In a pilot study on the safety of BlueCQ 50 adult males in the villages of Dembéléla, Dénissa Marka, Dénissa Mossi, and Lei received 3 mg/kg MB per day in the form of BlueCQ. Reported side effects included initial drowsiness, increased appetite, and the observation of blue urine up to 4 days after the last dose of MB. As a laboratory parameter, there was a tendency of rising hemoglobin values on day 5. (Coulibaly 2004, Merkle 2004). Currently clinical trials with Blue CQ which are generously supported by the DSM Dream Action Award are directed by Drs. Olaf Müller, Wolfgang Schiek and Bocar Kouyaté (see chapter 2.2.1 in this volume).

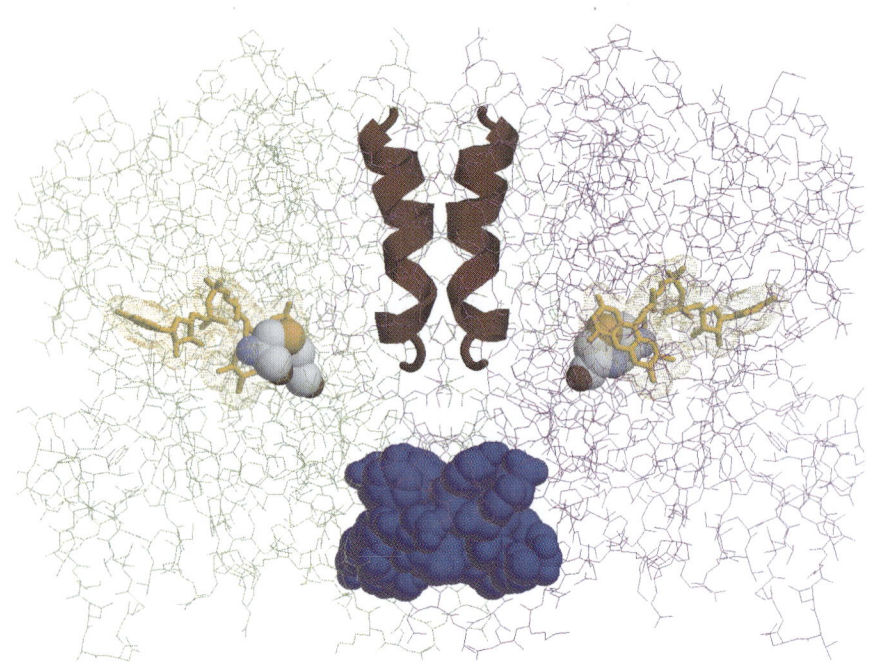

Figure 3: Submolecular drug target sites in glutathione reductase. Shown in red are the subunit interface helices 11 and 11´, in yellow the reactive cysteine residues at the two catalytic sites and in blue the cavity at the subunit interface where methylene blue and other tricyclic drugs bind.

The 2-wavelengths procedure, an alternative for the determination of methemoglobin

Anemia, reflecting a hemoglobin (Hb) concentration of less than 10.5 g/dL blood, is very common worldwide (Cook and Zumla 2003). There are numerous clinical situations where Hb must be determined. For instance, a rapid decrease in Hb is typical for severe childhood malaria. The standard procedure for Hb determination requires hazardous chemical reagents including potassium cyanide. At many health care centers worldwide, this method is therefore associated with safety problems and relatively high costs. At the CRNS we use a different procedure. We exploit the facts, that most forms of hemoglobin have very similar absorption coefficients at 340 nm and that, in blood samples, practically all absorbance at 340 nm is due to Hb (Becker et al. 1991). In a rapid, very sensitive, and inexpensive procedure, hemoglobin is determined according to the formula

$$\text{Hb concentration [g/dL]} = 0.054 \times \text{absorption at 340 nm}.$$

Methemoglobin (Hi) is a pathological form of hemoglobin. It contains iron in the ferri(III) form and cannot bind O_2. What is even worse, if there is only one Hi molecule in tetrameric hemoglobin, it blocks oxygen release from the other three subunits.

Hi formation plays a role in many clinical conditions. It has also been reported to be a complication of malaria-associated anemia in children (Anstey et al. 1996). Thus treatment of malaria with methylene blue may – apart from its direct antiparasitic action - prevent a fatal complication of the disease. The standard method for determining blood Hi has a number of shortcomings, including again the use of reagents like potassium cyanide. As detailed by Coulibaly (2004), we recently established a procedure which is based on absorption measurements at 340 nm and 630 nm and thus is designated as the "2-

wavelengths method". The ratio Hi-concentration / total Hb concentration is calculated using the equation

$$\frac{\text{Concentration of Hi}}{\text{Concentration of total Hb}} = \frac{c(Hi)}{c(Hb_T)} = \left(\frac{\Delta A_{630\,nm} \times 18.7}{\Delta A_{340\,nm}} - 0.14 \right) \times 64\%$$

As an example, for a blood sample the following absorbances were determined: ΔA_{340} = 93.4 and ΔA_{630} = 1.56. (All values are corrected for dilution.). Using these values we obtain cHi/cHb = (1.56 × 18.7 / 93.4 – 0.14) × 64% = 11%. That is, the percentage of Hi is 11% of total Hb. Since the total Hb concentration is 0.054 × 93.4 = 5.0 g/dL, the absolute Hi concentration is 0.55 g/dL blood.

The procedure requires only 50 µl blood even when total hemoglobin is as low as 5 g/dl. The tests were applied to blood samples of adult persons with mild malaria at the CRSN. 28 samples exhibited cHi/cHb$_{total}$ values below 1%, 14 between 1% and 2%, and 15 samples showed values between 2.0 and 3.3%. Values above 2% are considered to be pathological.

Coulibaly's 2-wavelengths method is independent of additional reagents, and it is suitable for anemic blood. In addition, using this procedure the absolute values for both total Hb and Hi are determined, not only the ratio of these two important values (Coulibaly 2004). Nevertheless the procedure is much less expensive than the standard Hi determination according to Evelyn and Malloy which entails forbiddingly high prices for the patients in many countries.

G6PD deficiency, a central issue of health care

Like in other parts of the world where malaria has been endemic, G6PD deficiency, an X-chromosome linked condition, is common in Burkina Faso. We determined the prevalence of aberrant genes to be approx. 20% in the male population, and this balanced G6PD polymorphism occurs in all ethnic groups – it was found in the communities of Bourasso (Bwaba), Dembéléla (Fulani), Dénissa Marka (Marka), in Dénissa Mossi (Mossi), and in Lei (Samo) (Schirmer et al. 2003). There is now compelling evidence that the balanced G6PD polymorphism offers relevant protection from severe malaria and thus has a selective advantage for malaria-exposed populations (Ruwende et al. 1998, Cook and Zumla 2003). On the other hand, persons with certain forms of G6PD deficiency may not tolerate oxidative antimalarial drugs like primaquine, dapsone, or methylene blue. Do these drugs represent a risk when used in Burkina Faso? An answer was given by Mandi et al. (2004) who reported that G6PD deficient men in the Nouna district did not develop hemolysis when they were exposed to methylene blue.

G6PD deficiency can manifest itself in acute bacterial diseases, especially when these are treated with oxidative drugs. Furthermore, in newborn boys G6PD deficiency increases the risk of hyperbilirubinemia and kernikterus. Following the health care principles established in Singapore, the G6PD status of the whole population should be assessed and be a focal point of health care.
We have established a screening test for G6PD which represents a miniaturization of the Beutler-Mitchell test (Scheiwein 2001, Coulibaly 2004). This "dry test" is based on demonstrating NADPH fluorescence on paper under the influence of G6PD. In our modified form, 10 µl pre-diluted blood sample is added to 100 µl screening mixture, and a spot of this mixture is made on filter paper. After 5 and 10 minutes, respectively, two further spots are applied. In normal samples, the first spot fluoresces slightly and the following spots brightly under the uv-lamp. G6PD deficient samples show little or no

fluorescence in any spot. A normal G6PD control sample and a deficient G6PD sample were always examined side by side with the unknown patient samples.

The first trial, conducted in the village of Bourasso with 750 participants, revealed the presence of *P. falciparum* parasitemia in 79.3% of the individuals. G6PD deficiency prevalence was found to be 16.9% in the male population and 7.6% in females; the latter value is twice as high as expected for an X-chromosome linked polymorphism. When differentiating according to age, the frequency for degree-1 G6PD deficiency was 3.7% in females and 17.7% in males under 5 years of age; for persons over 5 years, the values were found to be 9.0% for females and 16.7% for males. The apparent "over-diagnosis" in females over 5 years remains to be studied. The diagnosis of G6PD deficiency was confirmed for 62 male persons using the Brewer test, again in miniaturized version. In this test which is based on exposing the cells to nitrite and methylene blue, no tendency towards immediate hemolysis was observed for the G6PD-deficient erythrocytes (Coulibaly 2004).

Glutathione reductase deficiency is often an indicator of vitamin B$_2$ deficiency and malnutrition.

Glutathione reductase deficiency has similar effects as G6PD deficiency *in vivo*. Glutathione reductase is a vitamin B$_2$-dependent flavoenzyme catalyzing the reaction

$$NADPH + GSSG + H^+ \rightarrow NADP^+ + 2\ GSH.$$

Erythrocytes lacking this enzyme activity can fulfill their physiological functions but they do not serve as host cells of the malarial parasite *P. falciparum*. Consequently we searched for glutathione reductase deficiency in the village of Bourasso where malaria is holoendemic. The NADPH-fluorescence test on paper proved to be well suited also for this enzyme. 6.2% of the population was found to be deficient in glutathione reductase. Is this deficiency caused by genetic mutation of the enzyme or by vitamin deficiency? For differentiating between genetic mutation and riboflavin (vitamin B$_2$) deficiency as the cause of enzyme deficiency the EGRAC test was applied.

The principle of this test is as follows: *In vivo* glutathione reductase is not fully saturated with is prosthetic group FAD but the inactive apoenzyme can be completed *in vitro* according to the equation apoGR + FAD → holoGR. This is the basis for the determination of the erythrocyte glutathione reductase activation coefficient (EGRAC) which is operationally defined as the ratio of FAD-stimulated to unstimulated activity of erythrocytic glutathione reductase (Becker et al. 1991).

$$EGRAC = \frac{\text{Enzyme activity in the presence of excess FAD}}{\text{Enzyme activity without added FAD}}$$

We found that all glutathione reductase-deficient patients with one exception had EGRAC values above 1.3 indicative of vitamin B$_2$ deficiency (Table 1). This result has led to new questions:

a) Does malnutrition–based glutathione reductase deficiency also lead to some protection from severe malaria, as it was originally postulated by Anderson et al. (1994)?
b) How can persons with riboflavin deficiency be fed adequately?

Riboflavin deficiency *per se* is a clinical problem mainly in and around pregnancy. On the basis of our results we can state that riboflavin deficiency is prevalent in Burkina Faso and that it is probably an indicator of general malnutrition. This is so because vitamin B$_2$ occurs mainly in high quality foodstuffs such as milk, eggs, meat, and nuts; riboflavin is scarce in most cereals and other plant nutrients. It is often overlooked that riboflavin is transformed by visible light to a compound which is yellow but has no vitamin activity; in addition, it is toxic. Riboflavin containing liquids – for instance milk and vitamin-containing infusions but also a number of cell culture media – must be protected from light by using dark receptacles.

Table 1. Glutathione reductase deficiency in Bourasso. According to the NADPH fluorescence test, 48 out of 750 persons (6.2%) had glutathione reductase deficiency. (Scheiwein 2001; Coulibaly 2004).

EGRAC values	Females	Males	**Total**
<1.4	4	2	**6**
>1.4	12	13	**25**
not determined	9	8	**17**
Total	**25**	**23**	**48**

Conclusions

By miniaturization of Beutler´s methods, paper fluorescence ("dry") tests for identifying persons with G6PD deficiency and glutathione reductase deficiency were developed. For the latter enzyme, the EGRAC test was applied in order to distinguish between nutritional vitamin B_2 deficiency and hereditary apoenzyme deficiency.

The gene frequency for G6PD deficiency is approximately 17% in rural Burkina Faso and does not appear to be a contraindication against administering methylene blue as an antimalarial drug. Glutathione reductase deficiency is observed in 6.2% of the population but it is caused by inadequate vitamin B_2 intake. Methemoglobin formation as a potential complication of malaria – and thus as an additional target of methylene blue – can be assessed also in anemic patients by using the 2-wavelengths procedure introduced here. In a pilot study on BlueCQ, methylene blue (3 mg/kg per day) was well tolerated by fifty adult male G6PD-sufficient persons. The side effects of methylene blue appear to be mild and include also positive aspects such as the concomitant therapy of methemoglobinemia, a rise in hemoglobin levels, and increased appetite.

References

Anderson BB, Scattoni M, Perry GM, Galvan P, Giuberti M, Buonocore G, Vullo C (1994) Is the flavin-deficient red blood cell common in Maremma, Italy, an important defense against malaria in this area? *Am J Hum Genet* 55: 975-980.
Anstey NM, Hassanali MY, Mlalasi J, Manyenga D, Mwaikambo ED (1996) Elevated levels of methaemoglobin in Tanzanian children with severe and uncomplicated malaria. *Trans R Soc Trop Med Hyg* 90: 147-151.
Becker K, Krebs B, Schirmer RH (1991) Protein-chemical standardization of the erythrocyte glutathione reductase activation test (EGRAC test). Application to hypothyroidism. *Int J Nutr Res* 61:180-187.
Becker K, Rahlfs S, Nickel C, Schirmer RH (2003) Glutathione – function and metabolism in the malarial parasite *Plasmodium falciparum*. *Biol Chem* 384: 551-566.

Brewer GJ, Tarlov AR, Alving AS (1962) The methemoglobin reduction test for primaquine-type sensitivity of erythrocytes. A simplified procedure for detecting a specific hypersusceptibility for drug hemolysis. *JAMA* 180: 386-388.

Cook GC, Zumla A (2003) MANSON's TROPICAL DISEASES. Twenty-first edition. *WB Saunders-Elsevier Science Ltd, Edinburgh.*

Coulibaly B (2004) Malaria-related studies on enzymopathies, methemoglobin, and methylene blue. PhD thesis, Heidelberg University

Eubel J, Coulibaly B, Davioud-Charvet E, Becker K, Schirmer RH (2004) Interactions of methylene blue with the glutathione redox system of *Plasmodium falciparum*. *Intern J Med Microbiol* 293 Suppl.38: 84-85.

Ginsburg H (2003) Redox metabolism in malaria: from genes, through biochemistry and pathology, to drugs. *Redox Rep* 8:231-233

Guttmann P, Ehrlich P (1891) Über die Wirkung von Methylenblau bei Malaria. *Berl Klin Wochenschr 28*, 953-956

Kanzok S, Fechner A, Bauer H, Ulschmid JK, Botella JA, Schneuwly S, Müller HM, Schirmer RH, Becker K (2001) The thioredoxin system substitutes for glutathione reductase in *Drosophila melanogaster*. *Science 291*, 643-646

Krauth-Siegel RL, Bauer H, Schirmer RH (2004) Dithiol proteins as guardians of the intracellular redox milieu in parasites. Old and new drug targets in trypanosomes and malaria-causing plasmodia. *Angewandte Chemie International Edition English, in press*

Mandi G, Witte S, Meissner P, Coulibaly B et al. (2004) Safety of the combination of chloroquine and methylene blue in healthy adult men with G6PD deficiency from rural Burkina Faso, *in press*

Merkle H (2004) Redox-aktive Thiol-Proteine als Drug Targets. Beiträge zur Pathophysiologie und Chemotherapie der Malaria. *MD thesis, Heidelberg University*

Ruwende C, Hill A (1998) Glucose-6-phosphate dehydrogenase deficiency and malaria. *J Mol Med* 76:581-588.

Sarma GN, Savvides SN, Becker K, Schirmer M, Schirmer RH, Karplus PA (2003) Glutathione reductase of the malarial parasite *Plasmodium falciparum*: Crystal structure and inhibitor development. *J Mol Biol* 328: 893-907

Scheiwein M (2001) Pathophysiologische und chemotherapeutische Mechanismen der Glutathionreduktase-Inaktivierung bei Malaria. *MD thesis, Heidelberg University*

Schirmer RH (2002) Der Parasit ohne Gnade: Der Malariaerreger und seine Masken. *development company for television program dctp, Düsseldorf*, 45 min; EAS 07.04.02 SAT 1

Schirmer RH, Coulibaly B, Stich A, Scheiwein M, Merkle H, Eubel J, Becker K, Becher H, Müller O, Zich T, Schiek W, Kouyaté B (2003) Methylene blue as an antimalarial agent. *Redox Report 8, 272-275*

Ziebuhr W, Xiao K, Coulibaly B, Schwarz R, Dandekar T (2004) Pharmacogenomic strategies against resistance development in microbial infections. *Pharmacogenomics (2004) 5, 361-379*

5.2 Methylene blue as an antimalarial agent

SCHIRMER RH, COULIBALY B, STICH A, SCHEIWEIN M, MERKLE H, EUBEL J, BECKER K, BECHER H, MULLER O, ZICH T, SCHIEK W, KOUYATE B.

Redox Rep. 2003;8(5):272-5.

Reprinted with permission from Maney & Son Ltd.

Short refereed paper

Methylene blue as an antimalarial agent

R. Heiner Schirmer[1], Boubacar Coulibaly[1,2], August Stich[3], Michael Scheiwein[1,2], Heiko Merkle[1,2], Jana Eubel[1], Katja Becker[4], Heiko Becher[5], Olaf Müller[5], Thomas Zich[6], Wolfgang Schiek[6], Bocar Kouyaté[2]

[1]Biochemistry Center, Heidelberg University, Heidelberg Germany
[2]Centre de Recherche en Santé de Nouna (CRSN), Burkina Faso
[3]Medical Mission Institute, Department of Tropical Medicine and Epidemic Control, Würzburg, Germany
[4]Interdisciplinary Research Center, Justus-Liebig-University, Giessen, Germany
[5]Department of Tropical Hygiene and Public Health, Ruprecht-Karls-University, Heidelberg, Germany
[6]DSM Fine Chemicals Austria, Linz, Austria

Methylene blue has intrinsic antimalarial activity and it can act as a chloroquine sensitizer. In addition, methylene blue must be considered for preventing methemoglobinemia, a serious complication of malarial anemia. As an antiparasitic agent, methylene blue is pleiotropic: it interferes with hemoglobin and heme metabolism in digestive organelles, and it is a selective inhibitor of *Plasmodium falciparum* glutathione reductase. The latter effect results in glutathione depletion which sensitizes the parasite for chloroquine action. At the Centre de Recherche en Santé de Nouna in Burkina Faso, we study the combination of chloroquine with methylene blue (BlueCQ) as a possible medication for malaria in endemic regions. A pilot study with glucose-6-phosphate dehydrogenase-sufficient adult patients has been conducted recently.

INTRODUCTION

Methylene blue was introduced as an antimalarial medication in 1891. It was the very first synthetic, rather than natural, compound ever used in clinical therapy: indeed the paper by Guttmann and Ehrlich marks the advent of chemotherapy as we know it today.[1] Methylene blue became a lead structure which resulted in numerous other drugs including the tricyclic antidepressant agents. As an antimalarial, methylene blue has been replaced by its derivatives, mepacrine and chloroquine.

Received 13 March 2003
Accepted 14 March 2003

Correspondence to: Heiner Schirmer, Biochemie-Zentrum, Universität Heidelberg, Im Neuenheimer Feld 504, D-69120 Heidelberg, Germany
Tel: +49 6221 544165; Fax: +49 6221 545586;
E-mail: heiner.schirmer@gmx.de
or to Boubacar Coulibaly, Centre de Recherche en Santé de Nouna (CRSN), Nouna, Burkina Faso
Tel/Fax: 00226 53 70 55; E-mail: bocar.crsn@fasonet.bf

METHEMOGLOBIN REDUCTION BY LEUKOMETHYLENE BLUE

The major clinical indications for methylene blue are the treatment of most forms of methemoglobinemia[2,3] and, in cancer therapy, the prevention of ifosfamide-induced neurotoxicity.[4,5] Methemoglobin formation can occur as a severe manifestation of the malaria infection itself.[6] Methemoglobinemia complicating anemia is potentially fatal; the pathophysiological basis for this is that in methemoglobinemia the O_2-binding curve of hemoglobin is shifted to the left. It remains to be studied whether methylene blue can prevent this serious complication of malaria anemia.[6]

Methemoglobin reduction by methylene blue is understood at the biochemical level.[3,6,7] In this process, electrons flow from glucose-6-phosphate via the enzyme glucose-6-phosphate dehydrogenase (G6PD) to NADP, then from NADPH via flavin reductase to methylene blue forming leukomethylene blue, and from leukomethylene blue to methemoglobin resulting in hemoglobin formation.[7] NADPH can also reduce methylene blue directly (Fig. 1). The apparent rate of this chemical reaction (7.5 $M^{-1}s^{-1}$ at

37°C) was found to be practically independent of the dioxygen concentration in the environment.

The oxidation of NADPH by methylene blue has to be accounted for in assay systems containing both methylene blue and NADPH, for instance when testing methylene blue as an inhibitor of *Plasmodium falciparum* glutathione reductase.[8] The reaction between methylene blue and NADPH may play a role also *in vivo* since it depletes the cytosolic NADPH pool at a rate of 1–5 µM/min unless NADPH is replenished.[9]

EFFECTS OF METHYLENE BLUE ON MALARIAL PARASITES

In view of the spreading resistance of *P. falciparum* to mainstay antimalarial drugs like chloroquine and sulfadoxine-pyrimethamine, methylene blue has been revisited as an antimalarial agent by the groups of Vennerstrom[10] and Ginsburg.[9,11] Based on cell culture studies, Vennerstrom *et al*.[10] stated that methylene blue is notable for both its unusually high antimalarial potency (IC_{50} = 4 nM) and selectivity (with a cytotoxicity index of 450); no cross-resistance with chloroquine was observed for methylene blue. The latter result is consistent with Thurston's (often misquoted) finding[12] that 'resistance of *Plasmodium berghei* in mice after 4 months' exposure to methylene blue was less marked, and this strain retained its normal sensitivity to the other antimalarials that were tested. The resistance factor for methylene blue after 4 months was not higher than 2.3.' Ginsburg's group confirmed these results and contributed further important biochemical and pharmacological data on methylene blue, some of which are given in the caption of Figure 1.[11]

The lack of observable drug resistance indicates that methylene blue is either pleiotropic or/and that it has no unique target encoded in the parasite genome.[13] This is consistent with the finding that methylene blue interferes with the polymerisation of heme, a toxic product of hemoglobin degradation, into hemozoin.[11]

Cell-biochemical observations of Akompong *et al*.[14] suggested to us that methylene blue may inhibit parasite growth also by inhibiting (met)hemoglobin degradation. These authors presented evidence that methemoglobin, rather than hemoglobin, is the substrate of the parasite's proteases and that compounds like reduced riboflavin[7] exert their antiparasitic effect by preventing or reverting the oxidation of hemoglobin to methemoglobin in the parasite's digestive organelles.[14] At present, we are testing the hypothesis that leukomethylene blue has the effects reported for reduced riboflavin. Leukomethylene blue, the NADPH-reduced uncharged form of methylene blue, easily crosses membranes separating cells or cell organelles.

Apart from its effects on hemoglobin and heme metabolism, methylene blue is a non-competitive inhibitor of *P. falciparum* glutathione reductase which catalyses the reaction:[15–19]

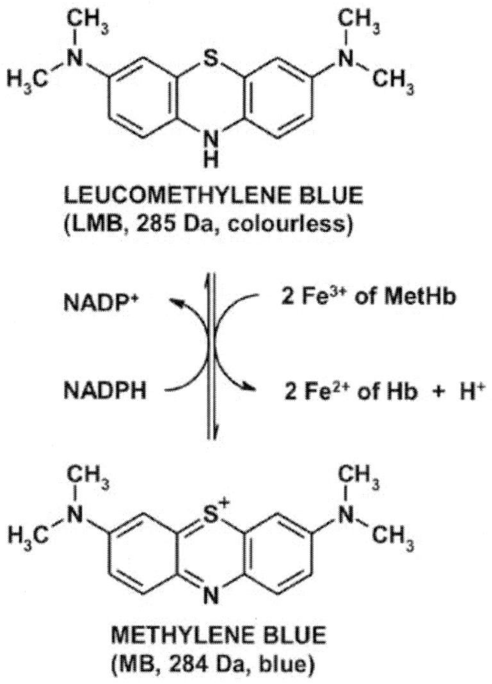

$$NADPH + GSSG + H^+ \rightarrow NADP + 2\ GSH \qquad Eq.\ 1$$

and indirectly leads to glutathione depletion in the cytosol.[18,20–22] Low glutathione levels in turn favour the activity of chloroquine.[23,24] Thus methylene blue might sensitize the parasite for chloroquine and even revert chloroquine resistance when grade I and grade II tolerance prevail. In order to guarantee the action of methylene blue as a glutathione reductase inhibitor, the plasma concentration of the drug should be high. The required concentration range remains to be established because

Fig 1. Methylene blue and leukomethylene blue at pH 7.3. When studying the spontaneous reaction methylene blue + NADPH -> leukomethylene blue + NADP$^+$ under various conditions, the oxidation of NADPH was measured at 340 nm, the ε-value being 6220 M^{-1}cm^{-1}. At pH 7.3 and 25°C, the apparent rate constant k was found to be 3.6 M^{-1}s^{-1} under air and 2.8 M^{-1}s^{-1} under a nitrogen atmosphere with less than 0.01% dioxygen. methylene blue concentrations above 60 µM were avoided in these experiments as methylene blue dimerizes, the K_{ass} being 4000 M^{-1}.[10,34] The ε-value of methylene blue at 662 nm was found to be as high as 45 mM^{-1}cm^{-1}. Other data for methylene blue were adopted form the literature. methylene blue has one pK value between 0 and 1, leukomethylene blue two pK values between 5 and 6 whereas the one electron-reduced cation of methylene blue has a pK value between 8 and 9.[10,11] The redox potential for the couple methylene blue/leukomethylene blue at pH 7.0 and 25°C is –210 mV.[11] Leukomethylene blue as a drugable compound has favourable Lipinski characteristics including a log p value between 4 and 5.[35,36] Methylene blue is a non-competitive inhibitor of *P. falciparum* glutathione reductase with a K_i-value of 6 µM.[15] Production costs for 1 g methylene blue (GMP grade) could be less than 5 UScents.

leukomethylene blue and methylene blue become concentrated in parasitized red blood cells.[11]

PATIENT STUDIES

In his classical book on chemotherapy and drug resistance in malaria, Peters refers to toxic episodes following methylene blue medication.[25] This toxicity of the drug appears to be restricted to persons with certain types of G6PD deficiency. In order to identify the risk group, we established an on-site screening test for G6PD deficiency.[26] This is a miniaturisation of the 'NADPH fluorescence test on paper' according to Beutler and Mitchell.[27] Before the actual test, the fingerprick blood sample was diluted with phosphate buffered saline to give 4 g Hb/dl. This standardization is necessary since in malaria-endemic regions children often have severe anemia.[6] For hemoglobin determination, we recommend the cyanide-independent photometric method.[28] The NADPH fluorescence test was validated using Brewer's methemoglobin reduction method[29] as a standard procedure.[26]

A total of 1018 randomly chosen persons from 5 villages of the Nouna region were tested; 138 of them (13.6%) were found to be G6PD-negative. Similar data, based on gene sequencing, have recently been reported for a homogeneous population in Nigeria.[30]

Our study illustrates that the entire population could be screened for G6PD status using fingerprick blood samples, and that individual patients can be pretested on-site prior to administering drugs which are not well tolerated by individuals with G6PD deficiency.[31,32]

A pilot study with 56 G6PD-sufficient adult patients based on the combination of chloroquine and methylene blue (BlueCQ) as a possible antimalarial medication was recently conducted in Burkina Faso. The results have not been analyzed yet, but here we can answer a most frequently asked question – Yes, the urine was indeed blue, and methylene blue is excreted, without being metabolised, as a mixture of methylene blue and leukomethylene blue (see also Peter et al.,[4] Atamna et al.[11] and Thurston[12]).

OUTLOOK

Apart from its own intrinsic antiparasitic activity, methylene blue may protect the efficacy of chloroquine when given together with this outstanding antimalarial drug. BlueCQ would be an affordable drug combination. It is obvious that methylene blue can be combined with other currently used and developed antimalarials.[13,33] Of special interest are agents that, like methylene blue, target redox reactions.[10] The potential of methylene blue to prevent methemoglobinemia as a complication of malarial anemia[6] remains to be studied.

ACKNOWLEDGEMENTS

This work was supported by the Deutsche Forschungsgemeinschaft (SFB 544 'Control of Tropical Infectious Diseases' and Grant BE 1540/7-1) and by the DSM Dream Action Award 2002. The patient studies were approved by the Ethical Boards of the CRSN, Burkina Faso, and of Heidelberg University.

REFERENCES

1. Guttmann P, Ehrlich P. Über die Wirkung des Methylenblau bei Malaria. *Berl Klin Wochenschr* 1891; **28**: 953–956.
2. Mansouri A, Lurie AA. Concise review: methemoglobinemia. *Am J Hematol* 1993; **42**: 7–12.
3. Coleman MD, Coleman NA. Drug-induced methaemoglobinaemia. Treatment issues. *Drug Saf* 1996; **14**: 394–405.
4. Peter C, Hongwan D, Kupfer A, Lauterburg BH. Pharmacokinetics and organ distribution of intravenous and oral methylene blue. *Eur J Clin Pharmacol* 2000; **56**: 247–250.
5. Pelgrims J, De Vos F, Van den Brande J, Schrijvers D, Prove A, Vermorken JB. Methylene blue in the treatment and prevention of ifosfamide-induced encephalopathy: report of 12 cases and a review of the literature. *Br J Cancer* 2000; **82**: 291–294.
6. Anstey NM, Hassanali MY, Mlalasi J, Manyenga D, Mwaikambo ED. Elevated levels of methaemoglobin in Tanzanian children with severe and uncomplicated malaria. *Trans R Soc Trop Med Hyg* 1996; **90**: 147–151.
7. Quandt KS, Hultquist DE. Flavin reductase: sequence of cDNA from bovine liver and tissue distribution. *Proc Natl Acad Sci USA* 1994; **91**: 9322–9326.
8. Färber PM, Becker K, Müller S, Schirmer RH, Franklin RM. Molecular cloning and characterization of a putative glutathione reductase gene, the *PfGR2* gene, from *Plasmodium falciparum*. *Eur J Biochem* 1996; **239**: 655–661.
9. Atamna H, Pascarmona G, Ginsburg H. Hexose-monophosphate shunt activity in intact *Plasmodium falciparum*-infected erythrocytes and in free parasites. *Mol Biochem Parasitol* 1994; **67**: 79–89.
10. Vennerstrom JL, Makler MT, Angerhofer CK, Williams JA. Antimalarial dyes revisited: xanthenes, azines, oxazines, and thiazines. *Antimicrob Agents Chemother* 1995; **39**: 2671–2677.
11. Atamna H, Krugliak M, Shalmiev G, Deharo E, Pescarmona G, Ginsburg H. Mode of antimalarial effect of methylene blue and some of its analogues on *Plasmodium falciparum* in culture and their inhibition of *P. vinckei petteri* and *P. yoelii nigeriensis* in vivo. *Biochem Pharmacol* 1996; **51**: 693–700.
12. Thurston JP. The chemotherapy of *Plasmodium berghei*. Resistance to drugs. *Parasitology* 1953; **43**: 246–252.
13. Ridley RG. Medical need, scientific opportunity and the drive for antimalarial drugs. *Nature* 2002; **415**: 686–693.
14. Akompong T, Ghori N, Haldar K. *In vitro* activity of riboflavin against the human malaria parasite *Plasmodium falciparum*. *Antimicrob Agents Chemother* 2000; **44**: 88–96.
15. Färber PM, Arscott LD, Williams Jr CH, Becker K, Schirmer RH. Recombinant *Plasmodium falciparum* glutathione reductase is inhibited by the antimalarial dye methylene blue. *FEBS Lett* 1998; **422**: 311–314.

16. Gilberger TW, Schirmer RH, Walter RD, Müller S. Deletion of the parasite-specific insertions and mutation of the catalytic triad in glutathione reductase from chloroquine-sensitive *Plasmodium falciparum* 3D7. *Mol Biochem Parasitol* 2000; **107**: 169–179.
17. Sarma GN, Savvides SN, Becker K, Schirmer M, Schirmer RH, Karplus PA. Glutathione reductase of the malarial parasite *Plasmodium falciparum*: crystal structure and inhibitor development. *J Mol Biol* 2003; In press.
18. Becker K, Rahlfs S, Nickel C, Schirmer RH. Glutathione – function and metabolism in the malarial parasite *Plasmodium falciparum*. *J Mol Biol* 2003; In press.
19. Luond RM, McKie JH, Douglas KT, Dascombe MJ, Vale J. Inhibitors of glutathione reductase as potential antimalarial drugs. Kinetic cooperativity and effect of dimethyl sulphoxide on inhibition kinetics. *J Enzyme Inhib* 1998; **13**: 327–345.
20. Davioud-Charvet E, Delarue S, Biot C *et al*. A prodrug form of a *Plasmodium falciparum* glutathione reductase inhibitor conjugated with a 4-anilinoquinoline. *J Med Chem* 2001; **44**: 4268–4276.
21. Ginsburg H. A double-headed prodrug that overcomes chloroquine resistance. *Trends Parasitol* 2002; **18**: 103.
22. Zhang YA, Hempelmann E, Schirmer RH. Glutathione reductase inhibitors as potential antimalarial drugs. Effects of nitrosoureas on *Plasmodium falciparum in vitro*. *Biochem Pharmacol* 1988; **37**: 855–860.
23. Dubois VL, Platel DF, Pauly G, Tribouley-Duret J. *Plasmodium berghei*: implication of intracellular glutathione and its related enzyme in chloroquine resistance *in vivo*. *Exp Parasitol* 1995; **81**: 117–124.
24. Müller S, Gilberger TW, Krnajski Z, Lüersen K, Meierjohann S, Walter RD. Thioredoxin and glutathione system of malaria parasite *Plasmodium falciparum*. *Protoplasma* 2001; **217**: 43–49.
25. Peters W. *Chemotherapy and Drug Resistance in Malaria*. London: Academic Press, 1970.
26. Scheiwein M. *Pathophysiologische und chemotherapeutische Mechanismen der Glutathionreduktase-Inaktivierung bei Malaria*. MD thesis, Heidelberg, Germany: Heidelberg University 2001.
27. Beutler E, Mitchell M. Special modifications of the fluorescent screening method for glucose-6-phosphate dehydrogenase deficiency. *Blood* 1968; **32**: 816–818.
28. Becker K, Krebs B, Schirmer RH. Protein-chemical standardization of the erythrocyte glutathione reductase activation test (EGRAC test). Application to hypothyroidism. *Int J Nutr Res* 1991; **61**: 180–187.
29. Brewer GJ, Tarlov AR, Alving AS. The methemoglobin reduction test for primaquine-type sensitivity of erythrocytes. A simplified procedure for detecting a specific hypersusceptibility for drug hemolysis. *JAMA* 1962; **180**: 386–388.
30. Ademowo OG, Falusi AG. Molecular epidemiology and activity of erythrocyte G6PD variants in a homogeneous Nigerian population. *East Afr Med J* 2002; **79**: 42–44.
31. Ruwende C, Hill A. Glucose-6-phosphate dehydrogenase deficiency and malaria. *J Mol Med* 1998; **76**: 581–588.
32. Beutler E. G6PD deficiency. *Blood* 1994; **84**: 3613–3636.
33. Rieckmann K, Cheng Q. Pyrimethamine-sulfadoxine resistance in *Plasmodium falciparum* must be delayed in Africa. *Trends Parasitol* 2002; **18**: 293–294.
34. Antonov L, Gergov G, Petrov V, Kubista M, Nygren J. UV-Vis spectroscopic and chemometric studies on the aggregation of ionic dyes in water. *Talanta* 1999; **49**: 99–106.
35. Lipinski CA. Drug-like properties and the causes of poor solubility and poor permeability. *J Pharmacol Toxicol Methods* 2000; **44**: 235–249.
36. Schirmer RH, Müller JG, Krauth-Siegel RL. Disulfide-reductase inhibitors as chemotherapeutic agents: the design of drugs for trypanosomiasis and malaria. *Angew Chem Int Edn* 1995; **34**: 141–154.

AUTHOR QUERIES

17. Sarma GN, Savvides SN, Becker K, Schirmer M, Schirmer RH, Karplus PA. Update?
18. Becker K, Rahlfs S, Nickel C, Schirmer RH. Update?

5.3. Pharmacogenomic strategies against resistance development in microbial infections

WILMA ZIEBUHR[1], KE XIAO[2], BOUBACAR COULIBALY[3], ROLAND SCHWARZ[4], THOMAS DANDEKAR[4,5,*]

[1] Institut für Molekulare Infektionsbiologie, Röntgenring 11, 97070 Würzburg, Germany

[2] Biochemiezentrum, Haus 3, Im Neuenheimer Feld 504, 69120 Universität Heidelberg, Germany

[3] Centre de Recherche en Santé de Nouna, BP2, Nouna, Burkina-Faso

[4] Lehrstuhl für Bioinformatik, Biozentrum, Am Hubland, 97074 Universität Würzburg, Germany

[5] European Molecular Biology Laboratory, Postfach 102209, 69120 Heidelberg, Germany

Tel.: ++49 931-888-4551

Email: dandekar@biozentrum.uni-wuerzburg.de

Abstract

Selected examples review several promising new strategies to antagonize resistance development in microbial infections. After reviewing typical experimental and bioinformatical strategies to study the impact of infectious challenges on host-pathogen interaction, we examine several new approaches and sources for new pharmaceutical strategies against resistance development. Genomics reveals promising new targets by (i) a better understanding of cellular pathways, (ii) identification of new pathways and (iii) identification of new intervention areas such as phospholipids, glycolipids, innate immunity, and antibiotic peptides. Additional antibiotic resources come from new genomes including marine organisms, lytic phages and probiotic strategies. A system perspective regards all interactions between host pathogen and environment to develop new pharmacogenomic strategies against resistance development.

Introduction

Pharmacogenomics and pharmacogenetics developed into fast growing sciences and make now use of the latest techniques such as microarray analysis and computational genome wide analyses of DNA in sequencing projects such as the Human Genome Project. The concept of applying pharmacogenomics to analyze and to find strategies against emergence of antibiotic resistance in bacterial pathogens is still a new one (1, Davison and Barett 2003), but becomes more important because of the alarming rise in antibiotic resistance and increasing hospital mortality rates (2, Cosgrove et al. 2003). Pipelines for new antibiotics are under a rising threat to run dry (3, Clarke, 2003). Resistance develops not only in industrialized countries; but emerges also in the Southern hemisphere for which the spread of chloroquin resistant malaria plasmodia is only one example (4, Wootton et al., 2002).

Pharmacogenomics can help us to prevent, diagnose and treat infectious diseases caused by resistant pathogens (5, Hayney 2002), and gives us new tools to repress the emergence of antibiotic resistances.

The following review focuses on such new pharmacogenomic strategies. Their development require novel targets, novel pathways or completely new strategies such as the use of lytic phages.

Are antibiotics from genome data the most powerful strategy to counter resistance development (6, Alekshun, 2001)? At least systematic bioinformatical screening and the exploitation of databases (7, Clarke, 2003b) open up possibilities exceeding previous capabilities by far.

After summarizing some of the adaptation strategies and countermeasures which microbes develop against antibiotics, we will next examine how conventional strategies against infections can be boosted by pharmacogenomics and then, which genome-based novel pharmacological strategies for antibiotic development can be tapped for future development. Having compared in this way the attacking and defense lines we finally want to give a comprehensive perspective to better prevent resistance development in microbial infections. Such systems-based approaches hold big promise for the future also in other areas of genome based biomedicine (8, Ghaemmaghami et al., 2003; 9, Hood and Galas, 2003).

Pharmacogenomic analysis of resistance in microbes

Selection for antibiotic resistance and genetic mechanisms. Analyzing the current resistance status in bacteria worldwide, the situation in the community is different from that in hospital settings. Resistance problems outside of hospitals comprise mainly respiratory tract infections caused by multidrug-resistant mycobacteria, penicillin-resistant pneumococci and ß-lactamase producing *Haemophilus influenzae* (10, Felmingham, et al., 2002). Moreover, multidrug-resistant diarrrhoegenic bacteria such as *Salmonella* and *Shigella* cause concern, specifically in developing countries (11, Parry, 2003; 12, Threlfall, et al., 2000). In contrast, the main focuses in nosocomial infections are clearly multiresistant gram positive cocci such as staphylococci and enterococci as well as antibiotic-resistant *Pseudomonas aeruginosa* and enterobacteria (13, Vincent, 2003; 14, Witte, 1999).

Often used mechanisms of antibiotic defense in microbes. Albeit numerous different resistant genes have been recognized so far their encoded functions can be subsumed into a few major mechanisms. Thus, bacteria can get resistant by (i) inactivation of the attacking antibiotic, by (ii) modification of the antibiotic target within the bacterial cell, (iii) by an increased antibiotic transport out of the cell, or (iv) by prevention of antibiotic uptake.

Key Conclusions

Without going into the full detail of the extensive review published elsewhere (Ziebuhr W, Xiao K, Coulibaly B, Schwarz R, Dandekar T. Pharmacogenomic strategies against resistance development in microbial infections. Pharmacogenomics. 2004 Jun;5(4):361-79.) here is a summary of our key conclusions:

- To combat antibiotic resistance pharmacogenomics including bioinformatics becomes critical for rapid detection, target information and modeling of involved pathways.

- Resistance evolution and adaptation mechanisms in microbes exploit genetic exchange and a complex battery of specific adaptation mechanisms

- Specific resistance mechanisms often involve an antibiotic uptake block, antibiotic secretion, inactivation or detoxification.

- Antibiotic strategies should broaden, including further pathways such as lipid and carbohydrate metabolism, innate immunity and antibiotic peptides.

- Further resources to explore include antibiotics from marine organisms, soil bacteria, bacteriophages and revisiting old drugs improved by pharmaco-design and network analysis.

- The interaction between host, microbe and controlling factors shows that further non-antibiotic and pro-biotic strategies help to preserve the efficiency of antibiotics

Outlook

The rich amount of different pharmacogenomic strategies against resistance development in microbial infections underlines that currently there is no lack of strategies, but great demand for implementations and more scientific research in these directions. In effect, without the new possibilities from pharmacogenomic research, both, the target detection process as well as its implementation into new drugs to fight resistance development is in high danger. Good practice of medical treatment and restricted use of "sharp" weapons against infections such as antibiotics are critical as well as ecological and population genetics insights into the dynamics of pathogen and resistance evolution. The new strategies from innate immunity, marine resources and drugs blocking new pathways will only work if they are not jeopardized by malpractice of drug administration or misuse (e.g. in animal husbandry as is practice for current antibiotics). New processes and new sources for antibiotics are very important as well as to understand more about probiotics and to combat infections by evolutionary or ecological strategies.

Bibliography

Davison DB, Barrett JF: Antibiotics and pharmacogenomics. *Pharmacogenomics 4(5), 657-665 (2003)*

Cosgrove SE, Sakoulas G, Perencevich EN, Schwaber MJ, Karchmer AW, Carmeli Y: Comparison of mortality associated with methicillin-resistant and methicillin-susceptible Staphylococcus aureus bacteremia: a meta-analysis. *Clin. Infect. Dis. 36(1), 53-9 (2003)*

Clarke T: Drug companies snub antibiotics as pipeline threatens to run dry. *Nature 425(6955), 225 (2003).*

Wootton JC, Feng X, Ferdig MT *et al.*: Genetic diversity and chloroquine selective sweeps in Plasmodium falciparum. *Nature 418(6895), 320-3 (2002).*

Hayney MS: Pharmacogenomics and infectious diseases: impact on drug response and applications to disease management. *Am. J. Health Syst. Pharm. 59(17), 1626-31 (2002)*

Alekshun MN: Beyond comparison--antibiotics from genome data? *Nat. Biotechnol. 19(12), 1124-5 (2001).*

Clarke T: Biologists deploy database to quash drug-resistant bacteria. *Nature 422(6934), 791 (2003).*

Ghaemmaghami S, Huh WK, Bower K *et al.*: Global analysis of protein expression in yeast. *Nature 425(6959), 737-41 (2003).*

Hood L, Galas D: The digital code of DNA. *Nature 421(6921), 444-8 (2003)*

Felmingham D, Feldman C, Hryniewicz W, Klugman K, Kohno S, Low DE, et al.: Surveillance of resistance in bacteria causing community-acquired respiratory tract infections. *Clin. Microbiol. Infect. 8 Suppl. 2, 12-42 (2002).*

Parry CM: Antimicrobial drug resistance in Salmonella enterica. *Curr. Opin. Infect. Dis. 16, 467-472 (2003).*

Threlfall EJ, Ward LR, Frost JA, Willshaw GA: The emergence and spread of antibiotic resistance in food-borne bacteria. *Int. J. Food Microbiol. 62, 1-5 (2000).*

Vincent JL: Nosocomial infections in adult intensive-care units. *Lancet 361, 2068-2077 (2003).*

Witte W: Antibiotic resistance in gram-positive bacteria: epidemiological aspects. *J. Antimicrob. Chemother. 44 Suppl. A, 1-9 (1999).*

Author index

Author	Chapter	Journal Article	Page
Baltussen van Zweeden, Anneke		2.2, 2.7	65, 89
Baltussen, Rob		4.4, 4.6	183, 209
Becher, Heiko	**0, 1.2, 3.1,**	2.2, 2.4, 2.6, 2.7, 3.2, 3.4, 3.5, 3.6, 3.7, 5.2	**XI, 17,** 65, 77, 83, 89, **99,** 105, 125, 135, 141, 149, 293
Becker, Katja		5.2	293
Binka, Fred	**1.3**		**21**
Böhler, Thomas	**2.1.2**		**55**
Boncongou Justine	**2.1.2**		**55**
Cairns, John		4.8, 4.9, 4.10	231, 241, 257
Chephn'eno Gloria		4.11	265
Coulibaly Boubacar	**2.1.2, 5.1, 5.3**	5.2	**55, 285,** 293, **299**
Dandekar, Thomas	**5.3**		**299**
Diallo, Diadier A		2.2	65
Diesfeld, Hans-Jochen	**1.1.1**		**1**
Dong, Hengjin		4.7, 4.8, 4.9, 4.10, 4.11, 4.12	219, 231, 241, 257, 265, 275
Ganamé, Jean	**2.1.2**		**55**
Garenne Michel		2.2, 2.6, 2.7	65, 83, 89
Gbangou, Adjima		2.2, 3.4, 3.7, 4.2, 4.3	65, 125, 149, 161, 171
Gromer, Stephan	**5.1**		**285**
Haddad, Pierre S		4.4	183
Hammer, Gael	**3.1**		**99**
Hofmann, Jennifer	**2.1.2**		**55**
Ido, Kolé		2.3	73
Jahn, Albrecht		2.4, 3.7	77, 149
Jana, Eubel	**5.1**	5.2	**285,** 293
Kielmann, Karina		0	XI
Konate, Amadou T		2.2	65
Kouyaté, Bocar	**0, 1.1.2, 1.4, 3.1**	0, 2.2, 2.5, 2.6, 2.7, 2.8, 3.4, 3.5, 3.6, 3.7, 4.3, 4.5, 4.7, 4.8, 4.9, 4.10, 4.11, 4.12, 5.2	**XI, 7, 33,** 65, 79, 83, 89, 95, **99,** 125, 135, 141, 149, 171, 191, 219, 231, 241, 257, 265, 275, 293
Kräusslich, Hans-Georg	**2.1.2**		**55**
Krickeberg, Klaus	**1.5**		**43**
Kynast-Wolf, Gisela	**3.1**	3.4, 3.5, 3.7	**99,** 125, 135, 149
Merkle, Heiko		5.2	293
Mugisha, Frederick		4.3, 4.7, 4.9, 4.11, 4.12	171, 219, 241, 265, 275

Author	Chapter	Journal Article	Page
Müller, Olaf	**1.4, 2.1.1**	2.2, 2.3, 2.4, 2.5, 2.6, 2.7, 2.8, 3.2, 3.3, 3.6, 3.7, 5.2	**33**, **55**, 65, 73, 77, 79, 83, 89, 95, 105, 115, 141, 149, 293
Nagabila, Youssouf	**2.1.2**		**55**
Okrah, Jane		3.3	115
Pale, Augustin		3.3	115
Reitmeier, Pitt		2.7	89
Sankoh, Osman	**1.3**	3.2, 3.4, 3.5	**21**, 105, 125, 135
Sanon, Mamadou		4.5, 4.6	191, 209
Sarker, Malabika	**2.1.2**		**55**
Sauerborn, Rainer	**1.1.2**	3.2, 4.2, 4.3, 4.4, 4.5, 4.7, 4.8, 4.9, 4.10, 4.11, 4.12	**7**, 105, 161, 171, 183, 191, 219, 231, 241, 257, 265, 275
Scheiwein, Michael		5.2	293
Schiek Wolfgang		5.2	293
Schirmer, Heiner	**5.1**	5.2	**285**, 293
Schmidt, Christof M		4.2	161
Schwarz, Roland	**5.3**		**299**
Snow, Rachel C	**2.1.2**	4.7	**55**, 219
Somé, Florent	**3.1**		**99**
Sommerfeld, Johannes		3.3, 4.5, 4.6	115, 191, 209
Stich, August		5.2	293
Stieglbauer, Gabriele	**1.2**		**17**
Tebit, Denis Manga	**2.1.2**		**55**
Traoré, Corneille		0, 2.3, 2.4, 2.5, 2.8, 3.3, 3.6	XI, 73, 77, 79, 95, 115, 141
Würthwein, Ralph		4.2, 4.6	161, 209
Xiao, Ke	**5.3**		**299**
Yé, Yazoume	**1.2**	2.2, 3.2, 4.4	**17**, 65, 105, 283
Zich, Thomas		5.2	293
Ziehbur Wilma	**5.3**		**299**

Authors of new book chapters given in bold

Adresses of authors of chapters

Prof. Dr. Heiko Becher
Universität Heidelberg
Abteilung Tropenhygiene und öffentliches Gesundheitswesen
Im Neuenheimer Feld 324
69120 Heidelberg
Germany

Prof. Dr. Fred Binka
INDEPTH Network
Communications and External Relations
PO Box KD 213 Kanda
Accra
Ghana

Justine Boncongou
Centre de Recherche en Santé de Nouna
BP 02 Nouna
Burkina Faso

Dr. Thomas Böhler
Med. Dienst d. Krankenversicherung
Adenauerplatz 1
69115 Heidelberg
Germany

Boubacar Coulibaly
Centre de Recherche en Santé de Nouna
BP 02 Nouna
Burkina Faso

Prof. Dr. Joachim Diesfeld
Leopold Str. 6
82319 Starnberg
Germany

Prof. Dr. Thomas Dandekar
Universität Würzburg
Lehrstuhl für Bioinformatik, Biozentrum
Am Hubland
97074 Würzburg
Germany

Jana Eubel
CRSN
and
Biochemie-Zentrum der Universität Heidelberg (BZH)
Im Neuenheimer Feld 504
69120 Heidelberg
Germany

Jean Ganamé
Centre de Recherche en Santé de Nouna
BP 02 Nouna
Burkina Faso

PD Dr. Stephan Gromer
Biochemie-Zentrum der Universität Heidelberg (BZH)
Im Neuenheimer Feld 504
69120 Heidelberg
Germany

Dr. Gael Hammer
Universität Heidelberg
Abteilung Tropenhygiene und öffentliches Gesundheitswesen
Im Neuenheimer Feld 324
69120 Heidelberg
Germany

Jennifer Hofmann
Universität Heidelberg
Abteilung Virologie
Im Neuenheimer Feld 324
69120 Heidelberg
Germany

Dr. Bocar Kouyaté
Centre de Recherche en Santé de Nouna
BP 02 Nouna
Burkina Faso

Prof. Dr. Klaus Krickeberg
Le Chatelet
63270 Manglieu
France

Prof. Dr. Hans-Georg Kräusslich
Universität Heidelberg
Abteilung Virologie
Im Neuenheimer Feld 324
69120 Heidelberg
Germany

PD Dr. Olaf Müller
Universität Heidelberg
Abteilung Tropenhygiene und öffentliches Gesundheitswesen
Im Neuenheimer Feld 324
69120 Heidelberg
Germany

Youssouf Nagabila
Centre de Recherche en Santé de Nouna
BP 02 Nouna
Burkina Faso

Dr. Osman Sankoh
INDEPTH Network
Communications and External Relations
PO Box KD 213 Kanda
Accra
Ghana

Malabika Sarker
Universität Heidelberg
Abteilung Tropenhygiene und öffentliches Gesundheitswesen
Im Neuenheimer Feld 324
69120 Heidelberg
Germany

Prof. Dr. Rainer Sauerborn
Universität Heidelberg
Abteilung Tropenhygiene und öffentliches Gesundheitswesen
Im Neuenheimer Feld 324
69120 Heidelberg
Germany

Prof. Dr. Heiner Schirmer
Biochemie-Zentrum der Universität Heidelberg (BZH)
Im Neuenheimer Feld 504
69120 Heidelberg
Germany

Roland Schwarz
Universität Würzburg
Lehrstuhl für Bioinformatik, Biozentrum
Am Hubland
97074 Würzburg
Germany

Prof. Dr. Rachel Snow
Universität Heidelberg
Abteilung Tropenhygiene und öffentliches Gesundheitswesen
Im Neuenheimer Feld 324
69120 Heidelberg
Germany

Gabriele Stieglbauer
Universität Heidelberg
Abteilung Tropenhygiene und öffentliches Gesundheitswesen
Im Neuenheimer Feld 324
69120 Heidelberg
Germany

Ke Xiao
Universität Heidelberg
Biochemiezentrum
Im Neuenheimer Feld 504
69120 Heidelberg
Germany

Yazoume Yé
Universität Heidelberg
Abteilung Tropenhygiene und öffentliches Gesundheitswesen
Im Neuenheimer Feld 324
69120 Heidelberg
Germany

PD Dr. Wilma Ziehbur
Universität Würzburg
Institut für Molekulare Infektionsbiologie
Röntgenring 11
97070 Würzburg
Germany